GW00725388

Baillière's
CLINICAL
GASTROENTEROLOGY

INTERNATIONAL PRACTICE AND RESEARCH

Editorial Board
M. J. P. Arthur (UK)
Ian A. D. Bouchier (UK)
David C. Carter (UK)
W. Creutzfeldt (Germany)
John Dent (Australia)
Michael Gracey (Australia)
G. N. J. Tytgat (The Netherlands)

Baillière's

CLINICAL

GASTROENTEROLOGY

INTERNATIONAL PRACTICE AND RESEARCH

Volume 10/Number 2
July 1996

Viral Hepatitis

A. ALBERTI MD
Guest Editor

Baillière Tindall
London Philadelphia Sydney Tokyo Toronto

This book is printed on acid-free paper.

Baillière Tindall   24–28 Oval Road
W.B. Saunders   London NW1 7DX, UK
Company Ltd
The Curtis Center, Independence Square West,
Philadelphia, PA 19106–3399, USA

55 Horner Avenue
Toronto, Ontario M8Z 4X6, Canada

Harcourt Brace & Company
Australia
30–52 Smidmore Street, Marrickville, NSW 2204, Australia

Harcourt Brace & Company
Japan Inc
Ichibancho Central Building,
22–1 Ichibancho, Chiyoda-ku, Tokyo 102, Japan

Whilst great care has been taken to maintain the accuracy of the information contained in this issue, the authors, editor, owners and publishers cannot accept any responsibility for any loss or damage arising from actions or decisions based on information contained in this publication; ultimate responsibility for the treatment of patients and interpretation of published material lies with the medical practitioner. The opinions expressed are those of the authors and the inclusion in this publication of material relating to a particular product, method or technique does not amount to an endorsement of its value or quality, or of the claims made by its manufacturer.

ISSN 0950–3528

ISBN 0–7020–2094–X (single copy)

© 1996 W B Saunders Company Ltd. All rights reserved.

No part of this publication may be reproduced, stored in a retrieval system, or transmitted in any form or by any means, electronic, mechanical, photocopying, recording or otherwise, without the prior written permission of the Publisher, W B Saunders Company Ltd, 24–28 Oval Road, London NW1 7DX, UK.

Special regulations for readers in the USA. This journal has been registered with the Copyright Clearance Centre, Inc. Consent is given for copying of articles for personal or internal use, or for the personal use of specific clients. This consent is given on the condition that the copier pays through the Center the per-copy fee stated in the code on the first page of the article for copying beyond that permitted by Sections 107 or 108 of the US Copyright Law. The appropriate fee should be forwarded with a copy of the first page of the article to the Copyright Clearance Center, Inc, 27 Congress Street, Salem, MA 01970 (USA). If no code appears in an article the author has not given broad consent to copy and permission to copy must be obtained directly from the author.

This consent does not extend to other kinds of copying such as for general distribution, resale, advertising and promotion purposes, or for creating new collective works, special written permission must be obtained from the Publisher for such copying.

Baillière's Clinical Gastroenterology is published four times each year by Baillière Tindall. Prices for Volume 10 (1996) are:

TERRITORY	ANNUAL SUBSCRIPTION	SINGLE ISSUE
Europe including UK	£102.00 (Institutional) post free £87.00 (Individual) post free	£30.00 post free
All other countries	Consult your local Harcourt Brace & Company office	

The editor of this publication is Ian Bramley, Baillière Tindall, 24–28 Oval Road, London NW1 7DX, UK.

Baillière's Clinical Gastroenterology is covered in Index Medicus, Current Contents/Clinical Medicine, Current Contents/Life Sciences, the Science Citation Index, SciSearch, Research Alert and Excerpta Medica.

Baillière's Clinical Gastroenterology was published from 1972 to 1986 as Clinics in Gastroenterology

Typeset by Phoenix Photosetting, Chatham.
Printed and bound in Great Britain by the University Printing House, Cambridge, UK.

Contributors to this issue

ALFREDO ALBERTI MD, Professor, Clinica Medica II, University of Padova, Via Guistiniani 2, 35128 Padova, Italy.

JONATHAN C. L. BOOTH BSc, MRCP, Senior Registrar in Gastroenterology and Hepatology, Department of Medicine, St Mary's Hospital Medical School, London W2 1PG, UK.

FLAVIA BORTOLOTTI MD, Senior Lecturer, Clinica Medica II, University of Padova, Via Guistiniani 2, 35128 Padova, Italy.

CHRISTIAN BRECHOT MD, PhD, Professor, INSERM U370 and Liver Unit, CHU Necker, 156 rue de Vaugirard, 75015 Paris, France.

ALESSANDRA COLANTONI MD, Research Fellow, Transplant Center, Chandler Medical Center, University of Kentucky, 800 Rose Street, Suite C-439, Lexington, KY 40536, USA.

MASSIMO COLOMBO MD, Professor of Medicine, Institute Internal Medicine and FIRC—University of Milan Research Center for Liver Cancer, IRCCS Policlinic Hospital, Milan, Italy.

GARY L. DAVIS MD, Professor of Medicine, Director, Section of Hepatobiliary Disease, University of Florida, Gainesville, FL 32610, USA.

NICOLA DE MARIA MD, Research Fellow, Transplant Center, University of Kentucky, 800 Rose Street, Room C-439, Lexington, KY 40536, USA.

GEOFFREY M. DUSHEIKO FCP(SA), FRCP, Department of Medicine, Royal Free Hospital School of Medicine, Pond Street, London NW3 3QG, UK.

STEFANO FAGIUOLI MD, Assistant Professor, Department of Gastroenterology, University of Padova, Ospedale Civile—Monoblocco, Viale Guistiniani 21, Padova, Italy.

KRZYSZTOF KRAWCZYNSKI MD, PhD, Hepatitis Branch, Building 6, Room 157, Centers for Disease Control and Prevention, 1600 Clifton Road, Atlanta, GA 30333, USA.

ERIC E. MAST MD, MPH, Hepatitis Branch, Building 6, Room 157, Centers for Disease Control and Prevention, 1600 Clifton Road, Atlanta, GA 30333, USA.

MARGHERITA MELEGARI MD, PhD, Research Fellow in Medicine, Molecular Hepatology Laboratory, Massachusetts General Hospital, Harvard Medical School, 149 13th Street, Charlestown, MA 02129, USA.

PATRIZIA PONTISSO MD, Assistant Professor, Department of Clinical and Experimental Medicine, University of Padova, Via Guistiniani 2, 35128 Padova, Italy.

MICHAEL A. PURDY BSc, PhD, Hepatitis Branch, Building 6, Room 157, Centers for Disease Control and Prevention, 1600 Clifton Road, Atlanta, GA 30333, USA.

PIER PAOLO SCAGLIONI MD, Research Fellow in Medicine, Molecular Hepatology Laboratory, Massachusetts General Hospital Cancer Center, MCH East, 149 13th Street, Charlestown, MA 02129, USA.

DONALD B. SMITH PhD, Research Fellow, Department of Medical Microbiology, University of Edinburgh, Teviot Place, Edinburgh ED8 9AG, UK.

HOWARD C. THOMAS BSc, PhD, FRCP, FRCPath, Professor & Head, Department of Medicine, St Mary's Hospital Medical School, London W2 1PG, UK.

DAVID H. VAN THIEL MD, Medical Director, Transplantation Center, Chandler Medical Center, University of Kentucky, 800 Rose Street, Room C-439, Lexington KY 40536, USA.

JACK R. WANDS MD, Director, Molecular Hepatology Laboratory, Massachusetts General Hospital, Harvard Medical School, 149 13th Street, Charlestown, MA 02129, USA.

Contributors to this issue

Table of contents

PREVIOUS ISSUES

FORTHCOMING ISSUE

Preface

Human viral hepatitis is caused by a unique group of different hepatotropic viruses which currently form a list which ranges from A to G. These viruses include two agents (HAV and HEV) which cause acute but not chronic hepatitis and four agents (HBV, HCV, HDV and HGV) responsible for both acute and chronic liver damage. HFV has been used to identify fulminant hepatitis of a possible but still unproved viral aetiology.

HAV has been recognized as an enterically transmissible acute infection of the liver for more than 30 years and is caused by an RNA virus classified in the family *Picorna viridae*. Clinical features are well known and include asymptomatic infection, acute hepatitis of variable clinical expression and severity, and fulminant liver failure. Vaccines against HAV have been developed and proved to be effective in conferring protective immunity.

HEV is a more recently identified enterically transmitted hepatotropic virus. Chapter 3 describes the main concepts of the biology of HEV and its peculiar epidemiology and summarizes how our understanding of the diagnosis and the clinical course of this infection has developed recently.

HBV is the prototype of parenterally transmitted hepatotropic viruses, which include HCV, HDV and HGV. In contrast with HAV and HEV, these agents are responsible for not only acute hepatitis of variable severity, but also for a chronic carrier state with a wide spectrum of hepatic lesions, ranging from minimal histological changes to chronic hepatitis of variable activity and evolution, cirrhosis and hepatocellular carcinoma. The biology of HBV has attracted the interest of many laboratories during the last 25 years, and research still remains extremely active in this field as HBV and the hepadnavirus family represent a unique and a most interesting model in virology. The different mechanisms of virus entry into hepatocytes and of intracellular replication and expression have been characterized in detail and represent clues to the better understanding of the clinical course of the disease and for designing more rational therapeutic interventions. A detailed review of the molecular biology of HBV is provided in Chapter 2.

HCV is currently the major cause of chronic liver disease, cirrhosis and hepatocellular carcinoma in many parts of the world. This virus exists as a family of distinct genotypes and within each virus strain discrete genomic heterogeneity has been described. This variability, described in Chapter 4, has attracted interest not only in the study of phylogenesis and epidemiology of HCV, but also in relation to the hypothesis that the virus type could play a central role in determining the pathogenesis of liver disease, its clinical course and its response to antivirals and interferons. Much debate has occurred in recent years in this field, with areas of consensus and controversy (Chapters 5 and 6).

Among the most debated and as yet uncertain aspects of HCV is the natural course and long-term outcome of chronic infection, and the risk of progression to fatal sequelae such as decompensated cirrhosis and liver cancer. While there is no doubt that HCV may progress slowly and often indolently in 20–30% of patients who develop cirrhosis over a period of 10–20 years and who then may progress to fatal complications, we still cannot predict the outcome in each individual case. This makes the clinical management of HCV difficult and uncertain, particularly if we take into account that, for the time being, we cannot offer an effective therapy to all patients. Indeed, treatment with alpha interferon(s), the only drug licensed for the treatment of chronic HCV infection, is successful only in a minority, depending on a number of variables. The best results (described in Chapter 7) are obtained in young individuals without cirrhosis and in patients infected by HCV genotypes other than HCV-1. Unfortunately, HCV-1 predominates in many parts of the world and this explains the low rates of success of treatment described in most studies.

There is certainly an extremely urgent need to identify new drugs for patients who are not treatable with interferon alone. Chapter 8 provides a comprehensive and up-to-date review on new compounds and strategies which are currently being evaluated for the treatment of chronic hepatitis, not only for HCV, but also for HBV. Successful interferon therapy is also limited to a minority of patients with chronic HBV, and there is a need for a more efficacious antiviral agent.

Chapter 1 describes long-term course of viral hepatitis in children and discusses the different settings, clinical features and response to antiviral therapy in those chronically infected with HBV, HDV or HCV.

One of the most threatening long-term consequences of chronic infection by HBV and HCV is the development of hepatocellular carcinoma (HCC). There is now doubt that viral hepatitis is the major cause of HCC worldwide and Chapter 9 is an excellent overview of the basic concepts needed for the understanding of the role of HBV and HCV in the genesis of the tumour.

Liver transplantation is the last chance that can be offered to patients with end-stage chronic liver disease and in many of them this procedure has to be taken while the infection by hepatotropic viruses is still in an active and productive phase. This represents an additional concern for the long-term success of the transplant as viral hepatitis often occurs in the new liver. The state of the art of this aspect and of the perspectives for improving further the results achieved with liver transplantation in end-stage chronic viral hepatitis is summarized in Chapter 10.

It may be surprizing to see that HGV is not covered in this issue. This is a deliberate omission, because, while there is no doubt that HGV has to be considered as a new parenterally transmitted RNA virus closely linked to HCV, it is still unclear what role, if any, this agent plays in causing acute and chronic hepatitis.

I would like to express my deep and sincere gratitude to all the authors and group leaders for collaborating in this issue and for contributing outstanding state-of-the-art reviews.

I hope that this issue of *Baillière's Clinical Gastroenterology* will provide readers with both stimulating basic concepts and useful clinical information on the current status and the future trends of our knowledge of viral hepatitis.

A. ALBERTI

1

Chronic viral hepatitis in childhood

FLAVIA BORTOLOTTI

Chronic infection with hepatitis viruses is a cause of considerable morbidity and mortality world-wide. Hepatitis B, C and D are the three recognized forms of chronic viral hepatitis, but other aetiologic agents, such as hepatitis G virus, are currently under investigation (Fry et al, 1995; Jeffers et al, 1995). In endemic areas, infection with hepatitis viruses, particularly hepatitis B virus (HBV), is a common cause of chronic liver disease in childhood. Vertical transmission and household spread are the main routes of infection in such areas. Chronic viral hepatitis tends to be an asymptomatic, mild and stable disease during childhood and adolescence, but hepatitis D leads to cirrhosis more frequently than do the other forms. Severe sequelae of long-term morbidity are more likely to appear in adult life. There is evidence that hepatitis B virus infection acquired early in life is a risk factor for the development of hepatocellular carcinoma (HCC) in adulthood. Vaccination against HBV, which, in turn, also protects against hepatitis D virus (HDV) infection, has proved to be highly efficient. Unfortunately, mass vaccination, capable of producing a rapid lowering of the endemicity, has been performed only in a limited number of countries. No vaccine has yet been developed for hepatitis C; however, the screening of blood donations is expected to reduce significantly the rate of new infections in developed countries. The role of interferon-alpha (IFN) in the treatment of chronic viral hepatitis in childhood is a debated issue. To date, few large-scale controlled studies in cases of hepatitis B and few pilot studies in children with hepatitis D or C have been conducted.

HEPATITIS B

The World Health Organization estimates that more than 300 million people are chronic HBV carriers world-wide (Maynard, 1990). Of these, about 25% are at risk for life-threatening complications of the associated liver disease. Thus, several years after the introduction of efficient HBV vaccines, infection with HBV and its long-term sequelae remain a world-wide public health problem.

185
Copyright © 1996, by Baillière Tindall
All rights of reproduction in any form reserved

Epidemiology

The prevalence of HBV carriers has significant geographical variations (Margolis et al, 1991). High rates (8–15%) of infection predominate in Asia, Africa, Pacific Islands and the Arctic. Eastern Europe and the Mediterranean basin are intermediate endemicity areas with prevalence rates of 2–7%, while North America and Western Europe are low prevalence areas (< 2%). The primary routes of infection, and consequently the prevalence of infection in infancy and childhood, vary with the endemicity of the disease.

Perinatal infection predominates in highly endemic areas where a high proportion of hepatitis B surface antigen (HBsAg)-positive women in childbearing age are hepatitis B e antigen (HBeAg)-positive and viraemic. About 90% of these women will infect their babies (Stevens et al, 1979). Conversely, in areas of intermediate endemicity mothers are often positive for antibody to HBeAg (anti-HBe). Only about 20% of them are viraemic and therefore capable of infecting their offspring (Lee et al, 1986). Recent investigations suggest that vertical transmission of HBV from anti-HBe-positive mothers may also depend on the presence, in the maternal serum, of a mixed viral population, including the wild-type virus capable of pro-ducing HBeAg (Raimondo et al, 1993).

Vertical transmission occurs through contact with maternal blood and other infectious fluids during labour, but rarely through placental trans-mission. In fact, of the mothers with acute hepatitis during pregnancy, only those who acquire infection late in the third trimester are likely to infect their babies (Tong et al, 1981).

Another major route of paediatric infection in areas of high and inter-mediate endemicity, such as Africa and the Mediterranean regions, respect-ively, is contact with HBsAg carriers, particularly siblings, during the first years of life. During the pre-vaccination era in Italy, we were able to see a heavy clustering of HBV infection within the families of chronically infected children, suggesting a high circulation of the virus through repeated, covert parenteral exposure (Bortolotti et al, 1988a). Horizontal transmission among playmates also seems to be important in highly endemic areas, while in intermediate or low endemicity regions spread of infection in the school or day-care centre is unlikely to play a relevant epidemiological role (Shapiro and Hadler, 1991).

In areas of low endemicity primary infection usually occurs in adolescents, following sexual intercourse or intravenous drug abuse. In USA only 1–3% of HBV infections are estimated to occur under 5 years of age (Margolis et al, 1991).

In recent years children adopted from high endemicity areas, such as South Asia and Rumania, have contributed to maintaining the pool of children with chronic HBV infection in low-endemicity areas and countries where mass vaccination is already under way, such as Italy (Hershow et al, 1987). In these children the source and the age of infection usually remain undefined. They often have high levels of HBV DNA in the serum and are highly infectious for non-vaccinated family contacts.

The likelihood of becoming chronically infected with HBV reflects the age at which infection occurs and the serological status of the mother. HBV transmitted from HBeAg-positive mothers results in HBV carriage in more than 90% of infants. This probably happens because of a tolerogenic effect of HBeAg (Milich et al, 1990). This low-molecular-weight, soluble viral protein can cross the placenta, inducing immunological tolerance in utero. The large HBeAg-positive viral inoculum from maternal blood or secretions can induce tolerance in the immunologically immature neonate. On the other hand, infection in infants born to anti-HBe-positive mothers is usually self-limited with asymptomatic seroconversion to anti-HBs or acute, rarely fulminant, hepatitis at the third or fourth month of life (Zanetti et al, 1982; Beasley and Hwang, 1983). This outcome seems to be the rule, even if the anti-HBe-positive mother has a mixed viral population, including the wild-type strain as a minor component. In these cases it was suggested that passively transmitted anti-HBe might neutralize the tolerogenic effect of HBeAg produced by wild-type HBV (Raimondo et al, 1993).

Infection acquired in the first few years of life becomes chronic in approximately 20–30% of cases, while infection acquired later persists in only 5–10%. Selective defects of immune response of IFN production could be implicated.

In recent years the improvement in living standards in several countries has induced a decrease in HBV endemicity. In Italy the incidence of acute hepatitis B has dramatically dropped since the mid 1980s and the prevalence of HBV carriers has decreased in both children and military recruits (D'Argenio et al, 1989; Stroffolini et al, 1989). Several social and sanitary events, including vaccination offered to the offspring of HBsAg-positive mothers and to family contacts of HBsAg carriers in several regions, along with AIDS prevention campaigns, have contributed to these changes. Universal vaccination of infants and 12-year old adolescents, started in 1991, is expected to control paediatric infection by the turn of the century.

Diagnosis

The diagnosis of chronic HBV infection relies on the detection of HBsAg in serum for more than 6 months. HBeAg and HBV DNA are the serological markers of active virus replication in the liver and are currently used to separate two phases of chronic infection: the early replicative phase and the later non-replicative, or low-replicative, phase. The highest levels of HBV DNA (over 1000 pg/ml) are found during the 'tolerant' phase of chronic infection, in children infected early in life in the absence of significant liver damage. Loss of HBeAg and subsequent anti-HBe seroconversion are usually associated with the disappearance of circulating HBV DNA by conventional hybridization techniques. Recently, however, the more sensitive polymerase chain reaction (PCR) amplification technique has allowed the detection of small amounts of HBV DNA even in anti-HBe-positive patients with normal alanine aminotransferase (ALT)

(Kaneko et al, 1990), but the clinical significance of this finding is, at present, unclear.

The observation that some anti-HBe-positive patients have high levels of viraemia and ongoing liver damage, and the availability of PCR sequencing techniques, have led to the identification of HBV variants with amino acid substitutions in the pre-core region which are unable to secrete HBeAg (Brunetto et al, 1989; Carman et al, 1989). These e-minus mutants are more common among HBsAg carriers in the Mediterranean area and have been associated with severe anti-HBe-positive hepatitis and the re-activation of chronic hepatitis after anti-HBe seroconversion. However, they are part of the natural course of chronic HBV infection and can be frequently detected as minor components of a mixed viral population. Barbera et al (1994a) found that 12 (40%) of 30 HBeAg-positive children with chronic hepatitis B circulated wild-type and e-minus mutant and that the pre-core mutant was associated with older age. The prognostic significance of these mutants and the reasons why, in some patients, they selectively accumulate during the course of infection remain to be clarified.

Alanine aminotransferase (ALT) is the most reliable serum test for monitoring liver disease. Conventionally, an ALT elevation lasting 6 months or more indicates chronic hepatitis. The rise in ALT levels is due to lysis of infected hepatocytes by cytotoxic lymphocytes. Therefore, high ALT levels are usually found during the immune clearance phase which precedes HBeAg-to-anti-HBe seroconversion.

Liver biopsy is helpful in defining the activity and stage of the disease and excluding other causes of liver damage such as metabolic or auto-immune disorders.

Natural history

Infection with HBV is usually asymptomatic in children. Acute icteric hepatitis is uncommon, and most patients come to observation for inter-current diseases leading to the detection of hepatomegaly or abnormal ALT, or following a family screening for HBV. Based on the biochemical, viro-logical and histological features, three phases of chronic HBV infection, reflecting different host–virus interactions, are recognized: the early repli-cative or immunotolerance phase, the late replicative or immuno-elimination or hepatitis phase and the non-replicative phase. Table 1 summarizes the most common features observed during these different phases in children.

As a rule the tolerance phase is sustained in patients infected during the perinatal period, such as Chinese children. Recently, Chan et al (1994) prospectively followed 111 infants, who had become chronic HBsAg carriers after perinatal infection, for a period of 8 to 10 years. Only 26% of these children had one or more episodes of ALT elevation during obser-vation (although this prevalence might be underestimated since ALT was determined only at annual intervals), and 33% lost HBeAg before the end of follow-up. Thus, children infected early in life are likely to seroconvert late during adolescence or adult life, when tolerance begins to break down

Table 1. The natural history of chronic hepatitis B and its different phases in children.

Feature	Tolerance phase	Immune clearance	Non-replicative phase
Duration			
perinatal infection	Several years	Few to several years	Long-lasting
post-natal infection	Few months to few years	Few to several years	Long-lasting
ALT	Normal	Elevated	Normal
HBeAg	Positive	Seroconversion rate: 15%/year	Negative
HBV DNA	Positive (>10^3 pg/ml)	Positive (<10^3 pg/ml)	Negative
Histology	Minimal hepatitis	Mild to moderate hepatitis	Normal liver, minimal hepatitis

spontaneously. We have followed two children born to mothers with acute hepatitis during pregnancy (Bortolotti et al, 1987) for 15 to 20 years and observed that ALT started to increase spontaneously at 14 and 17 years of age, respectively. Although tolerant children have sustained ALT normality, liver histology can discover inflammatory changes consistent with minimal hepatitis.

The tolerance phase is shorter in children infected after birth, and most of them come to observation when ALT abnormalities are already detectable. A wide range of histological lesions can be found in these patients, the most common consisting of mild to moderate chronic hepatitis (Bortolotti et al, 1990a). The spontaneous mean annual seroconversion rate is about 15%, and is similar to that observed in adults (Ruiz-Moreno et al, 1989; Bortolotti et al, 1990a). The results of the Padua Longitudinal study, started in 1976, indicate that up to 90% of children with chronic hepatitis B seroconvert to anti-HBe before reaching adulthood (Bortolotti et al, 1990a). A spontaneous ALT flare, sometimes higher than 20 times the upper normal range, is frequently seen to precede HBeAg-to-anti-HBe seroconversion if the patient is closely monitored. Males, children with a history of acute onset, those with high ALT levels and those with chronic active hepatitis, are likely to clear HBeAg earlier.

The non-replicative phase of chronic HBV infection is characterized by sustained ALT normalization, disappearance of histological features of necrosis and clearance of HBV DNA from serum. This apparently 'healthy carrier state' is long-lasting (Ruiz-Moreno et al, 1989; Bortolotti et al, 1990a; Zancan, et al, 1990). Few patients have occasional ALT alterations, usually below twice the normal. Only less than 2% per year will clear HBsAg during remission, some months to several years after anti-HBe seroconversion. Children infected after birth, with acute onset of illness and severe liver disease are more prone to become free of HBsAg.

Recent studies using PCR have disclosed the presence of small amounts of circulating HBV DNA in the majority of adults with chronic hepatitis B in remission after spontaneous or IFN-induced anti-HBe seroconversion (Loriot et al, 1992). We were able to confirm these data in 39 children followed for a mean period of 8 years after anti-HBe seroconversion. HBV DNA was detected in 87% of patients within 5 years of seroconversion and in 50% after 10 years (Bortolotti et al, 1995d). In particular, HBV DNA was persistently found in patients with late reactivation of liver disease and in one patient with cirrhosis who cleared HBsAg but later developed hepatocellular carcinoma. These low levels of HBV viraemia probably reflect low levels of virus replication. Persistent replication could support mild biochemical alterations and residual inflammatory liver lesions; it could also be responsible for late reactivation of liver disease and play a role in the development of hepatocellular carcinoma (HCC).

The long-term outcome of chronic hepatitis B and its complications in a series of 64 children with chronic hepatitis B are summarized in Table 2.

Table 2. Outcome of chronic hepatitis B in 64 untreated HBV DNA-positive children followed for longer than 10 years (median follow-up 13 years) in Padua (the large majority of patients had probably acquired infection in the post-natal period).

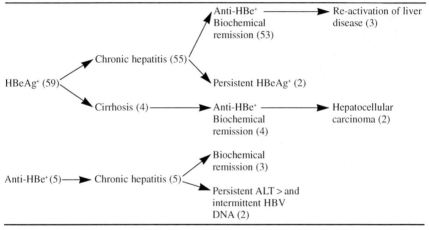

Cirrhosis and HCC

Severe forms of chronic hepatitis B are not commonly observed in childhood. During the replicative phase of the illness progression to cirrhosis has rarely been reported. In a large series of Italian and Spanish patients only 3% presented with cirrhosis, and progression of chronic hepatitis to cirrhosis during follow-up was uncommon (Bortolotti et al, 1986; Ruiz-Moreno et al, 1989). Cirrhosis is more often observed in males, infected early in life and with acute onset or high ALT levels at presentation. Patients with cirrhosis usually have a short-term replicative phase and are more prone to clear HBsAg. Two of four children with cirrhosis in our long-term follow-up study cleared HBsAg and seroconverted to anti-HBs.

Complications such as liver failure, ascites or oesophageal varices are rare during the paediatric age. Nevertheless, close monitoring of alphafetoprotein (every 6 months) and hepatic ultrasonography (every 12 months) is mandatory in cirrhotic children. In fact, cirrhosis may be a risk factor for HCC: in our longitudinal study, two of four children with cirrhosis have already developed HCC, 9 and 16 years after first observation, respectively, versus no patient with chronic hepatitis. At the time of diagnosis, both cases were asymptomatic. Alpha-fetoprotein levels were exceedingly high in one, but only slightly abnormal in the other. Hepatic ultrasonography showed a unique resectable lesion in both cases. Early diagnosis allowed successful resection, and both patients are still alive 1 and 6 years after diagnosis, respectively.

In parallel with the low prevalence of cirrhosis, HCC associated with HBV infection is rare in children from the Mediterranean area. Giacchino et al (1987) reported only three cases over a series of 325 chronically infected Italian children followed for 18 years. In one patient, who had seroconverted to anti-HBs, HCC was demonstrated in the absence of cirrhosis. In this patient, integrated sequences of HBV DNA were found in the tumour tissue, but not in the non-neoplastic tissue, suggesting that HBV DNA integration into the host's genome might have been important for HCC development. The largest series of children with HCC come from high endemicity areas such as the Far East. Hsu et al (1987) described 42 cases of HCC in children observed over three decades in Taiwan. Of them, 74% were cirrhotic, including 95% of those below 9 years of age. Most of these children had probably been infected in the perinatal period, and males predominated. The authors demonstrated that HCC could reach an advanced stage in children as young as 4 years.

Re-activation

Re-activation of hepatitis is usually defined by the re-appearance of HBV DNA in serum and the increase of ALT after a period of remission following anti-HBe seroconversion. Sometimes this event is associated with the re-appearance of HBeAg and sometimes with the persistence of anti-HBe positivity. During the Padua Longitudinal Study, annual visits and biochemical and virological tests were performed after anti-HBe seroconversion in 64 children or adolescents. Re-activation was observed in three females (aged 13 to 25 years) 3 to 9 years after anti-HBe seroconversion (Bortolotti, 1994). Only one patient was mildly symptomatic and complained of asthenia; thus, re-activation could have been missed in two cases if patients had not been regularly followed-up. ALT levels increased up to 25 times the normal, and seroreversion to HBeAg was observed in two cases.

The role of pre-core mutants in the re-activation of hepatitis B is still a matter of debate because either the e-minus variant or the wild-type population may be prevalent in the single patient. In fact, in our patients, direct HBV DNA sequencing (by courtesy of Dr M.R. Brunetto, Turin), showed the presence of a mixed viral population, including wild-type and e-minus mutants in all cases, with a prevalence of the mutant population only in the girl who remained anti-HBe positive.

Few children develop anti-HBe-positive hepatitis. In a follow-up study of 22 children with anti-HBe-positive chronic hepatitis at presentation, all but two achieved sustained biochemical remission within 4 years of follow-up (Bortolotti et al, 1990b). During the last 15 years, we have been able to identify only four children with long-lasting chronic hepatitis. All had fluctuating ALT, intermittent, low levels of viraemia, features of mild to moderate chronic hepatitis and no propensity for spontaneous remission.

Prevention

Numerous studies have documented the efficacy and safety of plasma-derived and recombinant hepatitis B vaccines. Both induce more than 95% protection against HBV in infants (Hsu et al, 1988). Recent long-term studies show that protection is sustained in a very high proportion of cases, and suggest that a booster dose at school age would not significantly increase protection (Committee on Infectious Diseases, 1992; Coursaget et al, 1994). Infants born to HBsAg-positive women should receive specific immunoglobulin (HB Ig) and should be immunized, preferably within 12 hours, receiving the second and third dose of vaccine at 1 and 6 months of age. Vaccination of children born to HBsAg-negative mothers can be performed during regularly scheduled visits, concurrently with other routine vaccinations.

Universal infant vaccination was found to be cost-saving in controlling HBV infections, and has been implemented in several endemic areas in the world (Xu et al, 1995). Such an immunization programme has resulted in the interruption of HBV transmission among Native Alaskan children and has reduced the HBsAg carrier rate in infants from African countries by more than 90%. The following family history can help us to appreciate fully the invaluable benefits of prevention. In 1980 a young, non-consanguineous couple brought their elder child, a 2-year-old boy, to us for examination. Their younger son had just died of fulminant hepatitis B at 3 months of age. Both mother and elder son were found to be HBsAg carriers, the mother being anti-HBe-positive. The child had already developed cirrhosis, which eventually progressed to HCC 9 years later. Meanwhile, the couple had had two further children: the first one treated with HB Ig at birth, and later vaccinated, and the second vaccinated and treated with HB Ig at birth. Both are free of infection.

Treatment

In recent years, IFN has been the drug of choice for the treatment of chronic hepatitis B in recent years, owing to its antiviral and immunomodulatory effect (Lok, 1994).

The long-term persistence of virus replication, particularly in those children who acquire HBV infection at birth, and the possibility that progression to a more severe liver disease may occur later in life, have prompted the use of IFN in an attempt to shorten the replicative phase of the illness and possibly prevent integration of the virus into the host genome. Candidates for treatment are HBeAg- and HBV DNA-positive children with abnormal ALT, preferably greater than twice the normal.

The *efficacy of therapy* is measured by HBV DNA and HBeAg clearance, and normalization of ALT. Different types of IFN and different treatment schedules have been used (Table 3). The results of controlled studies indicate that IFN-alpha is capable of enhancing the spontaneous anti-HBe seroconversion rate by twice to thrice in Caucasoid children, while in Chinese children with near-normal base-line ALT levels and low spontaneous seroconversion rate the effect is less appreciable. Ultimately the effect of IFN seems to be an acceleration of the spontaneous events occurring in children with chronic hepatitis B, with a significant increase in the seroconversion rate during treatment and subsequent months.

Table 3. IFN-alpha treatment of chronic hepatitis B in children.

Author	Number of cases	ALT IU/l	Schedule	HBe clearance (%)	Follow-up after therapy (months)
Lai et al (1987)	12	12	10 MU/m² t.i.w./12 weeks	0	15
	12	13	no treatment	0	15
Ruiz-Moreno et al	12	155	10 MU/m² t.i.w./12 weeks	33	12
(1990)	12	149	no treatment	25	12
Ruiz-Moreno et al	12	147	10 MU/m² t.i.w./6 months	58	9
(1991a)	12	138	5 MU/m² t.i.w./6 months	42	9
	12	115	no treatment	17	9
Utili et al (1991)	10	138	3 MU/m² t.i.w./12 months	20	6
	10	130	no treatment	10	6
Sokal et al (1993)	29	113	9 MU/m² t.i.w./16 weeks	38	8
	25	58	no treatment	8	8
Barbera et al (1994b)	21	109	7.5 MU/m² t.i.w./6 months	30	12
	19	72	3 MU/m² t.i.w./6 months	21	12
	39	72	no treatment	13.5	12

Available data suggest that 5 to 10 MU/m² of IFN-alpha administered thrice weekly for 6 months is the standard therapy. In our clinical practice we use 5 MU/m² of lymphoblastoid IFN and 7.5 to 10 MU/m² of recombinant IFN.

In an attempt to improve the rate of response to IFN some authors have used a 4-week course of steroids before IFN treatment. In Asian children this approach was unsuccessful (Lai et al, 1989). In Caucasoid children, Utili et al (1994) found that steroid priming significantly increased the spontaneous seroconversion rate, however the authors did not include patients treated with IFN alone for comparison. Giacchino et al (1995) randomized 35 children to receive either prednisolone or placebo followed by lymphoblastoid IFN, and found quite a similar HBeAg clearance rate in both groups. Similar results were obtained by Gregorio et al (1995) in a large multicentre, three-armed study comparing the outcome of hepatitis B in untreated children, in patients treated with steroids and IFN and in those receiving placebo and IFN. The anti-HBe seroconversion rate at 15–18 months was 13, 35 and 40%, respectively. The combination of levamisole plus IFN produced severe side-effects and has been discouraged (Ruiz-Moreno et al, 1993).

Kinetics of response

In patients who respond to IFN, HBV DNA clearance usually precedes HBeAg clearance by a few weeks to some months; this is then followed by anti-HBe seroconversion within a few weeks or months. These latter events are often accompanied by an ALT increase. ALT flares of up to 30 times the normal, associated with moderate asthenia and requiring therapy withdrawal, are rarely observed. HBeAg-to-anti-HBe seroconversion can take place either during therapy or within a few months after withdrawal. Late HBsAg clearance occurs in a trivial minority of cases, usually after an ALT flare.

Predictors of response

The small number of children enrolled in individual studies prevents a correct statistical evaluation of predictive factors as well as the meta-analysis of cumulative results. Higher ALT levels, HBV DNA values lower then 1000 pg/ml, a higher histological activity index and focal distribution of hepatitis B core-antigen-stained hepatocytes have all been associated with a better chance of response in Caucasoid children (Barbera et al, 1994b; Ruiz-Moreno et al, 1995a). In Asian children infected early in life the results are controversial as a recent report suggests that they are poor responders even if selected for ALT greater than twice the normal (Sira et al, 1994). For practical purposes we prefer to follow-up HBV DNA-positive children with ALT below twice the normal and treat them only in the case of ALT increase.

Few data are still available on the *long-term efficacy of therapy*. We observed a sustained virological and biochemical remission in all children who had seroconverted to anti-HBe after successful therapy and had been followed for up to 5 years. None of the patients cleared HBsAg, suggesting that eradication of infection occurs less frequently than in adult patients or requires a longer time span.

The *adverse effects of IFN* are usually represented by a flu-like syndrome which occurs in almost all cases at the start of treatment and ameliorates or disappears within 2 weeks of treatment. Persistence of slight fever, anorexia, weight or hair loss and abdominal pain can be observed in a minority of cases. Some patients develop leukopenia or thrombocytopenia which disappears with tapering or temporary interruption of IFN. Major side-effects such as convulsions or severe thrombopenia require withdrawal of treatment.

HEPATITIS DELTA

HDV is a defective virus that causes hepatitis only in individuals with concurrent HBV infection. Hepatitis delta is endemic in the Mediterranean basin and in some tropical areas. In the mid 1980s we found that 16% of children with chronic HBV infection were anti-HDV-positive in Southern

Italy and 5% in Northern Italy (Bortolotti et al, 1988a). Recent epidemiological surveys, however, indicate that the prevalence of delta infection is decreasing in Southern Italy in parallel with the changing epidemiology of hepatitis B (Sagnelli et al, 1994).

The diagnosis of chronic HDV infection is currently based on the detection of antibodies to HDV, at titre >1:100 in dilution series, for more than 6 months in patients with chronic HBV infection. However, the standard for diagnosis is the detection of HDAg in the liver by immunostaining, or of HDV RNA in serum by molecular hybridization.

Hepatitis delta in children is generally more severe than hepatitis B. Farci et al (1985) demonstrated that four (12%) of 34 children with hepatitis delta had cirrhosis at first liver biopsy, as compared to five (2%) of 236 hepatitis B patients. In addition, children with hepatitis delta are unlikely to achieve spontaneous remission during follow-up. In a recent study we investigated the long-term outcome of chronic delta hepatitis in 23 Italian children followed for 5–12 years after diagnosis and found that only three persistently normalized ALT during observation (Bortolotti et al, 1993). However, although 26% of patients had cirrhosis when first evaluated, the clinical and biochemical features remained reasonably stable over the years, independently of IFN therapy, and liver histology worsened only in two out of 14 children. Thus, adverse events associated with delta infection acquired in childhood are more likely to appear in adult life.

Since the late 1980s attempts have been made to treat children with hepatitis delta with IFN, due to the severity of liver disease. Craxi et al (1991) treated 10 children with chronic HDV hepatitis with recombinant IFN-alpha at the dose of 5 MU/m^2 for 4 months, followed by 3 MU/m^2 for 8 months. All were HDV DNA-positive on entry, and four were HBV DNA-positive. At the end of treatment, average ALT had decreased, and HDV RNA was positive in only three cases and HBV DNA in none; however, liver histology had improved in only one case, and HDAg had disappeared from the liver in only two. At 18 months, HDV RNA positivity appeared in five additional children. Thus, no relevant clinical and histological improvement were observed, suggesting that liver damage in these children is sustained by HDV.

HEPATITIS C

In recent years the cloning of the hepatitis C virus (HCV) and the development of antibody tests for HCV infection has resulted in numerous reports on the epidemiology, natural history and therapy of hepatitis C.

Unlike the large amount of information available on adults, data on paediatric HCV infection are still incomplete, mainly because most paediatric studies focused on vertical transmission and the prevalence and outcome of infection in multitransfused children. More recent investigations, however, are accumulating information on the epidemiology and natural history of hepatitis C in otherwise healthy children and on IFN treatment of the disease in paediatric patients.

Epidemiology

Anti-HCV prevalence in the paediatric population of different geographical areas is reported in Table 4. In developed countries the prevalence rates are lower than those in the adult population, probably as a consequence of a lower rate of parenteral exposure. Instead, a high circulation of HCV among children has been reported in some tropical areas where the disease might be endemic.

HCV infection is an infrequent cause of chronic hepatitis in childhood, at least in the Mediterranean area. In a study performed in Italy before the discovery of HCV, including 196 consecutive children with chronic hepatitis, only 5% of cases were classified as non-A, non-B hepatitis (Bortolotti et al, 1988a). The proportion of non-A, non-B cases remained low even when only asymptomatic cases were considered.

Table 4. Prevalence of anti-HCV in the paediatric population in different geographical areas.

Country (ref)	Type of population	Anti-HCV (%)
Japan[a] (Tanaka et al, 1992)	Children aged 6–15 years	0
Taiwan (Chang et al, 1993)	Children aged 0–12 years	0.1
Cambodia (Thuring et al, 1993)	Healthy children	0
Cameroon[a] (Ngatchu et al, 1992)	School children in urban area	14.5
Saudi Arabia[a] (Al-Faleh et al, 1991)	Children aged 1–10 years	1
Somalia (Aceti et al, 1993)	Children with diseases other than hepatitis	0
Italy (Romanò et al, 1994)	Children and teenagers	0.3

[a] Anti-HCV detected by first-generation tests.

Routes of transmission of HCV in childhood include: exposure to blood or blood products, vertical transmission, household contact and inapparent parenteral exposure. The impact of these different modes of infection probably has geographical variations. In developed countries most children with recognized HCV infection have received *blood or blood products*. In a series of 77 consecutive children with chronic hepatitis C without systemic diseases observed in Italy and Spain, 60% recalled occasional blood transfusion, often received in the perinatal period for intercurrent disorders (Bortolotti et al, 1994a). The high risk connected with blood transfusions is well documented in children with underlying systemic diseases receiving multiple transfusions of blood or blood products. Blanchette et al (1991) found that 95% of haemophilic children transfused with unheated or dry-heat-treated clotting factors were infected as compared to none of the children treated with cryoprecipitate, single-donor blood products or vapour-heated factor VIII or IX concentrates. Consistent rates of HCV infection have been reported in thalassaemic children (Resti et al, 1992). Leukaemic children are also at high risk for blood-borne hepatitis C, but specific antibodies may remain undetectable or appear transiently after chemotherapy withdrawal, due to immunosuppression. In these cases infection can be documented by the detection of circulating HCV RNA (Locasciulli et al, 1993). Paediatric dialysis patients are also at risk for HCV infection, the most predictive risk factor being the length of time on haemodialysis (Jonas et al, 1992).

The existence and extent of *vertical transmission* of HCV have been a matter of debate. In fact, passively transmitted antibodies circulate for some months after birth, before falling to indeterminate levels, and on the other hand children with HCV viraemia may fail to develop anti-HCV. Based on the detection of HCV RNA and on the sequencing of viral genomes in mother–infant pairs, vertical transmission of infection has now been clearly documented. The risk of transmission seems to be correlated with the titres of HCV RNA in the mother: Ohto et al (1994) showed that babies born to mothers with high levels of viraemia ($\geq 10^6$ infectious units of HCV per millilitre) had a 50% rate of infection. However, at variance with hepatitis B, and probably in relation to the low levels of HCV viraemia in the general population, the overall efficiency of vertical transmission would be low, as shown in Table 5. Evidence against appreciable vertical transmission is also provided by a Japanese survey of 1442 children aged 6–15 years, none of whom were found to be seropositive (Tanaka et al, 1992). Regarding the HCV genotype and transmission, Zanetti et al (1995) found that mothers with different HCV types could transmit infection to their offspring.

Table 5. Rate of vertical transmission of HCV infection detected by analysis of circulating HCV RNA in the offspring of anti-HCV-positive mothers.

Author (ref)	Number of infants	Transmission rate (%)
Ohto et al (1994)	54	5.6
Roudot-Thoraval et al (1993)	18	0
Ercilla et al (1993)	38	5.2
Lam et al (1993)	66	6
Zanetti et al (1995)	116	6
Manzini et al (1995)	45	2

There is evidence that concurrent infection with human immuno-deficiency virus (HIV) may increase the rate of vertical transmission of HCV. It has been hypothesized that the immunosuppression secondary to HIV infection might lead to increased HCV viraemia. In their series of mother–infant pairs, Giovannini et al (1990) observed that all 11 children with HCV infection were also HIV co-infected, while only one of the 14 children who did not seroconvert to anti-HCV was HIV infected. Using second-generation antibody tests and HCV RNA, Ercilla et al (1993) found that 11% of children born to co-infected mothers had acquired HCV infection as compared with 5.6% of the offspring of HIV-negative mothers. Zanetti et al (1995) investigated 116 babies of anti-HCV-positive mothers and found that none of the infants whose mother had HCV alone acquired infection, while eight babies (36%) of mothers co-infected with HIV acquired HCV alone (five cases) or associated with HIV (three cases). Other authors, however, denied any association between maternal HIV status and transmission of HCV (Lam et al, 1993; Manzini et al, 1995). The route and timing of transmission of HCV infection (in utero, at delivery, in the post-natal period) is still controversial. Breast-feeding does not seem to be an efficient mechanism. Ogasawara et al (1993) tested for the presence of HCV RNA in the breast milk of 10 HCV-infected mothers and did not detect viraemia. Zanetti et al (1995) found that 71 babies of anti-HCV-positive mothers remained uninfected despite breast feeding.

Household contact is also likely to have a limited role in the spread of HCV infection in the paediatric age, although some studies have shown that the circulation of HCV is higher in the families of chronic HCV carriers than in the general population. Compared to the high circulation of hepatitis B virus among siblings we were unable to identify couples of siblings in a series of 77 children with chronic hepatitis C (Bortolotti et al, 1994a). Iorio et al (1993) were also unable to detect anti-HCV in the siblings of 13 children with chronic hepatitis C, thus confirming the low efficiency of household transmission. A small but not trivial proportion of anti-HCV-positive children have *no obvious route of infection* (Table 6). The mechanisms of transmission and the sources of infection remain obscure in these cases. Conversely, inapparent transmission could be more frequent in tropical areas, such as Cameroon, where the infection rate is high in childhood, increases with age, and is correlated with social factors (Ngatchu et al, 1992). Child-to-child transmission has been hypothesized in this setting.

Diagnosis

Identification of the molecular structure of HCV allowed the detection of virus-specific antibodies that develop in response to HCV infection.

Second- and third-generation tests employing structural and non-structural antigenic specificities are currently being used. These tests have greatly improved the efficiency of first-generation assays, which detected only antibodies to c100–3 specificity. In fact, in a small series of Italian children with chronic hepatitis C, only 53% were found to circulate antibodies to c100–3, as compared with 86% of adults in the same area, suggesting that antibody production to some HCV antigens was less efficient in subjects who acquired infection early in life (Bortolotti et al, 1994b).

Because of the low titres of circulating virus that are common in HCV infection, reliable detection of viral antigens has not yet been demonstrated. Therefore, the detection of HCV RNA in the serum by PCR represents a valid diagnostic alternative. In children with chronic hepatitis, viraemia is often fluctuating, and more than one serum sample taken at different time intervals may be needed to confirm the serological diagnosis. In the small series of children we recently examined, circulating HCV RNA was detected in 93% of patients when serial serum samples were tested. The frequent fluctuations of PCR positivity suggested low levels of viraemia in these patients. Overall, a good correlation was found between anti-HCV positivity and HCV viraemia, while only one of 10 children with anti-HCV-negative non-A, non-B hepatitis was transiently HCV RNA-positive in the same study (Bortolotti et al, 1994b).

Following the isolation of HCV in 1989, several strains of HCV have been cloned. Comparative analysis of viral sequences provided evidence of at least six different existing viral genotypes, termed 1 to 6, with different geographical distributions. The most prevalent in Europe are genotypes 1 and 2 (Simmonds et al, 1994). These variants may have important clinical implications, including a different response rate to IFN therapy. The investigation of HCV types by serotyping in a series of Italian and Spanish children with chronic hepatitis C confirmed the prevalence of genotype 1, and indicated an association between genotype 3 and maternal HCV infection often associated with drug abuse (Bortolotti et al, 1995c). Further studies by PCR amplification in both Spanish and Italian children have shown the presence of genotype 1b in about half of the cases (Bortolotti et al, 1995b; Ruiz-Moreno et al, 1995b).

Clinical aspects and natural history of hepatitis C in childhood

The clinical features and the evolution of post-transfusion and community-acquired hepatitis C in childhood have been described in retrospective studies.

Few paediatric patients with chronic hepatitis C recall an acute symptomatic onset of their illness. Accordingly, in a prospective Italian study we found that non-A, non-B hepatitis accounted for only 6% of symptomatic cases of acute viral hepatitis in childhood (Bortolotti et al, 1988b). Hsu et al (1991) observed 27 Taiwanese children with acute non-A, non-B hepatitis, representing 15% of all children hospitalized for hepatitis-like episodes over a 10-year period. Using first-generation ELISA, eight (38%) of 21 were anti-HCV-positive, and three (37.5%) progressed to chronicity. Indeed, the chronicization rate of HCV infection in childhood has not yet been established. Resti et al (1992) investigated 30 thalassaemic children with acute hepatitis C, of whom 57% progressed to chronicity, independently of acute-phase features. Lai et al (1993) analysed 66 thalassaemic patients with acute hepatitis C and found a chronic evolution in 80%. More recently, Chang et al (1994) prospectively studied 88 children at risk due to frequent blood transfusion or maternal HCV infection during pregnancy. Of 10 children who contracted primary infection, confirmed by the detection of circulating HCV RNA, six (60%) progressed to chronicity, including three with abnormal transaminases. Single prospective studies of vertically transmitted infection do not yet allow us to estimate the chronicization rate owing to the small number of infants included.

As with chronic hepatitis B, chronic hepatitis C in children is usually an asymptomatic disease, independently of the source of infection. In a retrospective study of 77 otherwise healthy children aged 1–14 years, we were unable to show significant clinical differences between post-transfusion and community-acquired cases (Bortolotti et al, 1994a). Only 22% of patients complained of mild symptoms, and two were jaundiced at presentation. Hepatomegaly was recorded in 48% of cases and spleno-megaly in 18%. At presentation, liver histology was consistent with mild to moderate chronic hepatitis in 32% of cases, and with chronic persistent, lobular or non-specific reactive hepatitis in the other cases. Only a few cases had wide ALT fluctuations during follow-up, suggesting relapses, while the majority had milder variations sometimes with values falling within the normal range. Conversely, the histological pattern of chronic hepatitis C was severe in a series of 78 Italian thalassaemic patients, with active disease in 12% of cases and cirrhosis in another 38% (Resti et al, 1992). A similar pattern, however, was found in seven anti-HCV-negative children, suggesting a multi-factorial aetiology of liver damage in these patients, including iron overload.

Hepatitis C is likely to have an indolent course throughout adolescence, as suggested by the observation of children on long follow-up. Unlike hepatitis B, however, hepatitis C has a low propensity for spontaneous biochemical remission. Over a mean observation period of 6 years, only 11% of patients in the Italian–Spanish series achieved a sustained ALT normalization and one asymptomatic patient had histological evidence of cirrhosis (Bortolotti et al, 1994a). Long-term prospective studies are necessary to evaluate the putative contribution of chronic hepatitis C acquired in childhood to the pool of adult HCV carriers and the relationship between HCV genotype and outcome of the disease.

The possibility that a *healthy HCV carrier state* exists has been debated. In most adult patients with normal ALT but HCV RNA positivity, liver histology has shown features of associated liver disease (Alberti et al, 1992). Thaler et al (1991) found persistent HCV RNA positivity in infants of HCV carrier mothers despite normal ALT levels and a lack of anti-HCV production, suggesting that the infection might remain unrecognized during childhood. Nevertheless, in most infants born of anti-HCV-positive mothers serological evidence of infection is associated with occasional or persistent ALT alterations (Lesprit et al, 1995).

Prevention and therapy

With the lack of specific vaccines, the prevention of HCV infection is essentially based on blood screening and general precautions in order to avoid the spread of infection. Anti-HCV screening of blood and blood products using a second-generation test is expected to reduce significantly the rate of new HCV infections in children in developed areas. In Taiwan, a recent prospective study of post-transfusion hepatitis in children who had undergone open-heart surgery failed to detect infection in 56 transfused children, whereas 4% of 198 children had been infected before the introduction of HCV screening of blood units (Ni et al, 1994).

IFN-alpha has been extensively used in the treatment of chronic hepatitis C in adult patients. Although chronic hepatitis C is a mild disease in childhood, approach to therapy should be considered and evaluated also in paediatric patients for different reasons: there is a low propensity of the disease to biochemical remission over the years and progression to a more severe liver disease in adult life cannot be ruled out; patients with shorter duration of infection would respond better to IFN therapy; IFN, even at high doses, proved to be well tolerated in children with chronic hepatitis B.

Candidates to treatment are patients with increased ALT, serological evidence of HCV infection and histological diagnosis of chronic hepatitis,

Table 6. Putative source of chronic HCV infection in children from Italy and Spain.

Putative exposure	Bortolotti et al (1994a) (77 cases) (%)	Iorio et al (1993) (13 cases) (%)
Blood transfusions	60	54
Other percutaneous (surgery, needlestick ...)	9	15
Anti-HCV+ mother	15.5	23
Unknown	15.5	7

after accurate exclusion of other potential causes of liver damage. Associated autoimmunity has to be carefully ruled out, because the detection of auto-antibodies, particularly liver–kidney microsomal auto-antibodies, seems to be frequent in chronically infected children (Bortolotti et al, 1995a).

To date, the results of few pilot studies are available. An uncontrolled study by Ruiz Moreno et al (1992) evaluated the efficacy of a 6-month course of IFN-alpha at a dose of 3 MU/m² thrice weekly in 11 HCV RNA-positive children, four anti-HCV-positive and five anti-HCV-negative. At the end of treatment, 36% had normal ALT and most were HCV RNA-negative, while 45% had normal enzymes at 24 months. HBV RNA status at the end of follow-up was not investigated.

Recently we concluded a pilot controlled study of 27 otherwise healthy children with biopsy-proven anti-HCV-positive hepatitis randomized for treatment with recombinant IFN-alpha for 12 months at a dose of 5 MU/m² thrice weekly versus no treatment (Bortolotti et al, 1995a). Twenty-two patients were HCV RNA-positive on entry. According to the protocol, treatment was stopped at 4 months in four cases because of an increase or low change of ALT values. At 12 months a sustained ALT normalization was found in 78% of all treated patients versus 7.6% of untreated cases. At 24 months 43% of treated children had persistently normal ALT and absence of circulating HCV RNA as compared with 7.6% of untreated children who had sustained ALT normality but who were HCV RNA-positive.

Fujizawa et al (1994) treated 12 children with chronic hepatitis C, who had serious underlying diseases, with IFN-alpha at a dose of 0.1 MU/kg daily and then three times a week for 22 weeks. At the end of treatment all children had cleared HCV RNA and 11 had normal ALT. During follow-up HCV RNA re-appeared in four cases and ALT increased again in four.

Vegnente et al (1994) investigated 21 otherwise healthy children and randomized 11 of them to receive lymphoblastoid IFN (3 MU/m² thrice weekly for 48 weeks) and 10 to receive no treatment. Three patients stopped treatment because of an ALT increase, and five of eight, who completed treatment, maintained biochemical remission at 24 months, while only one child in the control group had a protracted ALT normalization.

Clemente et al (1994) treated 51 thalassaemic children with recombinant IFN-alpha at a dose of 3 MU/m² thrice weekly for 15 months and observed a long-term response in 37% of treated versus none of 14 untreated children. Response correlated directly with the liver iron burden, and the authors concluded that therapy was worthwhile in patients with mild to moderate iron burden.

IFN was generally well tolerated, and side-effects were similar to those observed in HBsAg-positive children. Two cases have been reported who did not respond to IFN and developed an ALT flare with the appearance of previously undetectable liver–kidney–microsomal auto-antibodies (Ruiz-Moreno et al, 1991b; Bortolotti et al, 1995d).

The preliminary results of IFN treatment are encouraging but need to be supported in larger series in order to evaluate adequate treatment schedules and also potential predictors of response. Preliminary data would suggest that, as observed in adults, genotype 1b is associated with a poorer response (Ruiz-Moreno et al, 1995b).

Conversely, a pilot study including six children with chronic hepatitis C cured of paediatric malignancies and treated with a 12-month course of IFN showed a primary response in three cases but subsequent relapse in all, suggesting that conventional therapy may be less efficient in this particular group of previously immunosuppressed subjects (Cesaro et al, 1994).

SUMMARY

In endemic areas infection with hepatitis B virus is a common cause of chronic liver disease in childhood. High levels of viral replication and mild ALT abnormalities are the rule in children infected perinatally and many of them are likely to maintain viral replication through their youth. Conversely about 90% of children infected later in life clear HBeAg and achieve sustained remission of liver disease before reaching adulthood. The eventual outcome of infection and disease in these patients remains unpredictable as reactivation of liver damage and viral replication may occur after several years of sustained remission. Cirrhosis is a rare and early complication of chronic HBV infection in children, and a risk factor for hepatocellular carcinoma. IFN therapy can accelerate HBV DNA clearance, improving the spontaneous anti-HBe seroconversion rate in Caucasian children by two to three times.

Hepatitis delta is the most severe form of chronic viral hepatitis in childhood. Cirrhosis can be diagnosed in up to 26% of patients at presentation, and few cases respond to IFN therapy.

Hepatitis C is relatively rare in children. Before the discovery of HCV, blood transfusions were the most common source of infection. Hepatitis C is usually a mild, asymptomatic disease in otherwise healthy children, but has a poor propensity to spontaneous remission over the years. For this reason, and based on the experience in adults, IFN treatment is now being evaluated.

REFERENCES

Aceti A, Taliani G, Bruni R et al (1993) Hepatitis C virus infection in chronic liver disease in Somalia. *American Journal of Tropical Medicine and Hygiene.* **48:** 581–584.
Alberti A, Morsica G, Chemello L et al (1992) Hepatitis C Viremia and liver disease in symptom-free individuals with anti-HCV. *Lancet* **340:** 697–698.

Al-Faleh FZ, Ayoola EA, Al-Jeffry M et al (1991) Prevalence of antibody to hepatitis C virus among Saudi Arabian children: a community-based study. *Hepatology* **14:** 215–218.

Barbera C, Calvo P, Coscia A et al (1994a) Precore mutant hepatitis B virus and outcome of chronic infection and hepatitis in hepatitis B e antigen positive children. *Pediatric Research* **36:** 247–350.

Barbera C, Bortolotti F, Crivellaro C et al (1994b) Recombinant interferon α 2a hastens the rate of HBeAg clearance in children with chronic hepatitis B. *Hepatology* **20:** 287–290.

Beasley RP, Hwang LY (1983) Post-natal infectivity of hepatitis B surface antigen-carrier mothers. *Journal of Infectious Diseases* **147:** 185–190.

Blanchette VS, Vorstman E, Shore A et al (1991) Hepatitis C infection in children with hemophilia A and B. *Blood* **78:** 285–289.

Bortolotti F (1994) Chronic hepatitis B in childhood. Unaswered questions and evolving issues. *Journal of Hepatology* **21:** 904–909.

Bortolotti F, Calzia R, Cadrobbi P et al (1986) Liver cirrhosis associated with chronic hepatitis B virus infection in childhood. *Journal of Pediatrics* **108:** 224–227.

Bortolotti F, Cadrobbi P, Rude L et al (1987) Prognosis of hepatitis B transmitted from HBsAg positive mothers. *Archives of Disease in Childhood* **62:** 201–203.

Bortolotti F, Calzia R, Vegnente A et al (1988a) Chronic hepatitis in childhood: the spectrum of the disease. *Gut* **29:** 659–664.

Bortolotti F, Cadrobbi P, Armigliato M et al (1988b) Acute non-A, non-B hepatitits in childhood. *Journal of Pediatric Gastroenterology and Nutrition* **7:** 22–26.

Bortolotti F, Cadrobbi P, Crivellaro C et al (1990a) Long-term outcome of chronic type B hepatitis in patients who acquired hepatitis B virus infection in childhood. *Gastroenterology* **99:** 805–810.

Bortolotti F, Calzia R, Cadrobbi P et al (1990b) Long-term evolution of chronic hepatitis B in children with antibody to hepatitis B e antigen. *Journal of Pediatrics* **116:** 552–555.

Bortolotti F, Di Marco V, Vajro P et al (1993) Long-term evolution of chronic delta hepatitis in children. *Journal of Pediatrics* **122:** 736–738.

Bortolotti F, Jara P, Diaz C et al (1994a) Posttransfusion and community-acquired hepatitis C in childhood. *Journal of Pediatric Gastroenterology and Nutrition* **18:** 279–283.

Bortolotti F, Vajro P, Barbera C et al (1994b) Patterns of antibodies to hepatitis C virus and hepatitis C virus replication in children with chronic non-A, non-B hepatitis. *Journal of Pediatrics* **125:** 916–918.

Bortolotti F, Vajro P, Balli F et al (1995a) Non-organ specific autoantibodies in children with chronic hepatitis C. *Journal of Hepatology* **23 (supplement 1):** 106.

Bortolotti F, Vajro P, Balli F et al (1995b) Hepatitis C virus genotypes in children with chronic hepatitis C. Proceedings of the International Congress of Liver Diseases, Basel, p 95.

Bortolotti F, Jara P, Simmonds P et al (1995c) Hepatitis C serotypes in chronic hepatitis C of children. *International Hepatology Communications* **4:** 35–41.

Bortolotti F, Giacchino R, Vajro P et al (1995d) Recombinant interferon alpha therapy in children with chronic hepatitis C. *Hepatology* **22:** 1623–1627.

Bortolotti F, Wirth S, Crivellaro C et al (1996) Long-term persistence of hepatitis B virus DNA in the serum of children with chronic hepatitis B after hepatitis B e antigen to antibody seroconversion. *Journal of Pediatric Gastroenterology and Nutrition* **22:** 270–274.

Brunetto MR, Stemmler M, Shodel F et al (1989) Identification of HBV variants which cannot produce precore-derived HBeAg and may be responsible for severe hepatitis. *Italian Journal of Gastroenterology* **21:** 151–154.

Carman WF, Jacina MR, Hadziyannis S et al (1989) Mutation preventing formation of 'hepatitis B e antigen' in patients with chronic hepatitis B infection. *Lancet* **ii:** 588–590.

Cesaro S, Rossetti F, De Moliner L et al (1994), Interferon for chronic hepatitis C in patients cured of malignancy. *European Journal of Pediatrics* **153:** 659–662.

Chan C-Y, Lee SD, Yu M-Y et al (1994) Long-term follow-up of hepatitis B virus carrier infants. *Journal of Medical Virology* **44:** 336–339.

Chang MH, Lee CY & Chen DS (1993) Minimal role of hepatitis C virus infection in childhood liver diseases in an area hyperendemic for hepatitis B virus infection. *Journal of Medical Virology* **40:** 322–325.

Chang MH, Ni YH, Hwang LH et al (1994) Long-term clinical and virologic outcome of primary hepatitis C virus infection in children: a prospective study. *Pediatric Infectious Diseases* **13:** 769–773.

Clemente MG, Congia M, Lai ME et al (1994) Effect of iron overload on the response to recombinant interferon-alfa treatment in transfusion-dependent patients with thalassemia major and chronic hepatitis C. *Journal of Pediatrics* **125**: 123–128.

Committee on Infectious Diseases, American Academy of Pediatrics (1992) Universal hepatitis B immunization. *Pediatrics* **89**: 795–800.

Coursaget P, Leboulleux P, Soumare M et al (1994) Twelve-year follow-up study of hepatitis B immunization of Senegalese infants. *Journal of Hepatology* **21**: 250–254.

Craxi A, Di Marco V, Volpes R et al (1991) treatment with recombinant alpha-2b-interferon of chronic HDV hepatitis in children. *Progress in Clinical and Biological Research* **364**: 399–404.

D'Argenio P, Esposito D, Mele A et al (1989) Decline in the exposure to hepatitis A and B infections in children in Naples, Italy. *Public Health* **103**: 385–389.

Ercilla MG, Fortuny C, Roca A et al (1993) Mother to infant transmission of hepatitis C virus. Proceedings 4th International Symposium on HCV, Tokyo, p 31.

Farci P, Barbera C, Navone C et al (1985) Infection with the delta agent in children. *Gut* **26**: 2–7.

Fry KE, Linnen J, Zhang-Keck Z-Y et al (1995) Sequence analysis of a new RNA virus (Hepatitis G virus, HGV) reveals a unique virus in the Flaviviridae family. *Hepatology* **22**: 181A.

Fujisawa T, Ohkawa T, Inui A & Yokota S (1994) Effect of interferon therapy on serum hepatitis C virus RNA levels in children with chronic hepatitis C. *International Hepatology Communications* **2**: 316–320.

Giacchino R, Pontisso P, Navone C et al (1987) Hepatitis B virus (HBV)-DNA-positive hepatocellular carcinoma following hepatitis B virus infection in a child. *Journal of Medical Virology* **23**: 151–155.

Giacchino R, Main J, Timitilli A et al (1995) Dual-centre, double blind, randomized trial of lymphoblastoid interferon alpha with or without steroid pretreatment in children with chronic hepatitis B. *Liver* **15**: 143–148.

Giovannini M, Tagger A, Ribero ML et al (1990) Maternal–infant transmission of hepatitis C virus and HIV infections: a possible interaction. *Lancet* **335**: 1166.

Gregorio M, Jara P, Vegnente A et al (1995) Lymphoblastoid interferon alpha with or without steroid pre-treatment in children with chronic hepatitis B: a multicentre controlled trial. *Hepatology* **22**: 326A.

Hershow RC, Hadler SC & Kane MA (1987) Adoption of children from countries with endemic hepatitis B: transmission risks and medical issues. *Pediatric Infectious Diseases* **6**: 431–441.

Hsu HC, Wu MZ, Chang MH et al (1987) Childhood hepatocellular carcinoma develops exclusively in hepatitis B surface antigen carriers in three decades in Taiwan. *Journal of Hepatology* **5**: 260–267.

Hsu HM, Chen DS, Chuang CH et al (1988) Efficacy of a mass hepatitis B vaccination program in Taiwan *JAMA* **260**: 2231–2235.

Hsu SC, Chang MH, Chen DS et al (1991) Non-A, non-B hepatitis in children: a clinical, histological, and serological study. *Journal of Medical Virology* **35**: 1–6.

Iorio R, Guida S, Porzio S et al (1993) Chronic non-A, non-B hepatitis: role of hepatitis C virus. *Archives of Disease in Childhood* **68**: 219–222.

Jeffers LJ, Piatak M, Bernstein DE et al (1995) Hepatitis G virus infection in patients with acute and chronic liver disease of unknown etiology. *Hepatology* **22**: 182A.

Jonas MM, Zilleruelo GE, La Rue SI et al (1992) Hepatitis C infection in a pediatric dialysis population. *Pediatrics* **89**: 707–709.

Kaneko S, Miller RH, Di Bisceglie AM et al (1990) Detection of hepatitis B virus DNA in serum by polymerase chain reaction. *Gastroenterology* **99**: 799–804.

Lai CL, Lok ASF, Lin HJ et al (1987) Placebo-controlled trial of recombinant alpha 2-interferon in Chinese HBsAg carrier children. *Lancet* **ii**: 877–880.

Lai CL, Lok ASF, Lin HJ et al (1989) Use of recombinant alpha 2 interferon (r-IFN) with or without steroids in Chinese HBsAg carrier children: a prospective double blind controlled trial. *Gastroenterology* **96 (supplement A):** 618.

Lai ML, De Virgilis S, Argiolu F et al (1993) Evaluation of antibodies to hepatitis C virus in a long-term prospective study of post-transfusion hepatitis among thalassemic children: comparison between first and second generation assay. *Journal of Pediatric Gastroenterology and Nutrition* **16**: 458–464.

Lam JPH, McOmish F, Burns SM et al (1993) Infrequent vertical transmission of hepatitis C virus. *Journal of Infectious Disease* **167**: 572–576.

Lee S-D, Lo K-J, Wu J-C et al (1986) Prevention of maternal-infant hepatitis B transmission by immunization: the role of serum hepatitis B virus DNA. *Hepatology* **6**: 369–373.

Lesprit E, Dussaix E, Laurent J et al (1995) Mother-to-child transmission of hepatitis C virus: presentation, virological markers and outcome. *Hepatology* 22: 348A.

Locasciulli A, Cavalletto D, Pontisso P et al (1993) Hepatitis C virus serum markers and liver disease in children with leukemia during and after chemotherapy. *Blood* 82: 2564–2567.

Lok ASF (1994) Treatment of chronic hepatitis B. *Journal of Viral Hepatitis* 1: 105–124.

Loriot MA, Marcellin P, Bismuth E et al (1992) Demonstration of hepatitis B virus DNA by polymerase chain reaction in the serum and the liver after spontaneous or therapeutically induced HBeAg to anti-HBe or HBsAg to anti-HBs seroconversion in patients with chronic hepatitis B. *Hepatology* 15: 32–36.

Manzini P, Saracco G, Cerchier A et al (1995) Human immunodeficiency virus infection as risk factor for mother-to-child hepatitis C virus transmission; persistence of antihepatitis C virus in children is associated with the mother's anti-hepatitis C virus immunoblotting pattern. *Hepatology* 21: 328–332.

Margolis HS, Alter MJ & Hadler SC (1991) Hepatitis B: evolving epidemiology and implications for control. *Seminars in Liver Disease* 11: 84–92.

Maynard JE (1990) Hepatitis B: global importance and need for control. *Vaccine* 8 (supplement): 18–20.

Milich DR, Jones JE, Hughes JL et al (1990) Is a function of the secreted hepatitis e antigen to induce immunologic tolerance in utero? *Proceedings of the National Academy of Sciences of the USA* 87: 6599–6603.

Ngatchu T, Stroffolini T, Rapicetta M et al (1992) Seroprevalence of anti-HCV in an urban children population: a pilot survey in a developing area, Cameroon. *Journal of Tropical Medicine and Hygiene* 95: 57–61.

Ni YH, Chang MH, Lue HC et al (1994) Posttransfusion hepatitis C virus infection in children. *Journal of Pediatrics* 124: 709–713.

Ogasawara S, Kage M, Kosai K et al (1993) Hepatitis C virus RNA in saliva and breastmilk of hepatitis C carrier mothers. *Lancet* 341: 561.

Ohto H, Terazawa S, Sasaki N et al (1994) Transmission of hepatitis C virus from mothers to infants. *New England Journal of Medicine* 330: 744–750.

Raimondo G, Tanzi E, Brancatelli S et al (1993) Is the course of perinatal hepatitis B virus infection influenced by genetic heterogeneity of the virus? *Journal of Medical Virology* 40: 87–90.

Resti M, Azzari C, Rossi ME et al (1992) Hepatitis C virus antibodies in a long-term follow-up of beta-thalassemic children with acute and chronic non-A, non-B hepatitis. *European Journal of Pediatrics* 151: 573–576.

Romanò L, Azara A, Chiaramonte M et al (1994) Low prevalence of anti-HCV antibody among Italian children. *Infection* 22: 350–352.

Roudot-Thoraval F, Pawlotsky JM, Thiers V et al (1993) Lack of mother-to-infant transmission of hepatitis C virus in human immunodeficiency virus-seronegative women: a prospective study with hepatitis C virus RNA testing. *Hepatology* 17: 772–777.

Ruiz-Moreno M, Camps T, Garcia Aguado J et al (1989) A serological and histological follow-up of chronic hepatitis B infection. *Archives of Disease in Childhood* 64: 1165–1169.

Ruiz-Moreno M, Jimenez J, Porres JC et al (1990) A controlled trial of recombinant interferon-alpha in caucasian children with chronic hepatitis B. *Digestion* 45: 26–33.

Ruiz-Moreno M, Rua MJ, Molina J et al (1991a) Prospective, randomized controlled trial of interferon alpha in children with chronic hepatitis B. *Hepatology* 13: 1035–1039.

Ruiz Moreno M, Rua MJ, Carreno V et al (1991b) Autoimmune chronic hepatitis type 2 manifested during interferon therapy in children. *Journal of Hepatology* 12: 265–266.

Ruiz-Moreno M, Rua MJ, Castillo I et al (1992) Treatment of children with chronic hepatitis C with recombinant interferon-alpha: a pilot study. *Hepatology* 16: 882–885.

Ruiz-Moreno M, Garcia R, Rua MJ et al (1993) Levamisole and interferon in children with chronic hepatitis B. *Hepatology* 18: 264–269.

Ruiz-Moreno M, Castillo I, Bartolomé J et al (1994) HCV genotypes in children and response to interferon therapy. *Hepatology* 20: 392A.

Ruiz-Moreno M, Camps T, Jimenez J et al (1995a) Factors predictive of response to interferon therapy in children with chronic hepatitis B. *Journal of Hepatology* 22: 540–544.

Ruiz-Moreno M, Castillo I, Bartolomé J et al (1995b) Hepatitis C virus genotypes in serum and liver of children with chronic hepatitis C. *Hepatology* 22: 345A.

Sagnelli E, Stroffolini T, Ascione A et al (1994) The epidemiology of hepatitis delta infection in Italy. *Journal of Hepatology* 15: 211–215.

Shapiro CN & Hadler SC (1991) Hepatitis A and hepatitis B virus infections in day-care settings. *Pediatric Annual* **20:** 435–441.

Simmonds P, Alberti A, Alter HJ et al (1994) A proposed system for the nomenclature of hepatitis C viral genotypes. *Hepatology* **19:** 1321–1324.

Sira JK, Sleight E, Boxall E et al (1994) Treatment of hepatitis B virus carrier children in the UK. *Hepatology* **20:** 301A.

Sokal EM, Wirth S, Goyens P et al (1993) Interferon alfa-2b therapy in children with chronic hepatitis B. *Gut* **34 (supplement):** S87–S90.

Stevens CE, Neurath RA, Beasley RP & Szmuness W (1979) HBeAg and anti-HBe detection by radioimmuneassay. Correlation with vertical transmission of hepatitis B virus in Taiwan. *Journal of Medical Virology* **3:** 237–241.

Stroffolini T, Franco E, Romano G et al (1989) Changing pattern in the seroepidemiology of hepatitis B virus infection in Sardinia, Italy. *European Journal of Epidemiology* **5:** 202–206.

Tanaka E, Kiyosawa K, Sodeyama T et al (1992) Prevalence of antibody to hepatitis C virus in Japanese schoolchildren: comparison with adult blood donors. *American Journal of Tropical Medicine and Hygiene* **46:** 460–464.

Thaler MM, Park CK, Landers DV et al (1991) Vertical transmission of hepatitis C virus. *Lancet* **338:** 17–18.

Thuring EG, Joller-Jemelka HI, Sareth H et al (1993) Prevalence of markers of hepatitis A, B, C and of HIV in healthy individuals and patients of a Cambodian province. *Southeast Asian Journal of Tropical Medicine and Public Health* **24:** 239–249.

Tong MJ, Thursby M, Rakela J et al (1981) Studies on the maternal–infant transmission of the viruses which cause acute hepatitis. *Gastroenterology* **74:** 205–208.

Utili R, Sagnelli E, Galanti B et al (1991) Prolonged treatment of children with chronic hepatitis B with recombinant alpha 2a interferon: a controlled randomized study. *American Journal of Gastroenterology* **86:** 327–330.

Utili R, Sagnelli E, Gaeta GB et al (1994) Treatment of chronic hepatitis B in children with prednisone followed by alpha interferon: a controlled randomized study. *Journal of Hepatology* **20:** 163–167.

Vegnente A, Iorio R, Guida S et al (1994) Preliminary results of a trial with alpha lymphoblastoid interferon (a-Ly-INF) in 21 children with chronic hepatitis C (CHC). *Journal of Pediatric Gastroenterology and Nutrition* **19:** 365.

Xu Z-Y, Duan S-C, Margolis HS et al (1995) Long-term efficacy of active postexposure immunization of infants for prevention of hepatitis B infection. *Journal of Infectious Diseases* **171:** 54–60.

Zancan L, Chiaramonte M, Ferrarese N & Zacchello F (1990) Pediatric HBsAg chronic liver disease and adult asymptomatic carrier status: two stages of the same entity. *Journal of Pediatric Gastroenterology and Nutrition* **11:** 380–384.

Zanetti AR, Ferroni P, Magliano EM et al (1982) Perinatal transmission of the hepatitis B virus and of the HBV associated delta agent from mothers to offspring in Northern Italy. *Journal of Medical Virology* **9:** 139–148.

Zanetti AR, Tanzi E, Paccagnini S et al (1995) Mother-to-infant transmission of hepatitis C virus. *Lancet* **345:** 289–291.

2

Recent advances in the molecular biology of
hepatitis B virus

PIER PAOLO SCAGLIONI
MARGHERITA MELEGARI
JACK R. WANDS

Hepatitis B virus (HBV) is the prototype member of the hepadnavirus
family (Gust et al, 1986). This group of enveloped DNA-containing viruses
share similar genomic and structural organization. Other members of the
family are the woodchuck hepatitis virus (WHV) (Summers et al, 1978),
the ground squirrel hepatitis virus (GSHV) (Marion et al, 1980), the duck
hepatitis virus (DHBV) (Mason et al, 1980) and the heron hepatitis virus
(HHV) (Sprengel et al, 1988). In addition to these five members of the
hepadnavirus family, there are two recently identified new agents, namely,
the Ross's Goose hepatitis virus (RGHV) (Cullen et al, 1994) and arctic
squirrel hepatitis virus (ASHV) (Testut et al, 1995). All viruses display
structural homology, primarily infect the liver of their natural host, and
cause acute or chronic hepatitis. Moreover, chronic infection with the
mammalian hepadnaviruses is often associated with the development of
hepatocellular carcinoma (McLachlan, 1991; *Current Topics in Microbiology and Immunology*, 1991).

Cloning of the hepadnavirus genome has allowed an analysis of the
genomic organization and replication cycle and the characterization of the
viral gene products, and it has also contributed to a better understanding of
the biology of these viruses. Critical to these studies was the availability of
animal models and the generation of tissue culture systems that support
complete viral replication. This review will focus on selected aspects of the
HBV biology with particular emphasis on advances made at the molecular
level. Comparison will be made to the other hepadnaviruses where significant similarities exist or the corresponding information for HBV is not
available. For general reviews we refer the readers to recent publications in
this area (McLachlan, 1991; *Current Topics in Microbiology and
Immunology*, 1991; Ganem et al, 1994; Chisari and Ferrari, 1995; Wands et
al, 1996).

The HBV virion consists of an outer shell composed of the virus-
encoded envelope proteins and host-derived lipid components. The viral
nucleic capsid displays a T3 symmetry and consists of 180 subunits of the

Copyright © 1996, by Baillière Tindall
All rights of reproduction in any form reserved

viral core monomeric protein (McLachlan, 1991; *Current Topics in Microbiology and Immunology*, 1991). The viral genome is located inside the nucleocapsid and comprises a partially double-stranded relaxed circular DNA molecule of 3.2 kb in length that encodes the virus-specific polymerase necessary for replication in the hepatocyte. The level of the circulating virions during the natural course of infection is variable and ranges from 10^3 to 10^9 viral particles per millilitre of serum. More abundant molecular species are the 22 nm subviral particles, with a concentration varying between 10^6 and 10^{14} particles per millilitre. These spheres and filamentous forms are composed of the envelope proteins and host-derived lipid components. They lack viral DNA or RNA and are therefore not infectious. Despite the abundancy of such particles in serum, their role in the biology of viral infection is unknown. These subviral particles are highly immunogenic, and, for this reason, have been used in the generation of the first clinical effective HBV vaccines (Szmuness et al, 1980). There is

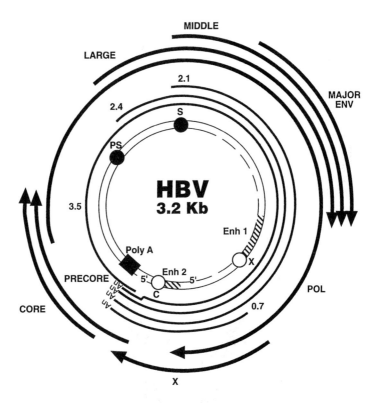

Figure 1. Diagram showing the molecular organization of HBV. The virus has a small compact 3.2 kb genome. The solid (●) and open circles (○) represent the promoter elements for pre-S and S envelope reading frames, and core and x open reading frames, respectively. The dashed bars represent the two enhancer regions. The symbol (■) represents the polyadenylation site. The thin lines of 3.5, 2.4, 2.1 and 0.7 kb in length represent the mRNA transcripts. The solid lines represent the various encoded viral structural proteins as indicated.

some speculation that the subviral particles absorb neutralizing antibodies and shield HBV virions from the host immune response but this hypothesis has not been substantiated by experimental data.

The host range of the hepadnaviruses is restricted. HBV has been shown to infect only man and chimpanzees (Maynard et al, 1971). In addition to the liver, HBV may infect a variety of other tissues, including skin, kidney, pancreas, peripheral blood lymphocytes and monocytes and spermatozoa (Dejan et al, 1984; Hadchouel et al, 1988; Pasquinelli et al, 1990). In view of the fact that HBV appear to replicate at very low levels in lymphocytes, it is not clear how these extra-hepatic sites contribute to the natural history of HBV infection or re-infection. Nevertheless, it has been proposed that extra-hepatic sites of HBV replication may contribute as a source of virus for re-infection of grafts following liver transplantation.

VIRAL ENTRY INTO HEPATOCYTES

The earliest molecular events that lead to viral entry into hepatocytes are poorly understood. It is generally believed that HBV interacts with specific cell-surface protein(s) followed by receptor-mediated endocytosis of virus into hepatocytes. However, lack of a tissue culture cell type that is susceptible to HBV infection has hampered progress in this area. The only in vitro system presently available for studies of HBV infection consists of primary human hepatocyte cultures, and results thus far are inconsistent and lack reproducibility (Gripon et al, 1988). However, primary duck hepatocyte cultures are consistently infectable by duck hepatitis B virus (DHBV) and provide a tissue culture system useful for the possible identification and cloning of DHBV receptor(s) on hepatocytes (Pugh and Summers, 1989). Moreover, the duck model allows for assays of infectivity that will be critical for functional evaluation of the candidate receptor proteins. At present, there is no convincing evidence that the HBV receptor protein(s) have been identified and characterized.

It is likely that hepadnavirus attachment to target cells will be mediated by the envelope proteins and, in the case of mammalian hepadnaviruses, three proteins named pre-S1, pre-S2 and s may be important in this regard. It is noteworthy that the avian hepadnavirus envelope protein lacks the pre-S2 component. With respect to HBV, it has not been established whether only one of the envelope proteins mediates the initial viral attachment to the hepatocyte membrane. Some evidence has been provided for involvement of the pre-S1 protein in binding to liver membranes, as well as to HepG2 hepatocellular carcinoma cells (HCC) and other cell lines (Neurath et al, 1986; 1990; Pontisso et al, 1989). It has also been reported that the pre-S2 protein may bind via polymerized human serum albumin to liver plasma membranes (Pontisso et al, 1989). Very recently it has been suggested that the pre-S2 protein may bind to fibronectin found in the liver sinusoids and facilitate HBV uptake into hepatocytes (Budkowska et al, 1995). In contrast, another report found that the HBV pre-S2 protein was not essential for HBV infectivity in vivo and in vitro (Fernholz et al, 1993).

Other investigations have proposed that the small s protein contains the putative binding sites for the hepatocyte receptor(s) (Hertogs et al, 1993; Mehdi et al, 1994). Finally, the interleukin-6 receptor has been proposed as the HBV binding protein (Neurath et al, 1992). Thus far, it has been difficult to establish firmly that such proteins play a role in viral entry into the hepatocyte, and further investigations in a cell culture system that is permissive for HBV infection will be required before firm conclusions are reached regarding the functional properties of these candidate receptor proteins.

On the other hand, there has been significant progress in the cloning of DHBV binding proteins. Two groups of investigation have independently identified and cloned a hepatocyte-derived glycoprotein that binds with high affinity to DHBV particles. Both studies have searched for proteins present in duck hepatocytes that were able to bind to the pre-S protein of DHBV since it was previously shown that this region is critical in mediating DHBV infection in primary duck hepatocyte cultures (Klingmüller and Schaller, 1993). This candidate DHBV receptor was identified as a novel member of the basic carboxypeptidase gene family and named gp170/180. The protein possesses some of the characteristics of a viral receptor (Kuroki et al, 1995; Tong et al, 1995). For example, it was expressed in tissues susceptible to DHBV infection and located on the cell surface. The interaction of gp170/180 with the pre-S protein was inhibited by 'wild type' DHBV virions in a dose-dependent manner. In addition, natural infection of duck hepatocytes with DHBV blocked the binding of a recombinant pre-S protein to gp170/180 and suggests that this molecule may be important during the life cycle of viral infection. Furthermore the binding site of pre-S to gp170/180 was mapped and found to coincide with known epitopes recognized by two neutralizing monoclonal antibodies that prevent DHBV infection of duck hepatocytes. Expression of gp170/180 in a non-DHBV infectable hepatoma cell lines resulted in viral attachment to the cell surface. Following attachment, however, viral replication was not detected. These experiments indicate that gp170/180 is an authentic DHBV binding protein but is not the only component(s) of a DHBV receptor complex (Kuroki et al, 1995). It seems likely that cellular uptake of DHBV may be mediated by a multistep process where multiple cellular proteins are involved. This is an active area of hepatitis B research, and identification of such viral receptor proteins would further stimulate efforts to design antiviral drugs aimed at blocking viral attachment to the hepatocyte membrane.

HEPADNAVIRUS REPLICATION

The cellular events following HBV entry into hepatocytes are unknown. The viral envelope is presumably removed by host factors and the nucleocapsid delivers the viral genome to the nucleus. Indeed, nucleocapsid proteins have been found both in the nucleus and cytoplasm of infected hepatocytes (McLachlan, 1991; *Current Topics in Microbiology and*

Immunology, 1991). It has been shown that the carboxyterminal region of the core protein contains a nuclear localization signal (Yeh et al, 1990) and nuclear localization of core proteins appears to be regulated by a phosphorylation event. For example, the phosphorylated form of the core protein is found predominantly in the nucleus, whereas the non-phosphorylated form is present both in the cytoplasm and circulating virions. (Machida et al, 1991; Liao and Ou, 1995). In addition, it has been reported that circulating HBV virions contain protein kinase activity (McLachlan, 1991). However, it is uncertain how viral DNA enters the nucleus since a recent study performed in HBV transgenic mice has shown that the nucleocapsids cannot be transported across intact nuclear membranes (Guidotti et al, 1994). This observation suggests that after viral entry into the cell and uncoating, the nucleocapsids are disassembled on the cytoplasmic side of the nuclear membrane. After this step, the viral DNA may enter the nucleus and initiate productive infection by unknown mechanism(s). This process seems to be conserved among the hepadnaviruses since DHBV nucleocapsids are found exclusively in the cytoplasm of infected hepatocytes (Pugh et al, 1989). Thus, according to present concepts of HBV replication, the encapsidation of viral nucleic acids probably occurs in the cytoplasm.

In the nucleus the partially double-stranded viral genome is converted into covalently closed circular DNA (cccDNA). The formation of cccDNA requires a series of enzymatic reactions. These include: (1) completion of positive plus (+) strand DNA synthesis; (2) removal of the bond that links the polymerase to the 5′ end of the negative (−) strand DNA; (3) removal of the RNA primer from the 5′ end of (+) strand DNA; and (4) ligation of the DNA ends. The observation that known inhibitors of viral DNA synthesis, such as foscarnet and 2′,3′-dideoxyguanosine, do not block the conversion of partially double-stranded DNA into cccDNA suggests that these steps may be mediated by cellular enzymes (*Current Topics in Microbiology and Immunology*, 1991; Kock and Schlicht, 1993). The cccDNA serves as the template for generation of viral transcripts, and therefore represent a key molecule in the hepadnaviral life cycle. It is organized as a viral minichromosome and is present in about 10–50 copies inside the nucleus of infected hepatocytes. The half-life is estimated to be 3–5 days (McLachlan, 1991; Summers et al, 1991; Civitico and Locarnini, 1994; Newbold et al, 1995). The copy number of DHBV cccDNA has been shown to be regulated by pre-S proteins. In this regard, infection of primary duck hepatocyte cultures with a mutant DHBV that was unable to synthesize pre-S proteins resulted in 20–30 times higher levels of both DHBV cccDNA and viral synthesis within the cells. Moreover, such mutant DHBV genomes were associated with a cytopathic effect in infected cells (Summers et al, 1991; Lenhoff and Summers, 1994). Hepatitis B viral genomes with equivalent mutations in the envelope genes produced similarly deregulated levels of viral DNA synthesis (Melegari, Scaglioni and Wands, unpublished results). Therefore, it appears that the envelope proteins not only play a role in virion uptake into the cell but may also be involved in the regulation of viral replication.

Hepadnaviruses replicate their DNA genomes by reverse transcription of an RNA intermediate, designated pre-genomic RNA (McLachlan, 1991; *Current Topics in Microbiology and Immunology*, 1991). This process has been analysed in great detail. Historically, the study of hepadnaviral replication has been hampered by the inability to synthesize an active viral polymerase enzyme in vitro. This problem has been solved since the discovery that active DHBV polymerase may be synthesized in a rabbit reticulocyte lysate system (Wang and Seeger, 1992). Subsequently, catalytically active HBV and DHBV polymerase have been produced in *Xenopus* oocytes, yeast and insect cells (Seifer and Standring, 1993; Tavis and Ganem, 1993; Landford et al, 1995).

The current model of HBV replication is based largely on data obtained with DHBV; however, it is believed that the same processes are probably conserved in the HBV replicative machinery as well. The pre-genomic RNA is generated by read-through transcription from the circular cccDNA as shown in Figure 2. This species of RNA is more than a full genome in length and contains a terminal redundancy region at the 5′ and the 3′ end of the transcript. Present in the terminal redundancy region are two key *cis*-acting motifs: (1) a direct repeat (DR1), comprising a 12-nucleotide-long element; (2) ε, an RNA stem–loop structure required for RNA packaging into the nucleocapsids. Of the two copies of ε, the 5′ end copy is the one used for encapsidation (Junker-Niepmann et al, 1990) since deletion of the 5′ end ε ablates RNA packaging and DNA replication, whereas deletion of the 3′ end ε allows both reactions to occur (Seeger and Maragos, 1990). The pre-genomic RNA is not only template for reverse transcription but also the messenger RNA of the polymerase gene (pol). Genetic studies have indicated that pol plays a key role both in RNA packaging and in priming DNA synthesis. Indeed, pol-deficient mutants will assemble morphologically normal nucleocapsids, but they are devoid of viral pre-genomic RNA (Hirsh et al, 1990). It has also been demonstrated that encapsidation of viral pol requires the presence of ε-containing RNA (Bartenschlager and Schaller, 1992). Therefore it may be concluded that packaging of RNA and pol activity within the nucleocapsids are tightly coupled molecular events.

After binding of pol to pre-genomic RNA, (−) strand DNA synthesis will occur. The 5′ end of (−) strand DNA maps within the DR1 region. Characterization of genetically marked GSHV and WHV genomes had previously suggested that reverse transcription proceeds from within the DR1 copy present at the 3′ end of the pre-genomic RNA (Seeger et al, 1986; Seeger and Maragos, 1990). However, recent studies have shown that reverse transcription initiates in the 5′ copy of ε in the pre-genomic RNA. The model that emerged supports the notion that pol binds to the 5′ copy of ε present on its own RNA template, and that this event is necessary to initiate both RNA packaging and DNA synthesis (Pollack and Ganem, 1994; Fallows and Goff, 1995). During this step, pol acts as primer of reverse transcription, synthesizing a four-nucleotide-long DNA oligonucleotide that becomes covalently linked to the amino-terminal region of pol (Zoulim and Seeger, 1994). Since DNA priming occurs also in the absence of core proteins, the four-nucleotide-long primer could be

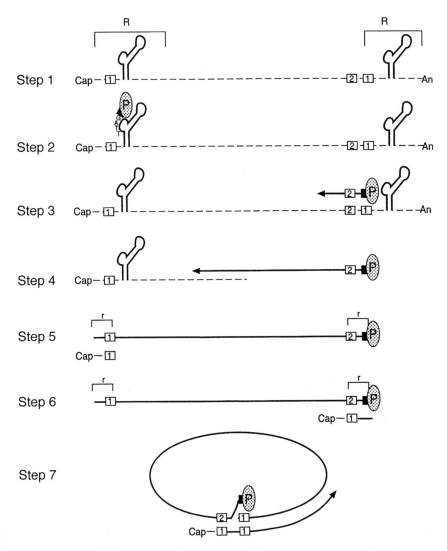

Figure 2. Model of HBV replication (1) Pre-genomic RNA (dashed line) is the template for reverse transcription. This molecule is more than one genome in length and bears a terminal redundancy (R) containing DR1 and a stem–loop structure defined as ε. The pre-genomic RNA is capped and polyadenylated (Cap and An respectively). (2) HBV polymerase (oval P) interacts with the ε present at the 5′ end of pre-genomic RNA and initiates reverse transcription, synthesizing the first four nucleotides of minus-strand DNA (GATT) using the ε bulge as template. The first nucleotide of minus-strand DNA is covalently bound to the polymerase terminal protein (black triangle). Pre-genomic RNA is packaged into viral nucleocapsids along with P through interaction with ε. (3) Inside the nucleocapsids, P is translocated to the copy of DR1 present at the 3′ end of pregenomic RNA. There, the previously synthesized GATT stretch anneals to DR1 and the minus-strand DNA is extended (upper solid line). (4) The pre-genomic RNA is degraded by the RNase H activity of P. (5) The 5′ end of pre-genomic template is left undegraded. (6) The RNA oligomer is transferred by virtue of its complementarity (r) to DR2, where it primes plus-strand DNA synthesis (lower solid line). (7) The sequence identity present in r allows circularization of the viral genome. Plus-strand DNA is extended to generate mature viral DNA.

synthesized either prior to, or concomitantly with, RNA packaging in vivo. Moreover, the *cis* preference that the polymerase exhibits in encapsidating the pre-genomic RNA from which it has been translated (and therefore, in replicating it) suggests that all these events may occur cotranslationally in vivo.

Following the synthesis of the first four nucleotides of (−) strand DNA, the polymerase–primer complex dissociates from the template and re-anneals with complementary sequences at the DR1 located near the 3′ end of the pre-genomic RNA where DNA synthesis will continue (Wang and Seeger, 1993). The molecular mechanism for this template switch is, at present, elusive. However, it is possible that the pre-genomic RNA complex constitutes the signal for the recruitment of core protein necessary to assemble the complete viral nucleocapsid structure and that the precise arrangement of polymerase and pre-genomic RNA inside the nucleocapsids accounts for the specificity of the transfer reaction.

The (−) strand DNA is elongated within the nucleocapsids. As DNA synthesis proceeds, the pre-genomic RNA is degraded by the pol derived RNAse H activity. When pol reaches the 5′ end of the RNA template, it leaves an undegraded 18-nucleotide-long RNA molecule. This RNA oligomer is then transferred onto DR2, the second 12-nucleotide-long element identical to DR1, that is located downstream from the 5′ end copy of DR1 on (−) strand DNA—from where it primes (+) strand DNA synthesis. During (+) strand DNA elongation, the circularization of (−) strand DNA will occur. However, in mature virions, (+) strand DNA is not extended to full length. The molecular mechanisms responsible for these events are unknown. It has been suggested that the structure of the nucleo-capsids provides the spatial arrangements required for the RNA oligomer transfer and circularization of the viral genome (McLachlan, 1991; *Current Topics in Microbiology and Immunology*, 1991).

TRANSCRIPTIONAL CONTROL OF HBV GENE EXPRESSION

Sequence analysis of the HBV genome reveals four open reading frames (ORF). These ORFs encode the core, envelope, polymerase (pol) and X genes as shown in Figure 1. The core ORF contains two in-frame translation initiation codons that allow for the synthesis of two distinct molecules, namely, the core and the hepatitis B e (HBe) proteins. The envelope ORF contains three in-frame translational initiation codons that direct the synthesis of the pre-S1, pre-S2 and s proteins. Thus, the compact HBV genome encodes, by partially overlapping ORFs containing transcriptional control elements, seven viral gene products. Moreover, HBV transcription not only serves as a source of the viral mRNAs, but also provides the RNA template necessary for reverse transcription into a (−) strand DNA molecule. As a molecular consequence of this organization, the hepadnaviruses displays a highly efficient transcriptional strategy that relies on the differential use of transcriptional initiation sites to synthesize both unspliced and spliced transcripts.

HBV infected hepatocytes express two classes of RNA transcript: (1) genomic transcripts of 3.5 kb, and (2) subgenomic transcripts of 2.4 and 2.1 kb. The 3.5 kb species serves as mRNA for the HBe, core and pol proteins as well as the template for reverse transcription into (−) strand DNA. The other two smaller species are templates for the envelope proteins. In addition to these species, a 0.7 kb transcript derived from the X gene region has been identified. We refer the readers to two reviews for a detailed description of the HBV transcripts, promoters and enhancer elements (McLachlan, 1991; *Current Topics in Microbiology and Immunology*, 1991). In addition to the above described transcripts, HBV also synthesizes at least two spliced RNA transcripts (*Current Topics in Microbiology and Immunology*, 1991). These transcripts may be encapsidated, reverse transcribed and present in a significant portion of the circulating virion population (Terré et al, 1991). The function of these spliced transcripts is not clear and appears not to be required for HBV replication. In vitro studies suggest that translation of spliced transcripts is associated with higher levels of core and HBe protein production (Wu et al, 1991; Rosmorduc et al, 1995; Melegari, Scaglioni and Wands, unpublished results). More important, the presence of reverse transcribed spliced transcripts in blood circulation as enveloped particles has been linked with persistent infection, and evaluation of the functional role of these defective particles during the natural course of disease is clearly warranted.

REGULATORY PROTEINS

Mammalian hepadnaviruses carry in their genome a short ORF that has been designated 'X'. The HBx gene encodes for a 154-amino-acid long gene product called hepatitis B x protein (HBx). The biochemical and functional characterization of this protein has proved to be difficult and, to date, no definitive function has been assigned to HBx. Since the X ORF is not present in the avian hepadnaviruses, it seems reasonable to propose that HBx may not be required for replication, but may play a regulatory role in the viral life cycle. Computer analysis of the X ORF reveals that HBx should be a hydrophobic non-secreted protein of 17 kDa. There are no motifs that would suggest a known function for the protein, and there is no sequence homology with other reported genes in the data base. Of note, however, are four consensus sites for protein phosphorylation in the protein. An mRNA transcript of 0.7 kb has been detected in tissue culture cells transfected with HBV DNA. It is important to emphasize that no studies have convincingly demonstrated the presence of the HBx in liver during natural infection. Nevertheless, indirect evidence suggests that HBx is produced during active HBV infection since several investigations have identified an anti-HBx immune response in individuals with acute and chronic disease (McLachlan, 1991).

In order to obtain levels of HBx protein that allow a biochemical characterization, many laboratories have expressed the X ORF in a variety of cell lines under the control of heterologous promoters. There is debate on the subcellular localization of HBx protein (McLachlan, 1991; Doria et al, 1995). Some studies have localized HBx exclusively to either the nucleus or cytoplasm, or both, as well as to other sites such as the nuclear membrane and cytoskeleton. This type of analysis has been hampered by two factors: (1) the lack of an antibody that consistently and specifically recognizes the HBx protein, and (2) investigators have rarely used the same cell line and experimental conditions. To overcome these limitations, we have studied the subcellular distribution of HBx using a high-affinity mouse monoclonal antibody (mAb) raised against a renatured recombinant HBx protein. A panel of cell lines were transiently transfected by an expression vector that allow the synthesis of 'wild type' HBx protein and subsequently stained with this mAb using indirect immunofluorescence and subcellular localization determined by confocal laser scanning microscopy. This type of analysis revealed that the subcellular distribution of HBx was cell-type-dependent. For example, in 293 kidney and HeLa cells, HBx was localized solely to the cytoplasm. In COS7 green monkey kidney and HuH-7 HCC cells, HBx appears associated with the nuclear membrane. Finally, HBx was localized to the nucleus of HepG2 human hepatoblastoma and LMH chicken hepatoma cells (Scaglioni, Melegari and Wands, unpublished results).

Many studies have suggested that HBx may play a role as a transcriptional regulator even though the protein does not bind to DNA directly (McLachlan, 1991; *Current Topics in Microbiology and Immunology*, 1991; Rossner, 1992; Doria et al, 1995). The activity of nearly all the promoter/enhancer combinations studied thus far have been reported to be affected by HBx. The regulatory elements included in these investigations are the HBV enhancer/core promoter, SV40 promoter/enhancer, HIV and RSV long terminal repeats (LTR), AP1 and NF-kB responsive elements. The HBx protein has also been reported to activate RNA polymerase II genes (Aufiero and Schneider, 1990; Wang et al, 1995). Very recently, it has been shown that HBx may bind to the RPB5 subunit of RNA polymerase II and stimulate the basal transcriptional machinery of eukaryotic cells (Cheong et al, 1995). Moreover, HBx also appears capable of interacting with TATA binding proteins and will stimulate transcriptional activity (Qadri et al, 1995; Wang et al, 1995). A direct interaction of HBx with so many protein partners seems promiscuous and highly unlikely, particularly when one considers the very low concentrations of HBx in HBV-infected liver (McLachlan, 1991). As an alternative hypothesis, one study suggested that HBx may exert a modulating function on cell growth related to activation of signal transduction pathways. One group of investigators has implicated the activation of protein kinase C as a candidate molecule to explain the pleiotropic activities of HBx (Kekulé et al, 1993). This finding, however, has not been confirmed by other groups (Lucito and Schneider, 1992; Murakami et al, 1994).

Most recently, the yeast two-hybrid screening method has been used to identify and clone proteins that interact with HBx. Such an approach has been successfully used in other systems to study protein–protein interactions and may ultimately contribute to the understanding of their biological function within the cell. Thus far, a gene encoding for DNA repair enzyme (Lee et al, 1995), two subunits of the proteasome complex (Fischer et al, 1995; Liang TJ, personal communication), and a novel leucine zipper containing protein (Melegari, Scaglioni and Wands, unpublished results) have been identified by this technique. Additional experiments will be required to evaluate the function of these HBx-interacting proteins. Despite numerous studies supporting the ubiquitous transcriptional activator properties of HBx, this function of the protein still remains controversial (Rossner, 1992). Most investigations have been based on transient transfection experiments using X ORF containing expression constructs together with reporter genes into cultured cells. The inherent variability of this approach in combination with lack of a reliable antibody to detect the HBx protein and its mutants has made interpretation of the findings regarding the transactivation properties of HBx difficult indeed.

Nevertheless, there is evidence to support the concept that, during productive viral infection, HBx may play a role in activating HBV gene transcription. This hypothesis is supported by both in vitro and in vivo experiments. Several groups have studied the effect of variant HBx produced by inactivating mutations of the X ORF and studied the mutant proteins in the context of HBV replication. The ability of HBV to replicate in a cell line that poorly supports HBx transactivation (i.e. HuH-7 HCC cells) was not affected by ablation of the X ORF. However, the capability of the same genome to replicate in a line that supports HBx transactivation (i.e. HepG2 HCC cells) was seriously compromised (Yaginuma et al, 1987; Blum et al, 1992, Nakatake et al, 1993; Zoulim et al, 1994). These results are supported by in vivo findings in woodchucks experimentally infected with WHV carrying several stop codons in the woodchuck X ORF. The mutant genomes were able to replicate in HepG2 cells although at reduced levels (Zoulim et al, 1994), but did not initiate a productive infection in the woodchuck liver (Chen et al, 1993; Zoulim et al, 1994).

The ability of the HBx protein to transactivate a variety of promoters of cellular genes involved in cell growth has led to the hypothesis that HBx may contribute to the development of hepatocellular carcinoma (HCC) in chronic HBV infected individuals. This hypothesis is supported by the finding that HBx has the ability to transform mouse hepatocytes in vitro (Hohne et al, 1990). Functional X gene sequences are also frequently found in the integrated forms of HBV DNA present in HCC tumour specimens (Wollersheim et al, 1988). It has been reported that transgenic mice expressing the X gene develop HCC (Kim et al, 1991). This observation implies a direct role for HBx in the pathogenesis of HCC. Unfortunately, these findings have not been confirmed by others despite repeated attempts, and no clear conclusions may be reached using this animal model system (Lee et al, 1990). Similarly, the reports that HBx interacts in vivo and in vitro with the p53 tumour suppressor protein and alters its functional capabilities has not been validated by other laboratories (Wang et al, 1994; Truant et al, 1995). Finally, the other viral protein reported to have transcriptional transactivator properties is a 3' truncated preS2/s molecule of HBV initially found in an integrated form of a HCC tumour specimen (McLachlan, 1991).

POST-TRANSCRIPTIONAL CONTROL OF HBV GENE EXPRESSION

By genetic and biochemical analysis, a novel *cis*-acting post-transcriptional regulatory element (PRE) which appears essential for high-level expression of the HBV gene products has been discovered. This element is located 3′ to the envelope coding region and is active at the post-transcriptional and RNA processing level (Huang and Liang, 1993). It has been proposed that PRE may inhibit the splicing process and facilitate the transport and utilization of HBV transcripts.

VIRAL ASSEMBLY AND SECRETION

Virion assembly is a series of complex events that takes place in the cytoplasm of HBV infected cells. Early steps involve the interaction of core proteins, DNA polymerase and pre-genomic RNA, and these components are assembled into nucleocapsids where viral DNA synthesis will take place. Interaction of the nucleocapsids with the viral envelope proteins occurs, but the domains on the preS/s proteins or on the nucleocapsids that mediate the interaction are not known. Virion budding or secretion through the secretory pathway has never been shown. The first step in virion assembly overlaps with the beginning of DNA replication and consists of the priming of DNA synthesis at the 5′ end of the pre-genomic RNA. This step does not require the presence of nucleocapsid proteins in vitro. However, transfer of the viral pol to the 3′ end containing DR1 region and completion of viral DNA synthesis requires the presence of the viral nucleocapsids. This structure consists of 180 core protein subunits arranged in an icosahedrical structure with $T = 3$ symmetry (McLachlan, 1991; *Current Topics in Microbiology and Immunology*, 1991) and will contain the viral nucleic acids and polymerase enzyme.

The core protein of HBV consists of an 187-amino acid polypeptide with two functional domains: an amino terminal region (from amino acid 1 to amino acid 144) necessary and sufficient for nucleocapsid oligomerization, and a carboxy terminal arginine-rich domain required for nucleic acid binding and viral DNA synthesis (Birnhaum and Nassal, 1990; McLachlan, 1991; *Current Topics in Microbiology and Immunology*, 1991; Nassal, 1992a). The current model for the nucleocapsid oligomerization (Zhou et al, 1992) is proposed as follows. Core protein homodimers are formed when a threshold concentration of core monomers is reached within the cytoplasm of the infected cell. These homodimers interact and form the spherical HBV capsid. Intermolecular disulphide bonds occurs between conserved cysteine residues present in the core protein subunits (Nassal, 1992b). These disulphide linkages are believed to stabilize the nucleocapsid structure, but are not required for assembly of replication competent core particles (Nassal, 1992b; Zhou and Standring, 1992).

The carboxy terminal arginine-rich portion of the core protein has the ability to bind viral and heterologous DNA and RNA probably on the basis of net positive charge (McLachlan, 1991; *Current Topics in Microbiology and Immunology*, 1991). Its functional role has been recently studied in the context of the entire HBV genome (Nassal, 1992a). Truncated mutants lacking this domain (core protein ending at amino acid 144) were able to assemble nucleocapsids, but were deficient in encapsidation of pre-genomic RNA. When the core protein ended at amino acid 164, pre-genomic RNA encapsidation and (–) strand DNA synthesis did occur; however, synthesis of (+) strand viral DNA was drastically reduced. Moreover, almost all of the DNA synthesized was in a double-stranded linear form, indicating that this truncated mutant core protein will not support the synthesis of relaxed circular (RC) viral DNA. Furthermore, addition of carboxy terminal residues to amino acid position 173 restored RC viral DNA synthesis to 'wild type' levels. The carboxy terminal region of the HBV core protein may be separated into two regions, each of which playing distinct roles in HBV nucleocapsid assembly and replication. The region from amino acid 144 to 163 is necessary for RNA encapsidation, whereas the region from amino acid 163 to 173 is required as an essential auxiliary component in HBV replication to allow viral DNA elongation and circularization. In this regard, it has been suggested that the carboxy terminal region of the HBV core acts as a single-stranded DNA-binding protein to arrange a favourable configuration for the completed (–) strand DNA inside the nucleocapsids and allow the viral DNA and polymerase correctly to initiate (+) strand synthesis at the DR2 region. There are additional cellular components that appear to participate in the nucleocapsid assembly process (Kann and Gerlich, 1994; Lingappa et al, 1994) and further characterization and identification of these factors is expected to improve the understanding of the molecular process(es) of virion assembly.

The HBV genome encodes for a second gene that has a primary sequence related to the core gene, namely, the pre-core protein. The pre-core ORF has an initiation codon in frame with the core ORF, and translation results in the synthesis of a core-related polypeptide (named p25) with a 29 amino acid extension at the N-terminus. The first 19 amino acids act as a signal peptide and directs the protein into the cell secretory pathway, and after amino and carboxy terminal processing, the protein is secreted from the cell in a soluble form. Processed pre-core protein or hepatitis B e antigen (HBeAg) has been found in the serum of HBV-infected patients and correlates with high levels of viraemia (McLachlan, 1991; *Current Topics in Microbiology and Immunology*, 1991). The observation that all the hepadnaviruses encode a pre-core protein suggests an evolutionary advantage for this molecule in the viral life cycle. However, HBV viruses lacking HBeAg production due to naturally occurring mutations display increased levels of viral replication in tissue culture cells (Lamberts et al, 1993). This finding is potentially important since HBV genomes harbouring mutations that produce stop codons in the pre-core region have been associated with outbreaks of fulminant hepatitis B (Liang et al, 1991).

NUCLEIC-ACID-BASED APPROACHES OF ANTIVIRAL THERAPY

Antisense oligonucleotides (ODNs) as well as ribozymes have been developed to target various regions of the HBV genome in an attempt to develop antiviral effects (Blum et al, 1991; von Weizsäcker et al, 1992). These molecules have been shown to inhibit HBV replication in vitro. Their clinical use will require the development of a cell-specific delivery system since accumulation of a high concentration of these compounds within the liver will be necessary to achieve antiviral effects. An alternative antiviral strategy is based on the design and use of dominant negative polypeptides that are able to interact and inhibit the function of their native counterparts. For example, cells overexpressing mutated forms of the HIV gag protein were unable to support 'wild type' HIV replication in cells (Trono et al, 1989).

We have recently identified and functionally characterized mutants of HBV and WHV core proteins that potently and specifically inhibit 'wild type' viral replication. Transient transfection experiments in hepatoma cell lines demonstrated that truncated core proteins fused in frame to the C-terminus of the envelope(s) protein were capable of inhibiting 'wild type' viral replication by 95% in both viral species. The antiviral effect was due to interference by the dominant negative mutant core protein of nucleocapsid assembly. As a molecular consequence, the process of pre-genomic RNA encapsidation was inhibited and viral DNA synthesis could not occur (Scaglioni et al, 1994). This class of mutant viral protein may prove useful as an antiviral approach when expressed at sufficient concentrations within HBV-infected hepatocytes. Indeed, such agents may be among the most potent inhibitors of HBV replication so far described. Moreover, since the dominant negative core mutants exert their effect by interacting with the functional domain of the 'wild type' viral core protein that mediates nucleocapsid oligomerization, selection of viral escape mutants, a phenomenon frequently observed with other antiviral regimens, should not occur.

Another approach to antiviral therapy of HBV is based on DNA immunization. This technique involves injection of plasmid DNA into the muscle tissue containing viral genes that encodes structural proteins under the control of the appropriate promoter elements. When such immunizations have been performed with DNA encoding for the small (s) envelope protein in mice, a major histocompatibility class I restricted cytotoxic T lymphocyte (CTL) response was observed (Schirmbeck et al, 1995). This type of immunization holds promise not only for viral prophylaxis, but also for use as therapeutic vaccines designed to induce or boost viral specific CTL activity against HBV structural proteins in an attempt to eradicate persistent viral infection from the liver.

SUMMARY

Hepatitis B virus (HBV) is an enveloped hepatotropic DNA virus. Acute and chronic HBV infection causes significant liver diseases such as acute hepatis, fulminant hepatitis and chronic active hepatitis that may lead to liver cirrhosis and the development of hepatocellular carcinoma. The use of molecular biological techniques has substantially improved our understanding of the HBV life cycle. In this review, we discuss recent advances that have contributed to a better understanding of HBV biology. Recent studies in the understanding of the life cycle of HBV such as viral entry, replication, transcriptional regulation, viral regulatory proteins, viral assembly and secretion, and nucleic acid based approaches to antiviral therapy will be emphasized. These advances in molecular biology and relationship to clinical disease will be instrumental in developing effective therapeutic approaches for the estimated 300 million individuals worldwide chronically infected with HBV.

Acknowledgement

This work was supported by grants CA-35711 and AA-08169 from the National Institute of Health.

REFERENCES

Aufiero B & Schneider RJ (1990) The hepatitis B virus HBx gene product transactivates both RNA polymerase II and III promoters. *EMBO Journal* **9:** 497–504.
Bartenschlager R & Schaller H (1992) Hepadnaviral assembly is initiated by polymerase binding to the encapsidation signal in the viral RNA pregenome. *EMBO Journal* **11:** 3413–3420.
Birnhaum F & Nassal M (1990) Hepatitis B virus nucleocapsid assembly: primary structure requirements in the core protein. *Journal of Virology* **64:** 3319–3330.
Blum HE, Galun E, von Weizsäcker F & Wands JR (1991) Inhibition of hepatitis B virus by antisense oligodeoxynucleotides. *Lancet* **337:** 1230.
Blum HE, Zhang ZS, Galun E et al (1992) Hepatitis B virus X protein is not central to the viral life cycle in vitro. *Journal of Virology* **66:** 1223–1227.
Budkowska A, Bedossa P, Groh F et al (1995) Fibronectin of human liver sinusoids binds hepatitis B virus: identification by an anti-idiotypic antibody bearing the internal image of the pre-S2 domain. *Journal of Virology* **69:** 840–848.
Chen HS, Kaneko S, Girones R et al (1993) The woodchuck hepatitis virus X gene is important for establishment of virus infection in woodchucks. *Journal of Virology* **67:** 1218–1226.
Cheong J, Yi M, Lin Y & Murakami S (1995) Human RPB5, a subunit shared by eucariotic nuclear RNA polymerases, binds human hepatitis B virus X protein and may play a role in x transactivation. *EMBO Journal* **14:** 143–150.
Chisari FV & Ferrari C (1995) Hepatitis B virus immunopathogenesis. *Annual Review of Immunology* **13:** 29–60.
Civitico GM & Locarnini S (1994) The half life of the duck hepatitis B virus supercoiled DNA in congenitally infected primary hepatocyte culture. *Virology* **203:** 81–89.
Cullen JM, Horton S, Shi HP & Newbold JE (1994) Ross's goose hepatitis virus: a novel avian hepadnavirus. Abstracts of the Congress: Molecular Biology of the Hepatitis B Viruses, Paris, France, October 3–6.
Dejan A, Lugassy C, Zafrani S et al (1984) Detection of hepatitis B virus DNA in the pancreas, kidney and skin of two human carriers of the virus. *Journal of General Virology* **65:** 651–656.
Doria M, Klein N, Lucito R & Schneider R (1995) The hepatitis B virus HBx protein is a dual specificity cytoplasmic activator of Ras and nuclear activator of transcription factors. *EMBO Journal* **14:** 4747–4757.

Fallows DA & Goff SP (1995) Mutations in the e sequences of human hepatitis B virus affect both RNA encapsidation and reverse transcription. *Journal of Virology* **69**: 3067–3073.

Fernholz D, Galle PR, Stemler M et al (1993) Infectious hepatitis B variant defective virus in Pre-S2 protein expression in a chronic carrier. *Virology* **194**: 137–148.

Fischer M, Runkel L & Schaller H (1995) HBx protein of hepatitis B virus interacts with the C-terminal portion of a novel human proteasome alpha-subunit. *Virus Genes* **10**: 99–102.

Ganem D, Pollack JR & Tavis J (1994) Hepatitis B virus reverse transcriptase and its many roles in hepadnaviral genomic replication. *Infectious Agents and Disease* **3**: 85–93.

Gripon P, Diot C, Theze N et al (1988) Hepatitis B virus infection of adult human hepatocytes cultured in the presence of dimethyl sulfoxide. *Journal of Virology* **62**: 4136–4143.

Guidotti LG, Martinez V, Loh YT et al (1994) Hepatitis B virus nucleocapsid particles do not cross the hepatocyte nuclear membrane in transgenic mice. *Journal of Virology* **68**: 5469–5475.

Gust ID, Burrell CJ, Coulepis AG et al (1986) Taxonomic classification of human hepatitis B virus. *Intervirology* **25**: 14–29.

Hadchouel M, Scotto J, Huret JL et al (1988) Presence of HBV DNA in spermatozoa: a possible vertical transmission of HBV via the germ line. *Journal of Medical Virology* **24**: 27–32.

Hertogs K, Leenders WP, Depla E et al (1993) Endonexin II, present on human liver plasma membranes, is a specific binding protein of small hepatitis B virus (HBV) envelope protein. *Virology* **197**: 549–557.

Hirsh RC, Lavine JE, Chang LJ et al (1990) Polymerase gene products of hepatitis B viruses are required for genomic RNA packaging as well as for reverse transcription. *Nature* **344**: 552–555.

Hohne M, Schaefer S, Seifer M et al (1990) Malignant transformation of immortalized transgenic hepatocytes after transfection with hepatitis B virus. *EMBO Journal* **9**: 1137–1145.

Huang J & Liang TJ (1993) A novel hepatitis B virus (HBV) genetic element with Rev response element-like properties that is essential for expression of HBV gene products. *Molecular and Cellular Biology* **13**: 7476–7486.

Junker-Niepmann M, Bartenschlager R & Schaller H (1990) Short cis acting sequence is required for hepatitis B virus pregenome encapsidation and sufficient for packaging of foreign RNA. *EMBO Journal* **9**: 3389–3396.

Kann M & Gerlich WH (1994) Effect of core protein phosphorylation by protein kinase C on encapsidation of RNA within core particles of hepatitis B virus. *Journal of Virology* **68**: 7993–8000.

Kekulé AS, Lauer U, Weiss L et al (1993) Hepatitis B virus transactivator HBx uses a tumor promoter signaling pathway. *Nature* **361**: 742–745.

Kim CM, Koike K, Saito I et al (1991) HBx gene of hepatitis B virus induces liver cancer in transgenic mice. *Nature* **351**: 317–320.

Klingmüller U & Schaller H (1993) Hepadnavirus infection requires interaction between the viral Pre-S2 domain and a specific hepatocellular receptor. *Journal of Virology* **67**: 7417–7422.

Kock J & Schlicht HJ (1993) Analysis of the earliest steps of hepadnavirus replication: genome repair after infectious entry into hepatocytes does not depend on viral polymerase activity. *Journal of Virology* **67**: 4867–4874.

Kuroki K, Eng F, Ishikawa T et al (1995) gp180, a host cell glycoprotein that binds duck hepatitis B virus particles, is encoded by a member of the carboxypeptidase gene family. *Journal of Biological Chemistry* **270**: 15 022–15 028.

Lamberts C, Nassal M, Velhagen I et al (1993) Precore-mediated inhibition of hepatitis B virus progeny DNA synthesis. *Journal of Virology* **67**: 3756–3762.

Landford RE, Notvall L & Beames B (1995) Nucleotide priming and reverse transcriptase activity of hepatitis B virus polymerase expressed in insect cells. *Journal of Virology* **69**: 4431–4439.

Lee TH, Finegold MJ, Shen RF et al (1990) Hepatitis B virus transactivator X protein is not tumorigenic in transgenic mice. *Journal of Virology* **64**: 5939–5947.

Lee TH, Elledge SJ & Butel JS (1995) Hepatitis B virus X protein interacts with a probable cellular DNA repair protein. *Journal of Virology* **69**: 1107–1114.

Lenhoff RJ & Summers J (1994) Construction of avian hepadnavirus variants with enhanced replication and cytopathicity in primary hepatocytes. *Journal of Virology* **68**: 5706–5713.

Liang TJ, Hasegawa K, Rimon N et al (1991) A hepatitis B virus mutant associated with an epidemic of fulminant hepatitis. *New England Journal of Medicine* **324**: 1705–1709.

Liao W & Ou JH (1995) Phosphorylation and nuclear localization of the hepatitis B virus core protein: significance of serine in the three repeated SPRRR motifs. *Journal of Virology* **69**: 1025–1029.

Lingappa JR, Martin RL, Wong ML et al (1994) An eukariotic cytosolic chaperonin is associated with high molecular weight intermediate in the assembly of hepatitis B virus capsid, a multimeric particle. *Journal of Cell Biology* **125:** 99–111.

Lucito R & Schneider RJ (1992) Hepatitis B virus X protein activates transcription factor NF-kappa B without a requirement for protein kinase C. *Journal of Virology* **66:** 983–991.

Machida A, Ohnuma H, Tsuda F et al (1991) Phosphorylation in the carboxyl-terminal domain of the capsid protein of hepatitis B virus: evaluation with a monoclonal antibody. *Journal of Virology* **65:** 6024–6030.

McLachlan A (1991) *Molecular Biology of the Hepatitis B Virus*. Boca Raton, FL: CRC Press.

Marion PI, Oshiro LS, Regnery DC et al (1980) A virus in Beechey ground squirrels that is related to hepatitis b virus in humans. *Proceedings of the National Academy of Sciences of the USA* **77:** 2941–2948.

Mason WS, Seal G & Summers J (1980) Virus of peckin ducks with structural and biological relatedness to human hepatitis B virus. *Journal of Virology* **36:** 829–835.

Maynard JE, Hartwell VW & Berquist KR (1971) Hepatitis associated antigen in chimpanzees. *Journal of Infectious Diseases* **123:** 660–667.

Mehdi H, Kaplan MJ, Anlar FY et al (1994) Hepatitis B virus surface antigen binds to apolipoprotein H. *Journal of Virology* **68:** 2415–2424.

Murakami S, Cheong J, Ohno S et al (1994) Transactivation of human hepatitis B virus X protein, HBx, operates through a mechanism distinct from protein kinase C and okadaic acid activation pathways. *Virology* **199:** 243–246.

Nakatake H, Chisaka O, Yamamoto S et al (1993) Effect of X protein on transactivation of hepatitis B virus promoters and on viral replication. *Virology* **195:** 305–314.

Nassal, M. (1992a) The arginine rich domain of the hepatitis B virus core protein is required for pregenome encapsidation and productive viral positive strand synthesis but not for virus assembly. *Journal of Virology* **66:** 4107–4117.

Nassal, M. (1992b) Conserved cysteine of the hepatitis B virus core protein are not required for assembly of replication competent core particles nor for their envelopment. *Virology* **190:** 499–505.

Nassal M, Ringer A & Steinau O (1992) Topological analysis of the hepatitis B virus core particle by cysteine-cysteine cross linking. *Journal of Molecular Biology* **225:** 1013–1025.

Neurath AR, Kent SBH, Strick N & Parker K (1986) Identification and chemical synthesis of a host receptor binding site on hepatitis B virus. *Cell* **46:** 426–432.

Neurath AR, Strick N, Sproul P et al (1990) Detection of receptors for hepatitis B virus on cells of extrahepatic origin. *Virology* **176:** 448–457.

Neurath AR, Strick & Li Y (1992) Cells transfected with human interleukin 6 cDNA acquire binding sites for the hepatitis B virus envelope protein. *Journal of Experimental Medicine* **176:** 1561–1569.

Newbold JE, Xin H, Tencza M et al (1995) The covalently closed duplex form of the hepadnavirus genome exists in situ as a heterogeneous population of viral minichromosomes. *Journal of Virology* **69:** 3350–3357.

Pasquinelli C, Melegari M, Villa E et al (1990) Hepatitis B virus infection of peripheral blood mononuclear cells is common in acute and chronic hepatitis. *Journal of Medical Virology* **31:** 135–140.

Pollack JR & Ganem D (1994) Site-specific binding by a hepatitis B virus reverse transcriptase initiates two distinct reactions: RNA packaging and DNA synthesis. *Journal of Virology* **68:** 5579–5587.

Pontisso P, Petit MA, Bankowski & Peeples ME (1989) Human liver plasma membranes contain receptors for the hepatitis B virus pre-S1 region and via polymerized human serum albumin, for the pre-S2 region. *Journal of Virology* **63:** 1981–1988.

Pugh JC & Summers J (1989) Infection and uptake of duck hepatitis B virus by duck hepatocytes maintained in the presence of dimethyl sulfoxide. *Virology* **172:** 564–572.

Pugh JC, Zweidler A & Summers J (1989) Characterization of the major duck hepatitis B virus core particle protein. *Journal of Virology* **63:** 1371–1376.

Qadri I, Maguire HF & Siddiqui A (1995) Hepatitis B virus transactivator protein X interacts with the TATA-binding protein. *Proceedings of the National Academy of Sciences of the USA* **92:** 1003–1007.

Rosmorduc O, Petit MA, Pol S et al (1995) In vivo and in vitro expression of defective hepatitis B virus particles generated by spliced hepatitis B virus RNA. *Hepatology* **22:** 10–19.

Rossner MT (1992) Review: hepatitis B virus X gene product: a promiscuous transcriptional trans-activator. *Journal of Medical Virology* **36**: 101–117.

Scaglioni PP, Melegari M & Wands JR (1994) Characterization of hepatitis B virus core mutants that inhibit viral replication. *Virology* **205**: 112–120.

Schirmbeck R, Bohm W, Ando K et al (1995) Nucleic acid vaccination primes hepatitis B virus surface antigen-specific cytotoxic lymphocytes in nonresponder mice. *Journal of Virology* **69**: 5929–5934.

Seeger C & Maragos J (1990) Identification and characterization of the woodchuck hepatitis virus origin of replication. *Journal of Virology* **163**: 16–23.

Seeger C, Ganem D & Varmus HE (1986) Biochemical and genetic evidence for the hepatitis B virus replication strategy. *Science* **232**: 477–484.

Seifer M & Standring DN (1993) Recombinant human hepatitis B virus reverse transcriptase is active in the absence of the nucleocapsid or the viral replication origin, DR1. *Journal of Virology* **67**: 4513–4520.

Sprengel R, Kaleta EF & Will H (1988) Isolation and characterization of hepatitis B virus endemic in herons. *Journal of Virology* **62**: 3832–3839.

Summers J, Smolec JM & Snyder R (1978) A virus similar to human hepatitis B associated with hepatitis and hepatoma in woodchucks. *Proceedings of the National Academy of Sciences of the USA* **75**: 4533–4539.

Summers J, Smith PM, Huang MJ & Yu M (1991) Morphogenetic and regulatory effects of mutations in the envelope proteins of an avian hepadnavirus. *Journal of Virology* **65**: 1310–1317.

Szmuness W, Stevens CE, Harley EJ et al (1980) Hepatitis B vaccine. *New England Journal of Medicine* **303**: 833–841.

Tavis JE & Ganem D (1993) Expression of functional hepatitis B virus polymerase in yeast reveals it to be the sole viral protein required for correct initiation of reverse transcription. *Proceedings of the National Academy of Sciences of the USA* **90**: 4107–4111.

Terré S, Petit MA & Brechot C (1991) Defective hepatitis B virus particles are generated by packaging and reverse transcription of spliced viral RNAs in vivo. *Journal of Virology* **65**: 5539–5543.

Testut P, Renard CA, Vitvitski-Trepo L et al (1995) A new hepadnavirus associated with liver cancer in arctic ground squirrels. Abstracts of the Congress: Molecular Biology of the Hepatitis B Viruses, San Diego, USA, July 23–27.

Tong S, Li S & Wands JR. (1995) Interaction between duck hepatitis B virus and a 170-kilodalton cellular protein is mediated through a neutralizing epitope of the pre-S region and occurs during viral infection. *Journal of Virology* **69**: 7106–7112.

Trono D, Feinberg MB & Baltimore D (1989). HIV-1 gag mutants can dominantly interfere with the replication of the 'wild type' virus. *Cell* **59**: 113–120.

Truant R, Antunovic J, Greenblatt J et al (1995) Direct interaction of the hepatitis B virus HBx protein with p53 leads to inhibition by HBx of p53 response element-directed transactivation. *Journal of Virology* **69**: 1851–1859.

Wands JR, Scaglioni PP & Melegari M (1996) *Hepatitis B Viral Variants*. Falk Foundation Symposium on Chronic Hepatitis (in press).

Wang GH & Seeger C (1992) The reverse transcriptase of hepatitis B virus acts as a protein primer for viral DNA synthesis. *Cell* **71**: 663–670.

Wang GH & Seeger C (1993) Novel mechanism for reverse transcription in hepatitis B viruses. *Journal of Virology* **67**: 6505–6512.

Wang XW, Forrester K, Yeh H et al (1994) Hepatitis B virus X protein inhibits p53 sequence-specific DNA binding, transcriptional activity, and association with transcription factor ERCC3. *Proceedings of the National Academy of Sciences of the USA* **91**: 2230–2234.

Wang HD, Yuh CH, Dang CV & Johnson D (1995) The hepatitis B virus X protein increases the cellular level of TATA binding protein, which mediates transactivation of RNA polymerase III genes. *Molecular and Cellular Biology* **15**: 6720–6728.

Wollersheim M, Debelka U & Hofschneider PH (1988) A transactivating function encoded in the hepatitis B virus X gene is conserved in the integrated state. *Oncogene* **3**: 545–552.

Wu HL, Chen PJ, Tu SU et al (1991) Characterization and genetic analysis of alternatively spliced transcripts of hepatitis B virus in infected human liver and transfected HepG2 cells. *Journal of Virology.* **65**: 1680–1686.

von Weizsäcker F, Blum HE & Wands JR (1992). Cleavage of hepatitis B virus RNA by three ribozymes transcribed from a single DNA template. *Biochemical and Biophysical Research Communications* **189**: 743–748.

Yaginuma K, Shirkata Y, Kobayashi M & Koike K (1987) Hepatitis B virus (HBV) particles are produced in a cell culture system by transient expression of transfected HBV DNA. *Proceedings of the National Academy of Sciences of the USA* **84:** 2678–2682.

Yee JK (1989) A liver specific enhancer in the core promoter region of human hepatitis B virus. *Science* **246:** 658–661.

Yeh CT, Liaw YF & Ou JH (1990) The arginine rich domain of hepatitis B virus precore and core proteins contain a signal for nuclear transport. *Journal of Virology* **64:** 6141–6147.

Yuh CH, Chang YL & Ting LP (1992) Transcriptional regulation of precore and pregenomic RNAs of hepatitis B virus. *Journal of Virology* **66:** 4073–4084.

Zhou S, Yang SQ & Standring DN (1992) Characterization of the hepatitis B virus capsid particle assembly in xenopus oocytes. *Journal of Virology* **66:** 3086–3092.

Zhou S & Standring DN (1992) Cys residues of the hepatitis B virus capsid protein are not essential for the assembly of viral core particles but can influence their stability. *Journal of Virology* **66:** 5393–5398.

Zoulim F, Saputelli J & Seeger C (1994) Woodchuck hepatitis virus X protein is required for viral infection in vivo. *Journal of Virology* **68:** 2026–2030.

Zoulim F & Seeger C (1994) Reverse transcription in hepatitis B viruses is primed by a tyrosine residue of the polymerase. *Journal of Virology* **68:** 6–13.

Current Topics in Microbiology and Immunology (1991) *Hepadnaviruses.* Vol. 168. Heidelberg, Germany: Springer-Verlag.

3

Hepatitis E

ERIC E. MAST
MICHAEL A. PURDY
KRZYSZTOF KRAWCZYNSKI

Hepatitis E virus (HEV) is the primary cause of enterically transmitted non-A, non-B hepatitis world-wide. Typical clinical signs and symptoms, and laboratory findings, of hepatitis E are similar to those of other types of viral hepatitis; however, fulminant hepatitis is more commonly associated with HEV infection among pregnant women. Areas of the world can be considered as HEV-endemic based on the occurrence of hepatitis E outbreaks, which have been reported over a wide geographical area in Asia, Africa, the Middle East and Central America, predominantly in developing countries with inadequate sanitation practices. Hepatitis E also accounts for a large proportion of sporadic hepatitis cases in many of these areas. In countries where hepatitis E outbreaks have not been documented to occur (non-endemic regions), hepatitis E cases have been reported primarily among travellers returning from HEV-endemic regions. In several of these countries, hepatitis E cases have been reported in patients with no history of travel to HEV-endemic areas; however, the mode of HEV transmission for these cases has not been determined.

During the past decade, much has been learned about the virology of HEV, and diagnostic tests for HEV infection have improved considerably. Increased surveillance for hepatitis E outbreaks and sporadic cases, and further information regarding the epidemiology and natural history of hepatitis E, will be needed to develop improved measures to prevent this disease.

VIROLOGY

HEV was first identified by immune electron microscopy (IEM) in the faeces of patients with enterically transmitted non-A, non-B hepatitis (Balayan et al, 1983; Kane et al, 1984). The agent is an icosahedral, non-enveloped virus about 32–34 nm in diameter (Figure 1), with a sedimentation coefficient of approximately 183S and a buoyant density of 1.29 g/ml in a potassium tartrate and glycerol gradient (Bradley, 1992).

Baillière's Clinical Gastroenterology—
Vol. 10, No. 2, July 1996
ISBN 0–7020–2094–X
0950–3528/96/020227 + 16 $12.00/00

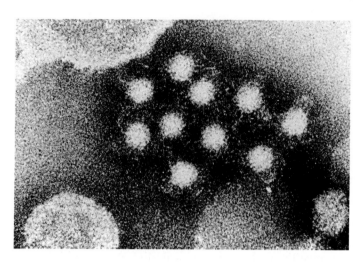

Figure 1. Electron micrograph of 32–34 nm HEV particles from stool.

The establishment of an animal model of disease in cynomolgus macaques led ultimately to the cloning and sequencing of HEV (Reyes et al, 1990). The HEV genome is a single-stranded, positive-sense, poly-adenylated RNA molecule, approximately 7.5 kilobases in length. Three open reading frames (ORFs) have been identified; ORF1 codes for non-structural proteins responsible for replication of the viral genome, ORF2 codes for structural protein(s), including the capsid protein, and ORF3 codes for a protein of unknown function. On the basis of similar structural and physicochemical properties to caliciviruses, HEV has been classified in the family Caliciviridae, genus *Calicivirus* (Cubitt et al, 1995). However, analysis of genomic sequences from ORF2 shows no similarity between the structural protein of HEV and that of prototypic caliciviruses, and HEV ORF1 sequences are more similar to those of rubella virus and plant furoviruses than to those of prototypic caliciviruses (Koonin et al, 1992; Purdy, 1994).

On the basis of available HEV RNA sequence data (Tsarev et al, 1992; Bi et al, 1993; Bradley et al, 1993; Yin et al, 1994), nucleotide variability among HEV isolates ranges from 1 to 8% among Asian isolates, and to as much as 25% between Mexican and Asian isolates. The variability in amino acid sequence ranges from 1 to 5% among various Asian isolates to 14% between Mexican and Asian isolates. Although genomic variability has been demonstrated among HEV isolates from various geographic regions, geographically distinct isolates have been shown to have at least one major cross-reactive epitope by IEM (Bradley et al, 1988), fluorescent antibody blocking assay (Krawczynski, 1991), Western blot analysis (Purdy et al, 1992), and enzyme immunoassay (Favorov et al, 1994).

DIAGNOSTIC TESTS

The first serological assays for antibody to HEV (anti-HEV) included IEM to detect native HEV antigen (HEVAg) on the surface of HEV particles in faecal specimens (Balayan et al, 1983; Kane et al, 1984) (Table 1). Subsequent developments in diagnostic methods included immunohisto-chemistry to identify HEVAg in liver tissue and a fluorescent antibody-blocking assay to detect anti-HEV reacting to HEVAg in serum specimens (Krawczynski and Bradley, 1989; Purdy et al, 1994). These assays involving identification of HEVAg are highly specific but have limited sensitivity; anti-HEV has been detected in only 50–70% of patients with acute hepatitis during hepatitis E outbreaks, and anti-HEV titres decline to subdetectable levels within several months of acute infection.

After HEV was cloned and sequenced, Western blot assays and enzyme immunoassays (EIAs) were developed to detect anti-HEV, using recombi-nant-expressed proteins or synthetic peptides representing immuno-dominant epitopes of the putative structural regions of HEV (ORFs 2 and 3) (Dawson et al, 1992; Favorov et al, 1992; Purdy et al, 1992; Tsarev et al, 1993a; Favorov et al, 1994; Li et al, 1994; Yarbough et al, 1994). Many of these assays have utilized antigenic domains from two geographically distinct HEV strains (e.g. cloned isolates from patients involved in hepatitis E epidemics in Myanmar [Burma] and Mexico). Several expression systems have been utilized to produce the recombinant proteins used in these tests, including *Escherichia coli* and recombinant baculovirus-infected insect cells.

The tests utilizing recombinant proteins are more sensitive than earlier assays and are able to detect anti-HEV in > 95% of patients with acute hepatitis during outbreaks of hepatitis E. However, few data are available to compare the sensitivity, specificity, and concordance of these assays. Differences may exist in the seroreactivity of recombinant proteins produced in different expression systems, used in different test formats (e.g.

Table 1. Diagnostic assays for HEV infection.

Assay	Specimen	Detection target/reagent
Anti-HEV		
Immune electron microscopy	Serum	HEV particles
Fluorescent antibody blocking assay	Serum	HEVAg in hepatocytes,
Western blot assay	Serum	Recombinant protein (ORF2[a])
Enzyme immunoassay	Serum	Recombinant protein (ORF2, 3) Synthetic peptides (ORF2, 3)
HEVAg		
Immunohistochemistry	Liver	FITC[b]-labelled convalescent IgG
Immune electron microscopy	Faeces	Convalescent serum
HEV RNA		
RT–PCR[c]	Serum, faeces, liver	HEV sequence-specific primers

[a] ORF = open reading frame.
[b] FITC = fluorescein isothiocyanate.
[c] RT–PCR = reverse transcriptase–polymerase chain reaction.

Western blot versus EIA), or derived from isolates from different geographical sources. Thus, the interpretation of seroprevalence studies using these assays is problematic. Tests for IgM anti-HEV based on recombinant HEV proteins have also been developed to differentiate acute from past infection. In outbreak settings, IgM anti-HEV has been detected in > 90% of patient sera obtained within 1 week to 2 months after illness onset (Bryan et al, 1994; Clayson et al, 1995a). However, IgM anti-HEV may not be detectable in some patients during the first week after illness onset, and titres decline rapidly, often to subdetectable levels, during early convalescence. In addition, these tests have not been well standardized to date, and their performance has not been determined for the diagnosis of acute hepatitis E in settings with a low incidence of disease.

In research laboratories, diagnostic tests are also available for detecting HEVAg in liver using an immunofluorescent probe prepared from convalescent-phase serum aggregating HEV particles (Krawczynski and Bradley, 1989). The specificity of this method has been documented in absorption studies, using a recombinant HEV peptide encoded by ORF2 (Purdy et al, 1994). HEV RNA has been detected in faeces, liver, and serum by reverse transcriptase–polymerase chain reaction (RT–PCR) (McCaustland et al, 1991; Schlauder and Mushahwar, 1994). Molecular analysis of genomic HEV RNA has been used as a diagnostic approach in an increasing number of clinical and experimental studies.

CLINICAL FEATURES

Clinical signs and symptoms in patients with symptomatic HEV infection are similar to those of other types of viral hepatitis, with a prodromal phase of about 1 week that is generally followed by an icteric phase (Figure 2, Table 2). The most commonly reported signs and symptoms include malaise (95–100%), anorexia (66–100%), nausea/vomiting (29–100%), abdominal pain (37–82%), fever (23–97%) and hepatomegaly (10–85%) (Morrow et al, 1968; Khuroo, 1980; Myint et al, 1985; Song et al, 1991). Other less frequent signs and symptoms include diarrhoea, arthralgia, pruritus, and urticarial rash. Laboratory findings in patients with hepatitis E are also similar to findings in patients with other forms of viral hepatitis and include elevated serum bilirubin, alanine aminotransferase (ALT), aspartate aminotransferase, alkaline phosphatase, and gamma-glutamyl transferase. Resolution of hyperbilirubinaemia and elevated aminotransferase levels generally occurs within 3 weeks (range 1–6 weeks) of the onset of illness.

In most hepatitis E outbreaks, the highest rates of symptomatic disease (jaundice) have been in young to middle-aged adults (Arankalle et al, 1988; Bryan et al, 1994; Mast et al, 1994). The ratio of clinical to subclinical infections has not been determined; however, lower disease rates for younger age groups may be the result of anicteric and/or subclinical HEV infections, which have been identified in several outbreak investigations (Arankalle et al, 1988; Bryan et al, 1994; Mast et al, 1994). For example, during an outbreak in India, only 13% of children 9–15 years of age with

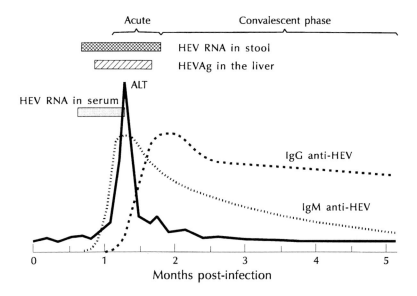

Figure 2. Typical clinical course following HEV infection.

Table 2. Clinical features of hepatitis E.

Incubation period:	mode (40 days); range (15–60 days)
Case-fatality rate:	overall (1–3%); pregnant women (5–25%)
Illness severity:	increases with age
Chronic sequelae:	none identified

elevated ALT levels had icterus, and less than half of persons who were positive for IgM anti-HEV had icterus during an outbreak in a refugee camp in Kenya.

Fulminant hepatitis is associated with HEV infection in infected pregnant women, among whom hepatitis E case-fatality rates of 5–25% have been reported (Khuroo et al, 1981; Kane et al, 1984; Song et al, 1991; Mast et al, 1994). Case-fatality rates have generally been highest among pregnant women infected during the third trimester.

Most patients with acute hepatitis E have a self-limited course. No evidence of chronic hepatitis has been detected among patients followed up clinically and among those who had liver biopsies after acute hepatitis E (Chuttani et al, 1966; Velázquez et al, 1990; Chadha et al, 1991; Khuroo et al, 1980). Treatment for hepatitis E is supportive. No data are available to evaluate the efficacy of antiviral agents or other specific therapies for the treatment of hepatitis E.

PATHOGENESIS OF HEPATITIS E

The pathogenic features associated with HEV infection have been characterized in human volunteer studies (Balayan et al, 1983; Chauhan et al, 1993) and by using experimental models of infection in non-human primates (Bradley et al, 1987; Krawczynski and Bradley, 1989; Soe et al 1989; Longer et al, 1993; Ticehurst et al, 1992a; Tsarev et al, 1993b). Infection in cynomolgus macaques has been the most reproducible and widely used experimental model. Experimental infection has also been demonstrated in other non-human primates, including chimpanzees, rhesus and owl monkeys, and tamarins; however, varying levels of virus excretion, liver enzyme elevations, and histopathological changes in liver have been demonstrated in these animals (Ticehurst, 1991). Experimental studies have shown that HEV infection is possible by both intravenous inoculation and oral ingestion. The incubation period in human volunteers after oral exposure was 4–5 weeks. Incubation periods of 15–60 days (mode = 40 days) have been reported during hepatitis E outbreaks (Viswanathan, 1957; Belabbes et al, 1985; Zhuang, 1992).

The mechanism(s) by which HEV initially reaches the liver from the intestinal tract are unknown. In cynomolgus macaques inoculated with HEV intravenously, HEVAg has been detected simultaneously in hepatocyte cytoplasm, bile, and faeces during the second or third week after inoculation, before and concurrently with the onset of ALT elevation and histopathological changes in the liver (Krawczynski and Bradley, 1989; Longer et al, 1993; Tsarev et al, 1993b). In this phase of infection, HEVAg has been detected in 70–90% of hepatocytes. These findings suggest that an initial highly replicative phase of infection occurs and that HEV may be released from hepatocytes into bile before the peak of morphological changes in the liver. The onset of ALT elevations and histopathological changes in the liver generally corresponds with the detection of anti-HEV in serum and with decreasing levels of HEVAg in hepatocytes. In addition, infiltrating lymphocytes in the liver have been found to have a cytotoxic/suppression immunophenotype (Soe et al, 1989). These findings suggest that liver injury may be largely immune-mediated and that both a cell-mediated immune mechanism and humoral immunity may be necessary for the development of liver lesions.

Histopathological features of HEV infection in liver tissue include both cholestatic hepatitis and standard (classic) acute viral hepatitis. In studies of patients involved in outbreaks in Delhi (1955–1956), Kashmir (1978–1979), and Ghana (1962–1963), a cholestatic or 'obstructive' type of morphological change, characterized by bile stasis in canaliculi and a gland-like transformation of parenchymal cells, was found in the majority of cases (Gupta and Smetana, 1957; Morrow et al, 1968; Khuroo, 1980). Degenerative changes of liver cells, including acidophilic bodies, and focal necrosis were seen less frequently. In serial biopsy specimens, glandular transformation of liver cell plates was observed, and lobular architecture was restored after liver function tests returned to normal. The 'standard' type of viral hepatitis was characterized by focal intralobular necrosis of hepatocytes, with accumulations of mononuclear macrophages, activated Kupffer cells, and lymphocytes. Ballooned hepatocytes, acidophilic degeneration of hepatocytes, and acidophilic body formation were frequently noted. In fatal cases, features of severe acute hepatitis, along with submassive and massive hepatic necrosis, were observed.

The pattern of HEV excretion in faeces has not been fully characterized. HEV has been detected in faeces by IEM beginning approximately 1 week before the onset of illness and persisting for less than 2 weeks (Balayan et al, 1983; Ticehurst et al, 1992b; Zhuang, 1992; Chauhan et al, 1993). The infectivity of faeces with HEV, detectable by IEM, has been demonstrated up to 1 week after the onset of illness based on transmission to non-human primates (Balayan et al, 1983; Chauhan et al, 1993). HEV RNA can be detected in the faeces of most patients with acute hepatitis E by RT–PCR for about 2 weeks (Aggarwal and Naik, 1992; Clayson et al, 1995a) and faecal HEV excretion of up to 52 days has been reported (Nanda et al, 1995); however, the correlation of HEV RNA detection with infectivity in stools has not been demonstrated.

In one study, viraemia was detected by RT–PCR in virtually all patients from whom sera were collected within 2 weeks of the onset of illness (Clayson et al, 1995a), and prolonged periods of viraemia (4–16 weeks) have been reported (Chauhan et al, 1993; Schlauder et al, 1993; Nanda et al, 1995).

The natural history of protective immunity after acute HEV infection has not been fully determined. In one study, the presence of pre-existing IgG anti-HEV was found to prevent hepatitis E in young adults (Bryan et al, 1994), which suggests that hepatitis E in this age group was the result of primary infection, rather than re-infection. In addition, non-human primates infected with HEV were immune to subsequent HEV challenge for up to 33 months (Arankalle et al, 1995a). IgG anti-HEV titres peak during early convalescence and markedly decline during the next several months. Virtually all patients have detectable IgG anti-HEV for at least 20 months after acute infection (Bryan et al, 1994); however, in one study, less than 50% of persons had detectable antibody approximately 14 years after infection (Khuroo et al, 1993). Whether the loss of detectable antibody over time reflects the sensitivity of available tests or a loss of immunity is not known.

EPIDEMIOLOGY

Occurrence of hepatitis E in endemic regions

Areas of the world can be classified as HEV-endemic based on the occurrence of hepatitis E outbreaks, which have been reported throughout Asia, Africa, the Middle East and Central America, predominantly in developing countries where sanitation practices are inadequate. Many hepatitis E outbreaks have consisted of several thousand cases; the largest reported to date, involving over 100 000 cases, occurred in northwest China in

1986–1988 (Zhuang, 1992). In population-based studies of hepatitis E outbreaks, clinical attack rates of 1–15% have been reported (Khuroo, 1980; Kane et al, 1984; Centers for Disease Control, 1987; Velázquez et al, 1990; Naik et al, 1992), ranging from 3 to 20% among adults and from 0.2 to 10% among children under 15 years of age. Classical features of these outbreaks include higher attack rates of clinically evident disease among persons 15–40 years of age compared with other age groups, high overall case-fatality rates, and high case-fatality rates among pregnant women.

Recurrent hepatitis E epidemics, with a periodicity of 5–10 years, have been observed in several parts of the world, including India, Northwest China, Indonesia, and the Central Asian Republics of the former Soviet Union (Favorov et al, 1986; Zhuang, 1992; Corwin et al, 1995). Reasons for this periodicity have not been determined. Several outbreaks have occurred in a seasonal pattern after heavy rains (Kane et al, 1984; Bile et al, 1994). For example, in Northwest China a distinctive seasonal peak has been described in October or November, a period in which heavy rains and flooding occur (Zhuang, 1992). However, outbreaks associated with faecally contaminated river water in Indonesia have occurred after periods of lower rainfall, suggesting that higher concentrations of virus in shallow, slow-moving rivers may have increased the risk of exposure (Corwin et al, 1995).

In many areas where hepatitis E outbreaks have been reported, HEV infection accounts for a substantial proportion of acute sporadic hepatitis in both children and adults (Hyams et al, 1992; Khuroo et al, 1994). Hepatitis E may also be endemic in several countries where outbreaks have not been reported, including Egypt, Hong Kong, Senegal, Taiwan and Turkey, based on a high incidence of sporadic hepatitis E in these countries (Goldsmith et al, 1992; Lok et al, 1992; Pillot et al, 1992; Coursaget et al, 1993; el-Zimaity et al, 1993).

In seroprevalence studies conducted in HEV-endemic countries, anti-HEV has been detected in as many as 5% of children under 10 years of age, and this ratio increases to 10–40% among adults over 25 years of age (Lok et al, 1992; Thomas et al, 1993; Arif et al, 1994; Paul et al, 1994; Arankalle et al, 1995b). By comparison, the prevalence of antibody to hepatitis A virus (anti-HAV) among children under 10 years of age in most HEV-endemic countries is more than 90% (Shapiro and Margolis, 1993). These findings suggest that HEV, unlike other enterically-transmitted agents, is infrequently transmitted among young children in developing countries. However, until the natural history of long-term anti-HEV persistence is defined, the true frequency of infection cannot be determined.

Occurrence of hepatitis E in non-endemic regions

In most countries where hepatitis E outbreaks have not been documented (non-endemic regions), hepatitis E accounts for fewer than 1% of reported cases of acute viral hepatitis. Most acute hepatitis E cases reported in these countries have been associated with travel to HEV-endemic regions (De Cock et al, 1987; Centers for Disease Control and Prevention, 1993). However, the geographical distribution of hepatitis E has not been fully determined because diagnostic tests for this illness have only recently become available, and the performance of these assays in seroprevalence studies and for the diagnosis of acute disease in non-endemic regions is unknown. Nevertheless, in several non-endemic countries, including Australia, Greece, New Zealand and the United States, acute hepatitis E cases have been reported among persons with no history of travel to disease-endemic countries (Munoz et al, 1992; Chapman et al, 1993; Zanetti et al, 1994; Coursaget et al, 1994; Tassopoulos et al, 1994; Sallie et al, 1994; Heath et al, 1995; Kwo et al, 1995). Thus, a reservoir of HEV may exist in these countries.

Few studies have assessed the risk of HEV infection among travellers to HEV-endemic regions. In a cohort of 328 US missionaries, more than three-fourths of whom lived in sub-Saharan Africa, no anti-HEV sero-conversions were detected during an average period of 7.3 years, but more than 5% had anti-HAV seroconversion (Smalligan et al, 1995). In a blinded seroprevalence study among Peace Corps volunteers who had recently returned from a 2-year tour of duty in Africa, 10% were found to be anti-HEV positive (Eng TR, personal communication), a prevalence that is substantially higher than the anti-HEV prevalence among blood donors in the United States (1–2%). However, no pre-travel sera were available from these persons for comparison.

Seroprevalence studies among blood donors in some non-endemic countries have found an anti-HEV prevalence of 1–5% (Dawson et al, 1992; Paul et al, 1994; Zanetti et al, 1994; Karetnyi et al, 1995; Moaven et al, 1995), which is relatively high compared with the low rate of clinically evident disease associated with HEV in these areas. Possible reasons for these findings may include subclinical and/or anicteric HEV infection, serological cross-reactivity with other agents, and false-positive tests.

Mechanisms and risk factors for HEV transmission

HEV is transmitted primarily by the faecal–oral route (Table 3). In most reported outbreaks, faecally contaminated drinking water has been identified as the likely vehicle of transmission. Food-borne transmission has been postulated to be the cause of some outbreaks (Zhuang, 1982), but investigations of these outbreaks did not include control groups or sero-logical testing. Risk factors for hepatitis E cases occurring in non-endemic regions among persons with no history of travel have not been determined.

Unlike HAV, which is also transmitted by the faecal–oral route, person-to-person transmission of HEV appears to be uncommon, even in settings with poor environmental sanitation, such as refugee camps (Viswanathan, 1957; Myint et al, 1985; Aggarwal and Naik, 1994; Mast et al, 1994). Reported secondary attack rates for households with hepatitis E cases have ranged from 0.7 to 2.2% compared with 50 to 75% among susceptible contacts in households with hepatitis A cases (Villarejos et al, 1982; Greco et al, 1986). In non-endemic regions, no secondary HEV transmission has been reported among household members of persons with travel-associated cases of hepatitis E, and sexual contact has not been identified as a risk

Table 3. Epidemiological features of hepatitis E.

Mode of transmission	Faecal–oral (person-to-person transmission uncommon)
Vehicle of transmission	In outbreaks—faecally contaminated water; for most sporadic cases—unknown
Occurrence in HEV-endemic regions	Large outbreaks, often involving thousands of cases; sporadic cases (> 50% in some areas)
Occurrence in non-endemic regions	Rare sporadic cases (primarily travellers to HEV-endemic regions)

factor for transmission in studies conducted in outbreak settings (Khuroo et al, 1980; Myint et al 1985; Aggarwal and Naik, 1994). However, nosocomial transmission, presumably by person-to-person contact, has been reported in South Africa (Robson et al, 1992).

During an outbreak in India, HEV transmission from mother to infant has been reported among pregnant women who recovered after infection during the third trimester; in this study, most infants recovered after transient hepatitis, but one infant died with massive hepatic necrosis (Khuroo et al, 1995).

Percutaneous blood exposures are a possible mode of HEV transmission, since a period of viraemia occurs in patients with acute hepatitis E. Administration of blood products manufactured from large plasma pools (e.g. coagulation factor concentrates) have also been suggested as a possible mode of HEV transmission because current methods of viral inactivation used for these products may not inactivate non-enveloped viruses (Mannucci et al, 1994). However, no studies have implicated these exposures in the transmission of HEV.

Reservoir of HEV

The reservoir of HEV is unknown. It is possible that an environmental reservoir may exist because hepatitis E outbreaks have been associated with faecally contaminated drinking water. HEV RNA has been detected in water by RT–PCR (Jothikumar et al, 1993), but the source of faecal contamination leading to hepatitis E outbreaks has not been determined. In addition, the stability of HEV in the environment is unknown, although HEV has been found to be labile when exposed to high concentrations of salt, freeze–thawing, and pelleting (Bradley, 1992). Another potential reservoir for HEV is serial transmission among susceptible individuals. In many countries where hepatitis E outbreaks have been reported, sporadic cases of hepatitis E account for a substantial proportion of acute viral hepatitis, and these sporadic infections may maintain transmission in endemic regions during interepidemic periods. A third possibility is that hepatitis E may be a zoonotic disease. Experimental HEV infection has been reported in several animal species, including pigs, sheep, cynomolgus macaques and chimpanzees (Balayan et al, 1990; Ticehurst, 1991; Usmanov et al, 1994). Moreover, in endemic regions, HEV has been detected in the faeces of pigs by RT–PCR, and anti-HEV has been detected in the serum of pigs, cattle and sheep (Clayson et al, 1995b; Favorov MO, personal communication). However, cross-species transmission of HEV has not been demonstrated, and the mechanisms by which such transmission may occur are unknown.

PREVENTION

Few studies have evaluated the efficacy of pre- or post-exposure immune globulin (Ig) prophylaxis for the prevention of hepatitis E. In studies in which Ig was prepared from donors in an HEV-endemic country (India) and administered in outbreak settings, no statistically significant difference in disease rates was found among persons who received and those who did not receive Ig (Tandon et al, 1982; Joshi et al, 1985; Khuroo and Dar, 1992). Ig prepared from plasma collected from donors in non-HEV-endemic areas is unlikely to contain sufficient levels of protective antibody and has not been effective in preventing clinical disease when administered before travel to HEV-endemic areas or during a hepatitis E outbreak (Molinié et al, 1988; Velázquez et al, 1990). In cynomolgus macaques, passive immunization with convalescent-phase plasma from an animal previously infected with HEV appeared to provide protection against clinical disease after intravenous challenge, but did not prevent infection (Tsarev et al, 1994).

The lack of a tissue culture system to propagate HEV in vitro has precluded the development of inactivated or live attenuated virus vaccines; however, several recombinant HEV proteins have been evaluated as potential candidates for a prototype hepatitis E vaccine, including *TrpE*-C2 fusion protein (derived from ORF2) expressed in *Escherichia coli* and baculovirus-expressed ORF2 protein. Studies with the recombinant protein vaccine constructs to date in cynomolgus macaques indicate that vaccine-induced antibody attenuates HEV infection, but does not prevent virus excretion in stools (Purdy et al, 1993; Tsarev et al, 1994; Krawczynski et al, in preparation). Further modifications of the recombinant immunogen, the use of more efficient adjuvants, and optimization of immunization schedules may all be necessary to induce satisfactory levels of neutralizing antibodies and prevent HEV infection. If a vaccine is developed, the epidemiology of hepatitis E will need to be defined further in order to determine whether vaccination strategies can be effectively used to prevent hepatitis E.

Because no products are available for preventing hepatitis E, prevention relies primarily on the provision of clean drinking water. Epidemiological data suggest that boiling water may inactivate HEV (Velázquez et al, 1990; Corwin et al, 1995). However, no data are available regarding the efficacy of chlorination of water in inactivating HEV, and studies are needed to identify other appropriate environmental control measures. Until such prevention measures are determined, the use of prudent hygienic practices may help to prevent hepatitis E and other enterically transmitted diseases among travellers to developing countries. Consistent with these practices, travellers should not consume drinking water (and beverages with ice) of unknown purity, uncooked shellfish, and uncooked fruits or vegetables that have not been peeled or prepared by the traveller.

SUMMARY

Hepatitis E has a world-wide distribution and causes substantial morbidity and mortality in some developing countries, particularly among pregnant women. Hepatitis E virus (HEV) has recently been cloned and sequenced, and new diagnostic tests have been developed. These tests have been used to begin to characterize the natural history and epidemiological features of HEV infection. Experimental vaccines have also been developed that offer the potential to prevent hepatitis E. However, much remains to be learned about HEV, including the mechanisms of transmission, the reservoir(s) of the virus, and the natural history of protective immunity in order to develop effective strategies to prevent this disease.

REFERENCES

Aggarwal R & Naik SR (1992) Fecal excretion of hepatitis E virus. *Lancet* **340:** 787.
Aggarwal R & Naik SR (1994) Hepatitis E: intrafamilial transmission versus waterborne spread. *Journal of Hepatology* **21:** 718–723.
Arankalle VA, Chadha MS, Mehendale SM & Banerjee K (1988) Outbreak of enterically transmitted non-A, non-B hepatitis among schoolchildren. *Lancet* **ii:** 1199–1200.
Arankalle VA, Chadha MS, Chobe LP et al (1995a) Cross-challenge studies in rhesus monkeys employing different Indian isolates of hepatitis E virus. *Journal of Medical Virology* **46:** 358–363.
Arankalle VA, Tsarev SA, Chadha MS et al (1995b) Age-specific prevalence of antibodies to hepatitis A and E viruses in Pune, India, 1982 and 1992. *Journal of Infectious Diseases* **171:** 447–450.
Arif M, Qattan I, Al-Faleh F & Ramia S (1994) Epidemiology of hepatitis E virus (HEV) infection in Saudi Arabia. *Annals of Tropical Medicine and Parasitology* **88:** 163–168.
Balayan MS, Andjaparidze AG, Savinskaya SS et al (1983) Evidence for a virus in non-A, non-B hepatitis transmitted via the fecal–oral route. *Intervirology* **20:** 23–31.
Balayan MS, Usmanov RK, Zamyatina NA et al (1990) Experimental hepatitis E infection in domestic pigs. *Journal of Medical Virology* **32:** 58–59.
Belabbes EH, Bouguermouh A, Benatallah A & Illoul G (1985) Epidemic non-A, non-B viral hepatitis in Algeria: strong evidence for its spreading by water. *Journal of Medical Virology* **16:** 257–263.
Bi SL, Purdy MA, McCaustland KA et al (1993) The sequence of hepatitis E virus isolated directly from a single source during an outbreak in China. *Virus Research* **28:** 233–247.
Bile K, Isse A, Mohamud O et al (1994) Contrasting roles of rivers and wells as sources of drinking water on attack and fatality rates in a hepatitis E epidemic in Somalia. *American Journal of Tropical Medicine and Hygiene* **51:** 466–474.
Bradley DW (1992) Hepatitis E: epidemiology, aetiology and molecular biology. *Reviews in Medical Virology* **2:** 19–28.
Bradley DW, Krawczynski K, Cook EH et al (1987) Enterically transmitted non-A, non-B hepatitis: serial passage of disease in cynomolgus macaques and tamarins and recovery of disease-associated 27- to 32-nm viruslike particles. *Proceedings of the National Academy of Sciences of the USA* **84:** 6277–6281.
Bradley DW, Andjaparidze A, Cook EH et al (1988) Aetiological agent of enterically transmitted non-A, non-B hepatitis. *Journal of General Virology* **69:** 731–738.
Bradley DW, Beach MJ & Purdy MA (1993) Molecular characterization of hepatitis C and E viruses. *Archives of Virology* **7 (supplement):** 1–14.

Bryan JP, Tsarev SA, Iqbal M et al (1994) Epidemic hepatitis E in Pakistan: patterns of serologic response and evidence that antibody to hepatitis E virus protects against disease. *Journal of Infectious Diseases* **170**: 517–521.

Centers for Disease Control (1987) Enterically transmitted non-A, non-B hepatitis—East Africa. *Morbidity and Mortality Weekly Report* **36**: 241–244.

Centers for Disease Control and Prevention (1993) Hepatitis E among U.S. travelers, 1989–1992. *Morbidity and Mortality Weekly Report* **42**: 1–4.

Chadha MS, Arankalle VA & Banerjee K (1991) Follow up of cases of enterically transmitted non-A, non-B hepatitis. *Journal of the Association of Physicians of India* **39**: 651–652.

Chapman BA, Burt MJ, Wilkinson ID, & Schousboe MI (1993) Community acquired viral hepatitis in New Zealand: a case of sporadic hepatitis E virus infection. *Australian and New Zealand Journal of Medicine* **23**: 722–723.

Chauhan A, Jameel S, Dilawari JB et al (1993) Hepatitis E virus transmission to a volunteer. *Lancet* **341**: 149–150.

Chuttani HK, Sidhu AS, Wig KL et al (1966) Follow-up study of cases from the Dehli epidemic of infectious hepatitis of 1955–6. *British Medical Journal* **ii**: 676–679.

Clayson ET, Myint KSA, Snitbhan R et al (1995a) Viremia, fecal shedding, and IgM and IgG responses in patients with hepatitis E. *Journal of Infectious Diseases* **172**: 927–933.

Clayson ET, Innis BL, Myint KSA et al (1995b) Detection of hepatitis E virus infections among domestic swine in the Kathmandu Valley of Nepal. *American Journal of Tropical Medicine and Hygiene* **53**: 228–232.

Corwin A, Jarot K, Lubis I et al (1995) Two years' investigation of epidemic hepatitis E virus transmission in West Kalimantan (Borneo), Indonesia. *Transactions of the Royal Society of Tropical Medicine and Hygiene* **89**: 262–265.

Coursaget P, Depril N, Yenen OS et al (1993) Hepatitis E virus infection in Turkey. *Lancet* **342**: 810.

Coursaget P, Depril N, Buisson Y et al (1994) Hepatitis type E in a French population: detection of anti-HEV by a synthetic peptide-based enzyme-linked immunosorbent assay. *Research in Virology* **145**: 51–57.

Cubitt D, Bradley DW, Carter MJ et al (1995) Caliciviridae. Virus Taxonomy. *Archives of Virology* **(supplement 10)**: 359–363.

Dawson GJ, Chau KH, Cabal CM et al (1992) Solid-phase enzyme-linked immunosorbent assay for hepatitis E virus IgG and IgM antibodies utilizing recombinant antigens and synthetic peptides. *Journal of Virological Methods* **38**: 175–186.

De Cock KM, Bradley DW, Sandford NL et al (1987) Epidemic non-A, non-B hepatitis in patients from Pakistan. *Annals of Internal Medicine* **106**: 227–230.

el-Zimaity DM, Hyams KC, Imam IZ et al (1993) Acute sporadic hepatitis E in an Egyptian pediatric population. *American Journal of Tropical Medicine and Hygiene* **48**: 372–376.

Favorov MO, Khukhlovich PA, Zairov GK et al (1986) Clinico-epidemiological characteristics and diagnosis of viral non-A, non-B hepatitis with fecal and oral mechanisms of transmission of the infection. *Voprosy Virusologii* **31**: 65–69.

Favorov MO, Fields HA, Purdy MA et al (1992) Serologic identification of hepatitis E virus infections in epidemic and endemic settings. *Journal of Medical Virology* **36**: 246–250.

Favorov MO, Khudyakov YE, Fields HA et al (1994) Enzyme immunoassay for the detection of antibody to hepatitis E virus based on synthetic peptides. *Journal of Virological Methods* **46**: 237–250.

Goldsmith R, Yarbough PO, Reyes GR et al (1992) Enzyme-linked immunosorbent assay for diagnosis of acute sporadic hepatitis E in Egyptian children. *Lancet* **339**: 328–331.

Greco D, De Giacomi G, Piersante GP et al (1986) A person to person hepatitis A outbreak. *International Journal of Epidemiology* **15**: 108–111.

Gupta DN & Smetana HF (1957) The histopathology of viral hepatitis as seen in the Delhi epidemic (1955–56). *Indian Journal of Medical Research* **45 (supplement)**: 101–113.

Heath TCB, Burrow JNC, Currie BJ et al (1995) Locally acquired hepatitis E in the Northern Territory of Australia. *Medical Journal of Australia* **162**: 318–319.

Hyams KC, Purdy MA, Kaur M et al (1992) Acute sporadic hepatitis E in Sudanese children: analysis based on a new Western blot assay. *Journal of Infectious Diseases* **165**: 1001–1005.

Joshi YK, Babu S, Sarin S et al (1985) Immunoprophylaxis of epidemic non-A, non-B hepatitis. *Indian Journal of Medical Research* **81**: 18–19.

Jothikumar N, Aparna K, Kamatchiammal S et al (1993) Detection of hepatitis E virus in raw and treated wastewater with the polymerase chain reaction. *Applied and Environmental Microbiology* **59**: 2558–2562.

Kane MA, Bradley DW, Shrestha SM et al (1984) Epidemic non-A, non-B hepatitis in Nepal: recovery of a possible etiologic agent and transmission studies in marmosets. *Journal of the American Medical Association* **252**: 3140–3145.

Karetnyi YV, Favorov MO, Khudyakova NS et al (1995) Serologic evidence for hepatitis E virus infection in Israel. *Journal of Medical Virology* **45**: 316–320.

Khuroo MS (1980) Study of an epidemic of non-A, non-B hepatitis. Possibility of another human hepatitis virus distinct from post-transfusion non-A, non-B type. *American Journal of Medicine* **68**: 818–824.

Khuroo MS & Dar MY (1992) Hepatitis E: evidence for person-to-person transmission and inability of low dose immune serum globulin from an Indian source to prevent it. *Indian Journal of Gastroenterology* **11**: 113–116.

Khuroo MS, Saleem M, Teli MR & Sofi MA (1980) Failure to detect chronic liver disease after epidemic non-A, non-B hepatitis. *Lancet* **ii**: 97–98.

Khuroo MS, Teli MR, Skidmore S et al (1981) Incidence and severity of viral hepatitis in pregnancy. *American Journal of Medicine* **70**: 252–255.

Khuroo MS, Kamili S, Dar MY et al (1993) Hepatitis E and long-term antibody status. *Lancet* **341**: 1355.

Khuroo MS, Rustgi VK, Dawson GJ et al (1994) Spectrum of hepatitis E virus infection in India. *Journal of Medical Virology* **43**: 281–286.

Khuroo MS, Kamili S & Jameel S (1995) Vertical transmission of hepatitis E virus. *Lancet* **345**: 1025–1026.

Koonin EV, Gorbalenya AE, Purdy MA et al (1992) Computer-assisted assignment of functional domains in the nonstructural polyprotein of hepatitis E virus: delineation of an additional group of positive-strand RNA plant and animal viruses. *Proceedings of the National Academy of Sciences of the USA* **89**: 8259–8263.

Krawczynski K (1991) Antigens and antibodies of hepatitis E virus infection in experimental primate models and man. In Hollinger FB, Lemon SM, Margolis HS (eds) *Viral Hepatitis and Liver Disease*, pp 517–521. Baltimore: Williams & Wilkins.

Krawczynski K & Bradley DW (1989) Enterically transmitted non-A, non-B hepatitis: identification of virus-associated antigen in experimentally infected cynomolgus macaques. *Journal of Infectious Diseases* **159**: 1042–1049.

Kwo P, Balan VJ, Carpenter H et al (1995) Acute hepatitis E acquired in the United States. *Hepatology* **22 (supplement)**: 182A.

Li F, Zhuang H, Kolivas S et al (1994) Persistent and transient antibody responses to hepatitis E virus detected by western immunoblot using open reading frame 2 and 3 and glutathione S-transferase fusion proteins. *Journal of Clinical Microbiology* **32**: 2060–2066.

Lok ASF, Kwan WK, Moeckli R et al (1992) Seroepidemiological survey of hepatitis E in Hong Kong by recombinant-based enzyme immunoassays. *Lancet* **340**: 1205–1208.

Longer CF, Denny SL, Caudill JD et al (1993) Experimental hepatitis E: pathogenesis in cynomolgus macaques (*Macaca fascicularis*). *Journal of Infectious Diseases* **168**: 602–609.

McCaustland KA, Bi S, Purdy MA & Bradley DW (1991) Application of two RNA extraction methods prior to amplification of hepatitis E virus nucleic acid by the polymerase chain reaction. *Journal of Virological Methods* **35**: 331–342.

Mannucci PM, Gringeri A, Santagostino E et al (1994) Low risk of transmission of hepatitis E virus by large-pool coagulation factor concentrates. *Lancet* **343**: 597–598.

Mast E, Polish L, Favorov M et al (1994) Hepatitis E among refugees in Kenya: minimal apparent person-to-person transmission, evidence for age-dependent disease expression and new serologic assays. In Nishioka K, Suzuki H, Mishiro S, Oda T (eds) *Viral Hepatitis and Liver Disease*, pp 375–378. Tokyo: Springer-Verlag.

Moaven L, van Asten M, Crofts N & Locarnini SA (1995) Seroepidemiology of hepatitis E in selected Australian populations. *Journal of Medical Virology* **45**: 326–330.

Molinié C, Saliou P, Roué R et al (1988) Acute epidemic non-A, non-B hepatitis: a clinical study of 38 cases in Chad. In Zuckerman AJ (ed.) *Viral Hepatitis and Liver Disease*, pp 154–157. New York: Alan R. Liss, Inc.

Morrow RH, Smetana HF, Sai FT & Edgcomb JH (1968) Unusual features of viral hepatitis in Accra, Ghana. *Annals of Internal Medicine* **68**: 1250–1264.

Munoz S, Bradley D, Martin P et al (1992) Hepatitis E found in patients with apparent fulminant non-A non-B hepatitis. *Hepatology* **16 (supplement)**: 76A.

Myint H, Soe MM, Khin T et al (1985) A clinical and epidemiological study of an epidemic of non-

A, non-B hepatitis in Rangoon. *American Journal of Tropical Medicine and Hygiene* **34**: 1183–1189.

Naik SR, Aggarwal R, Salunke PN & Mehrotra NN (1992) A large waterborne viral hepatitis E epidemic in Kanpur, India. *Bulletin of the World Health Organization* **70**: 597–604.

Nanda SK, Ansari IH, Acharya SK et al (1995) Protracted viremia during acute sporadic hepatitis E virus infection. *Gastroenterology* **108**: 225–230.

Paul DA, Knigge MF, Ritter A et al (1994) Determination of hepatitis E virus seroprevalence by using recombinant fusion proteins and synthetic peptides. *Journal of Infectious Diseases* **169**: 801–806.

Pillot J, Lazizi Y, Diallo Y & Leguenno B (1992) Frequent sporadic hepatitis E in west Africa evidenced by characterization of a virus-associated antigen in the stool. *Journal of Hepatology* **15**: 420–421.

Purdy MA (1994) Molecular Biology of HEV. *Interaction* **2**: 7–11.

Purdy MA, McCaustland KA, Krawczynski K et al (1992) Expression of a hepatitis E virus (HEV)-trpE fusion protein containing epitopes recognized by antibodies in sera from human cases and experimentally infected primates. *Archives of Virology* **123**: 335–349.

Purdy MA, McCaustland KA, Krawczynski K et al (1993) Preliminary evidence that a trpE-HEV fusion protein protects cynomolgus macaques against challenge with wild-type hepatitis E virus (HEV). *Journal of Medical Virology* **41**: 90–94.

Purdy MA, Carson D, McCaustland KA et al (1994) Viral specificity of hepatitis E virus antigens identified by fluorescent antibody assay using recombinant HEV proteins. *Journal of Medical Virology* **44**: 212–214.

Reyes GR, Purdy MA, Kim JP et al (1990) Isolation of a cDNA from the virus responsible for enterically transmitted non-A, non-B hepatitis. *Science* **247**: 1335–1339.

Robson SC, Adams S, Brink N et al (1992) Hospital outbreak of hepatitis E. *Lancet* **339**: 1424–1425.

Sallie R, Silva AE, Purdy M et al (1994) Hepatitis C and E in non-A non-B fulminant hepatic failure: a polymerase chain reaction and serologic study. *Journal of Hepatology* **20**: 580–588.

Schlauder GG & Mushahwar IK (1994) Detection of hepatitis C and E virus by the polymerase chain reaction. *Journal of Virological Methods* **47**: 243–253.

Schlauder GG, Dawson GJ, Mushahwar IK et al (1993) Viraemia in Egyptian children with hepatitis E virus infection. *Lancet* **341**: 378.

Shapiro CN & Margolis HS (1993) Worldwide epidemiology of hepatitis A virus infection. *Journal of Hepatology* **18 (supplement 2)**: S11–S14.

Smalligan RD, Lange WR, Frame JD et al (1995) The risk of viral hepatitis A, B, C, and E among north American missionaries. *American Journal of Tropical Medicine and Hygiene* **53**: 233–236.

Soe S, Uchida T, Suzuki K et al (1989) Enterically transmitted non-A, non-B hepatitis in cynomolgus monkeys: morphology and probable mechanism of hepatocellular necrosis. *Liver* **9**: 135–145.

Song DY, Zhuang H, Kang XC et al (1991) Hepatitis E in Hetian City: a report of 562 cases. In Hollinger FB, Lemon SM, Margolis HS (eds) *Viral Hepatitis and Liver Disease*, pp 528–529. Baltimore: Williams & Wilkins.

Tandon BN, Joshi YK, Jain SK et al (1982) An epidemic of non-A non-B hepatitis in north India. *Indian Journal of Medical Research* **75**: 739–744.

Tassopoulos NC, Krawczynski K, Hatzakis A et al (1994) Case report: role of hepatitis E virus in the etiology of community-acquired non-A, non-B hepatitis in Greece. *Journal of Medical Virology* **42**: 124–128.

Thomas DL, Mahley RW, Badur S et al (1993) Epidemiology of hepatitis E virus infection in Turkey. *Lancet* **341**: 1561–1562.

Ticehurst J (1991) Identification and characterization of hepatitis E virus. In Hollinger FB, Lemon SM, Margolis HS (eds) *Viral Hepatitis and Liver Disease*, pp 501–513. Baltimore: Williams & Wilkins.

Ticehurst J, Rhodes LL, Krawczynski K et al (1992a) Infection of owl monkeys (*Aotus trivirgatus*) and cynomolgus monkeys (*Macaca fascicularis*) with hepatitis E virus from Mexico. *Journal of Infectious Diseases* **165**: 835–845.

Ticehurst J, Popkin TJ, Bryan JP et al (1992b) Association of hepatitis E virus with an outbreak of hepatitis in Pakistan: serologic responses and pattern of virus excretion. *Journal of Medical Virology* **36**: 84–92.

Tsarev SA, Emerson SU, Reyes GR et al (1992) Characterization of a prototype strain of hepatitis E virus. *Proceedings of the National Academy of Sciences of the USA* **89**: 559–563.

Tsarev SA, Tsareva TS, Emerson SU et al (1993a) ELISA for antibody to hepatitis E virus (HEV) based on complete open-reading frame-2 protein expressed in insect cells: identification of HEV infection in primates. *Journal of Infectious Diseases* **168**: 369–378.

Tsarev SA, Emerson SU, Tsareva TS et al (1993b) Variation in course of hepatitis E in experimentally infected cynomolgus monkeys. *Journal of Infectious Diseases* **167**: 1302–1306.

Tsarev SA, Tsareva TS, Emerson SU et al (1994) Successful passive and active immunization of cynomolgus monkeys against hepatitis E. *Proceedings of the National Academy of Sciences of the USA* **91**: 10 198–10 202.

Tsega E, Hansson BG, Krawczynski K & Nordenfeldt E (1992) Acute sporadic viral hepatitis in Ethiopia: causes, risk factors, and effects on pregnancy. *Clinical Infectious Diseases* **14**: 961–965.

Usmanov RK, Balayan MS, Dvoinikova OV et al (1994) An experimental infection in lambs by the hepatitis E virus. *Voprosy Virusologii* **39**: 165–168.

Velázquez O, Stetler HC, Avila C et al (1990) Epidemic transmission of enterically transmitted non-A, non-B hepatitis in Mexico, 1986–1987. *Journal of the American Medical Association* **263**: 3281–3285.

Villarejos VM, Serra J, Anderson-Visoná K & Mosley JW (1982) Hepatitis A virus infection in households. *American Journal of Epidemiology* **115**: 577–586.

Viswanathan R (1957) Infectious hepatitis in Delhi (1955–56): a critical study: epidemiology. *Indian Journal of Medical Research* **45 (supplement)**: 1–29.

Wang CH, Flehmig B & Moeckli R (1993) Transmission of hepatitis E virus by transfusion? *Lancet* **341**: 825–826.

Wang JT, Lin JT, Sheu JC et al (1994) Hepatitis E virus and posttransfusion hepatitis. *Journal of Infectious Diseases* **169**: 229–230.

Yarbough PO, Tam AW, Gabor K et al (1994) Assay development of diagnostic tests for hepatitis E. In Nishioka K, Suzuki H, Mishiro S, Oda T (eds) *Viral Hepatitis and Liver Disease*, pp 367–370. Tokyo: Springer-Verlag.

Yin S, Purcell RH & Emerson SU (1994) A new Chinese isolate of hepatitis E virus: comparison with strains recovered from different geographical regions. *Virus Genes* **9**: 23–32.

Zanetti AR, Dawson GJ & The Study Group of Hepatitis E (1994) Hepatitis type E in Italy: a sero-epidemiological survey. *Journal of Medical Virology* **42**: 318–320.

Zhuang H (1992) Hepatitis E and strategies for its control. In Wen YM, Xu ZY, Melnick JL (eds) *Viral Hepatitis in China: Problems and Control Strategies. Monographs in Virology*, vol 19, pp 126–139. Basel: Karger.

4

Heterogeneity of hepatitis C virus

DONALD B. SMITH
PATRIZIA PONTISSO

Since the nucleotide sequence of hepatitis C virus was first reported in 1989, a great deal of information has accumulated on the extent of variation between samples from different infected individuals. However, as yet, rather little is known about the biological and clinical significance of this variation.

Hepatitis C virus (HCV) is a positive-stranded RNA virus with a genome that encodes a polyprotein from which the mature virus proteins are cleaved. The organization of the genome and phylogenetic comparison of nucleotide sequences suggest that HCV belongs within the flaviviridae in its own genus, although closely related to the pestivirus genus. Even more closely related to HCV are two viruses recently isolated from tamarinds inoculated with human serum (GVB-A and GVB-B, Simons et al, 1995a) and a virus identified directly in patients with liver disease (GVB-C, Simons et al, 1995b).

LEVELS OF VIRUS HETEROGENEITY

The variation existing between different HCV sequences occurs at several different levels:

1. Almost all known HCV samples can be classified into six distinct groups or types. These types differ by 31–34% of nucleotide positions over the entire virus genome (Tokita et al, 1994). This level of diversity is equivalent to that existing between serotypes of poliovirus or dengue, and so HCV types might be expected to have different serological and/or biological properties.
2. Each of the types of virus can be divided into several subtypes that differ by 20–23% in nucleotide sequence. There is presently no strong evidence for any significant biological differences between HCV subtypes.
3. The different viruses comprising each subtype do not have identical sequences, but are up to 10% divergent from each other. These differences are mainly silent nucleotide substitutions that do not affect the sequence of the encoded virus protein, and are probably mostly of little

Baillière's Clinical Gastroenterology—
Vol. 10, No. 2, July 1996
ISBN 0–7020–2094–X
0950–3528/96/020243 + 13 $12.00/00

243

Copyright © 1996, by Baillière Tindall
All rights of reproduction in any form reserved

significance. However, differences in the 'hypervariable' region of the E2 envelope glycoprotein may be important in the persistence of virus infection (Wiener et al, 1992; Taniguchi et al, 1993; Farci et al, 1995), while a particular region of NS5A (NS5A$_{2209-2248}$) has been correlated with resistance to interferon treatment (Enotomo et al, 1995a) (see below).

4. Viruses co-circulating within a single infected individual are not identical, but can differ by up to 1.5% (Martell et al, 1992; Murakawa et al, 1992; Okamoto et al, 1992a). These closely related but distinct viruses have been termed 'quasispecies', but their clinical significance is unknown, and it is possible that some of the sequence differences observed are artefacts produced during amplification and cloning of virus RNA. Similar levels of sequence diversity are observed when virus sequences from infected individuals are compared at two different time points (Ogata et al, 1991; Enotomo et al, 1995a) and this complicates the interpretation of sequence changes during chronic infection.

GENOTYPE NOMENCLATURE

The most widespread nomenclature for HCV variants is a two-tiered system that recognizes the existence of virus types, identified by arabic numerals, that are each divided into subtypes, termed by small alphabetic letters (Simmonds et al, 1994). Virus genotypes are assigned in order of discovery, so that the prototype strain is 1a and the distinct variant first described in Japan is 1b.

The basis for this classification system is that pairwise comparison of different HCV sequences generates values of sequence differences that fall into largely non-overlapping distributions (Simmonds et al, 1993a). These three distributions are approximately normally distributed and correspond to comparisons between HCV types, between subtypes, and within subtypes. The same three distributions are observed whichever region of the virus genome is used for comparison, although the separation of the distributions is reduced for less variable regions such as that encoding the core polypeptide (Mellor et al, 1995). Similar relationships between sequences are observed whether comparisons are based on entire genomic sequences or regions as small as 222 nucleotides ($< 2.5\%$ of the virus genome). The only regions that cannot be reliably used for classification of HCV are the highly conserved 5' non-coding region (5'NCR) (Simmonds et al, 1993a; Ohba et al, 1995), and the hypervariable region at the NH$_2$-terminus of the E2 glycoprotein which is extremely divergent even within virus subtypes. However, the 5'NCR contains several substitutions that are strongly associated with virus genotype (Smith et al, 1995) and these provide the basis for some typing assays (see below).

Following recent intensive analysis of HCV variants from around the world, the number of HCV genotypes has exploded, and the six genotypes now consist of more than 70 distinct subtypes. A recent complication to this classification system has been the discovery of HCV variants from South East Asia that are related to type 6, but which are more divergent from type 6a than are the subtypes comprising other HCV types (Tokita et al, 1994; Mellor et al, 1995; Sugiyama et al, 1995; Tokita et al, 1995). The classification of these variants is presently controversial, with some groups considering them as new types and subtypes (7a, 7b, 8a, 9a, etc.) while others consider them as divergent subtypes within a type 6 clade (Mellor et al, 1995, 1996). Similar issues arise with a divergent subtype of type 3 described from Indonesia (Apichartpiyakul et al, 1994; Tokita et al, 1996).

GEOGRAPHICAL DISTRIBUTION OF VIRUS GENOTYPES

Virus genotypes are not uniformly distributed around the world, but occur at different frequencies in different populations (Tokita et al, 1994, 1995; Bukh et al, 1995; Davidson et al, 1995; Mellor et al, 1995, 1996). In some regions, the range of HCV genotypes is limited to many different subtypes of a single virus type. Examples of this pattern are types 1 and 2 in Western Africa, type 3 in the Indian subcontinent, type 4 in Central Africa, and type 6 in South East Asia. This pattern of diversity is consistent with the transmission of HCV within these communities for long periods, by an unknown, but possibly exclusively parenteral route. A contrasting pattern is seen in other regions where several HCV types are present, but these are represented by only a few subtypes. In Western Europe, North America and Australia the most common HCV genotypes are 1a, 1b, 2a, 2b and 3a, while in Japan and China only types 1b, 2a and 2b are common. This pattern suggests relatively recent and limited introduction of HCV into groups newly at risk of infection. For example, HCV is associated with transmission by blood and blood products, and with needle-sharing by intravenous drug users. A third pattern has been described in Egypt, where type 4a is the dominant genotype (McOmish et al, 1994). The frequency of HCV infection is unusually high in Egypt but infected individuals do not have the usual parenteral risk factors (Darwish et al, 1993; Abdelwahab et al, 1994). This situation is suggestive of a recent epidemic of HCV infection, possibly associated with campaigns of mass immunization or treatment with anti-schistosomal agents.

Despite these strong geographical associations with virus genotypes, all six major types have been detected in Western Europe and North America (Murphy et al, 1994; van Doorn et al, 1995). The occurrence of 'exotic' genotypes at low frequency is sometimes the result of immigration, but may also result from international trade in blood, blood products and human tissue (Preston et al, 1995).

TYPING ASSAYS

The possibility that clinical differences exist between HCV genotypes makes it important to be able to distinguish between them, and this can be achieved by both genomic and serological assays. All the genomic typing assays begin with amplification of the virus RNA genome by reverse transcription followed by polymerase chain reaction amplification (RT–PCR). The presence of type-specific polymorphisms in the amplified DNA is then assessed by restriction analysis (McOmish et al, 1994; Murphy et al, 1994; Davidson et al, 1995) or by hybridization to type-specific probes (Nakao et al, 1991; Stuyver et al, 1993; Tisminetzky et al, 1994; Viazov et al, 1994), or by the presence of amplified products after amplification with type-specific primers (Okamoto et al, 1992b, 1993). The most extensive systems are those based on the 5'NCR (Stuyver et al, 1993; Davidson et al, 1994; Pontisso et al, 1995c) and have predicted accuracies of 90% or more in distinguishing virus types and in recognizing certain virus subtypes (Smith et al, 1995). However, the recent discovery of variants of type 6 (Tokita et al, 1994) that have 5'NCR sequences indistinguishable from those of type 1 viruses in these systems has necessitated the development of supplemental assays based on the core region (Stuyver et al, 1995; Mellor et al, 1996).

Virus genotype can also be deduced from the serological reactivities induced following infection, and serological assays have been developed using antigens derived from both the core and NS4 proteins (Machida et al, 1992; Simmonds et al, 1993c; Tanaka et al, 1994; Bhattacherjee et al, 1995). Infection with types 1–6 can be recognized with a peptide based NS4 assay (Bhattacherjee et al, 1995) but no discrimination is possible between virus subtypes. Serological assays have the advantage of being relatively cheap and simple to apply in a routine diagnostic laboratory, but are less effective for immunocompromised individuals, or in individuals prior to seroconversion.

Neither serological nor genotypic typing assays are completely accurate (Lau et al, 1995b) and so the definitive identification of virus genotype must be based on nucleotide sequence analysis of virus coding regions.

CLINICAL IMPLICATIONS

Screening

The prevention of HCV transmission following medical intervention depends on the efficacy of screening of blood, blood products and tissue donors for HCV infection. Current serological screening assays employ a variety of antigens derived from both structural and non-structural virus proteins and have significantly decreased post-transfusion HCV infection (van der Poel et al, 1994). However, all the antigens employed in such assays are derived from type 1a or 1b viruses, and the possibility exists that these assays may be less efficient in detecting individuals infected with non-type 1 viruses. In this context, it is noteworthy that most studies of the efficacy of screening have been conducted in regions where type 1 viruses predominate (Donahue et al, 1992; Kleinman et al, 1992; Mathiesen et al, 1993; Wang et al, 1995).

There is evidence that serological responses to the component antigens of current screening assays are genotype-dependent (Chan et al, 1991; McOmish et al, 1994; Zein et al, 1995) and this may affect the sensitivity of detection of antibody in samples from individuals infected with types 2 and 3 (Dhaliwal et al, 1996). In addition, the possibility remains that current screening assays may not detect anti-HCV antibodies in individuals infected with unidentified HCV genotypes.

Levels of virus replication

Studies on viraemic levels in individuals infected with different virus geno-types have yielded conflicting results. While some reports have suggested that virus levels are higher in individuals infected with type 1 (Yoshioka et al, 1992; Mahaney et al, 1994; Chan et al, 1995; Martinot-Peignoux et al, 1995), other studies have found no evidence for a significant difference (Lau et al, 1995a; Smith et al, 1996). To some extent these discrepancies may be explained by differences in the efficiency of virus quantification for different genotypes, since probes and primers have usually been designed to match type 1 virus sequences. For example, the branched DNA assay version 1.0 (Quantiplex™, Chiron Corporation) detects virus types 2 and 3 with an efficiency of only 0.3 and 0.5, respectively, relative to type 1 (Collins et al, 1995). Studies where this has been taken into account have found that no difference in virus level exists between different virus geno-types (Lau et al, 1995a; Smith et al, 1996). The effect of genotype on other quantification systems, such as the Roche Amplicor Assay (PCR) has not been measured.

Mixed genotype infections

Detailed analysis of large groups of HCV-infected individuals reveals that a small proportion are apparently infected with more than one virus geno-type. While mixed infection might be expected to have consequences for virus pathology and/or treatment, many reported mixed infections may actually represent mistyping. The typing system based on type-specific amplification of the core gene (Okamoto et al, 1992b, 1993) identifies as many as 20% of samples as containing type 1b and another genotype but, in these cases, amplification with the type 1b primers is usually erroneous (Lau et al, 1995b). Other typing methods suggest a much lower frequency (<1%) of mixed infection even though some systems could identify mixed infections when one of the two types is 100 times less represented than the other (Tisminetzky et al, 1995). On the other hand, higher frequencies of mixed infections are observed among certain multiply exposed groups such as haemophiliacs (Preston et al, 1995; Tagariello et al, 1995).

Clinical characteristics and pathogenetic implications

The influence of virus genotype on the pathology of HCV infection has been difficult to investigate because of the wide spectrum of clinical manifestations of disease, ranging from asymptomatic carriage of the virus to chronic hepatitis, eventually evolving to liver cirrhosis and hepatocellular carcinoma. Severity of disease may be influenced by several factors, including the duration of infection, mode of acquisition, host immunity and genetic factors, co-existing infections, or toxic agents such as alcohol.

For example, type 1b is associated more with end-stage liver disease, including liver cirrhosis and hepatocellular carcinoma (Dusheiko et al, 1994; De Mitri et al, 1995; Nousbaum et al, 1995), compared with other HCV types, suggesting a higher pathogenic effect of this viral type. However, the concurrent association of older age and longer duration of disease observed in these patients may be responsible, rather than a higher pathogenicity of the virus 'per se' (Nousbaum et al, 1995). In keeping with this interpretation is the finding of similar histological and clinical features in patients infected with type 1 and type 2, observed in series of chronically infected patients undergoing interferon treatment (Mahaney et al, 1994; Pontisso et al, 1995c). On the other hand, patients infected with type 3 are often younger, with a frequent history of drug abuse, indicating that this parenteral route has been one of the most important routes of virus spreading in Western Europe (Martinot-Peignoux et al, 1995; Pontisso et al, 1995c). These patients are reported to have higher mean ALT levels than patients infected with types 1 and 2 (Simmonds et al, 1993b; Tagariello et al 1995), and a higher incidence of past history of overt acute hepatitis (Pontisso et al, 1995c).

Clues about the potential pathogenetic role of different genotypes can also be derived from prospective clinical studies, but at present little information is available due to the slow progression of the disease (Kiyosawa et al, 1982). A unique model is offered by patients undergoing orthotopic liver transplantation: in most HCV-positive patients re-infection of the graft occurs, and about 50% of them show recurrence of disease within 5 years (Wright et al, 1992; Féray et al, 1994). It is interesting to note that this event has been more frequently observed in patients infected with HCV type 1b (Féray et al, 1995). Liver damage appears more severe and leads to a progressive liver disease more rapidly in type 1b infected patients, than in those infected with other viral types. However, a longitudinal survey in a cohort of 109 cirrhotic patients followed for 4–10 years has demonstrated that the cumulative probability of worsening of the disease, including Child's stage deterioration, development of hepatocellular carcinoma or death for complications of liver disease was not different in relation to the infecting genotype (Benvegnù et al, 1995).

Different findings have been described in asymptomatic HCV carriers, where cross-sectional studies on large series of Italian patients with normal transaminase profiles have often shown infection by HCV type 2 (Silini et al, 1994; Pontisso et al, 1995b). The occurrence of HCV type 2 infection has also been identified in most patients who remain viraemic after sustained biochemical remission with interferon therapy (Chemello et al, 1996), suggesting that selection of a less pathogenic viral strain associates with type 2 infection.

Immunological studies have indicated that HLA I-restricted, CD8[+] T cell mediated cytotoxicity may play a role in the pathogenesis of chronic HCV infection (Liaw et al, 1995). Several lines of evidence have identified both structural and non-structural viral antigens as the targets of this response (Koziel et al, 1992). Expression of interferon-inducible molecules, such as HLA-A, B, C and ICAM-1 molecules in infected livers by the endogenous interferon system is higher in patients infected with type 1, compared with patients infected with types 2 and 3 (Ballardini et al, 1995). These findings may contribute to knowledge on the different rates of response to exogenous interferon (see below) and add insight on the possible different mechanisms of liver damage during infection with different viral types.

Response to therapy

The first therapeutic agent showing beneficial effect in chronic hepatitis C was interferon alpha (Hoofnagle et al, 1986) and since then several randomized trials have been conducted. The sustained response rate ranges from 10% to more than 30% in different studies. Despite many differences in the design of the studies, the most important variables repeatedly found to predict a response are age, disease duration, liver histology, the infecting virus genotype and pretreatment HCV RNA levels (Conjeevaram et al, 1995).

A consistent finding obtained in several sudies, where different typing techniques have been used, is the better response rate obtained in individuals infected with viral type 2 or type 3, compared with that observed in patients infected with type 1 (Conjeevaram et al, 1995). Analysing the response rate in relation to type 1 subtypes, a higher rate of primary response has been reported in patients infected with subtype 1a, compared with 1b; however, the rate of sustained response does not differ between the two subtypes (Mahaney et al, 1994; Pontisso et al, 1995a). A dose-dependence of the response rate for types 1 and 3 has been reported, while values observed in type 2-infected individuals have not been found to improve with increasing dosages of interferon (Kohara et al, 1995). A randomized trial comparing three different regimens of interferon conducted in 174 Caucasian patients has shown rates of sustained response ranging from 9 to 28% in patients infected by type 1b, from 42 to 46% in those infected by type 2a/c, and from 67 to 100% in those infected by type 3, in relation to the lower or higher dose of interferon used, respectively (Chemello et al, 1995). In addition, responders with type 2 infection showed a much faster decrease in serum HCV RNA levels than did patients infected by type 1, and patients infected with the same genotype had similar rates of HCV reduction, independently of the starting viraemic level (Kohara et al, 1995). These findings support the possibility that type 2 has a higher intrinsic sensitivity than type 1 to exogenous interferon.

The relationship between viral load, infecting genotype and response to therapy is ambiguous, several studies indicating a clear association of viraemic levels with the response (Hagiwara et al, 1993; Yamada et al,

1995), while this finding has not been confirmed in others (Nousbaum et al, 1995). One point to be considered is that quantification by Quantiplex™(1.0) Chiron Corporation, underestimates values of viraemia in type 2-and type 3-infected sera (Collins et al, 1995; Lau et al, 1995a), and therefore misleading findings have been reported. The genotype dependence of other quantification methods is unknown. Since the geographic distribution of viral types is not homogeneous and HCV genotype has not always been taken into consideration in studies evaluating the effect of viral levels on the response to treatment, discrepant results may also be explained by differences in the relative proportion of different viral types in the populations studied.

The $NS5A_{2209-2248}$ region has been correlated with resistance to interferon treatment in patients infected with genotype 1b (Enotomo et al, 1995a). The close relationship between mutations within this region and decreased HCV-RNA levels suggests that it may play a role in virus replication (Enotomo et al, 1995b). In keeping with this hypothesis is the report that amino acid residues 2200–2250, encompassing this region, are essential for the phosphorylation of NS5A (Tanji et al, 1995).

Biological implications

The lack of suitable systems for growth of HCV has limited knowledge about the biological properties of HCV and the significance of genomic differences between genotypes. Recent studies indicate that, as in picornaviruses, the translation control elements of HCV are located in a portion of the 5'NCR sequence that folds into highly ordered secondary structures and whose presence directs cap-independent initiation of translation (Brown et al, 1991; Tsukiyama-Kohara et al, 1992; Wang et al, 1993). This secondary structure is remarkably conserved in the 5'NCR of all genotypes, despite some sequence variation (Smith et al, 1995). However, interesting data obtained from transcriptional studies performed in HeLa cell systems have shown that HCV type 2 has higher translational activity than type 1 (Tsukiyama-Kohara et al, 1992). Similar studies, in which plasmid constructions containing 5'NCR sequences not only of types 1 and 2 but also of type 3 were used, have shown an even lower efficiency of translation for type 3 (Gerotto, personal communication). These preliminary findings suggest potential biological differences for each genotype due to sequence variation, despite conservation of RNA secondary structure. Research is in progress to identify coding regions that could produce biological differences between virus genotypes.

Vaccination

The absence of a simple cell or animal system for the study of HCV replication makes it difficult to test the effect of variation between virus genotypes on virus neutralization or on the effectiveness of vaccination. However, there are several reasons for expecting that variation between genotypes will have to be taken into account in the eventual development of an effective vaccine.

The envelope proteins, identified as potential targets for virus neutralization (Choo et al, 1994) are the most variable region of the virus genome, differing by 25–40% of amino acids between virus types. Similar levels of variation in other viruses are sufficient to prevent cross-neutralization, suggesting that vaccination with one virus type may not protect against infection with a different type. Direct evidence for this possibility comes from the observation that individuals successively exposed to different HCV genotypes are not protected against infection by the initial exposure; this finding has not only been observed in polytransfused patients with haematological disorders (Jarvis et al, 1994; Lai et al, 1994), but also in individuals with a sustained clinical and virological response to interferon treatment (unpublished observation).

There is also evidence for the lack of an efficient immune protection, even in presence of the same viral type (Farci et al, 1995), perhaps reflecting virus evolution in response to immune pressure.

SUMMARY

A great deal of information on the molecular heterogeneity of hepatitis C virus (HCV) has been achieved since its discovery in 1989. However, little is known about the clinical significance of these variations.

Based on the degree of sequence variation, HCV has been classified into six major groups or types, differing by 31–34% at the nucleotide level over the entire virus genome. Each type is divided into several subtypes that differ by 20–23% in nucleotide sequence. Viruses within the same subtype are up to 10% divergent and, within infected individuals, vary by up to 1.5%. Genotype distributions are not homogeneous around the world and may reflect both historical and recent parenteral routes of transmission. The clinical implication of these genomic variations are not yet fully elucidated: genotype 1b has been associated with end-stage liver disease, including liver cirrhosis and hepatocellular carcinoma, but this finding might rather reflect its earlier introduction to the populations studied. Consistent evidence exists that types 2 and 3 have a higher response rate to interferon treatment than type 1, although the interplay between genotype and viral load in determining the response is still unclear. Immunohistochemical studies indicate a stronger activation of the endogenous interferon system in the liver of patients infected with type 1 compared to those infected with types 2 and 3, explaining, at least in part, its low responsiveness to exogenous interferon treatment. Biological, sequence-dependent variations of genotypes have been poorly investigated to date, but differential efficiency of translation activity of the $5'$ non-coding region has been reported. The availability of 'in vitro' systems for evaluating pathogenetic aspects and neutralization mechanisms will improve the present knowledge on this world-wide infectious disease and on the clinical usefulness of distinguishing between genotypes.

REFERENCES

Abdelwahab MF, Zakaria S, Kamel M et al (1994) High seroprevalence of hepatitis C infection among risk groups in Egypt. *American Journal of Tropical Medicine and Hygiene* **51:** 563–567.

Apichartpiyakul C, Chittivudikarn C, Miyajima H et al (1994). Analysis of hepatitis C virus isolates among healthy blood donors and drug addicts in Chiang Mai, Thailand. *Journal of Clinical Microbiology* **32:** 2276–2279.

Ballardini G, Groff P, Pontisso P et al (1995) Hepatitis C virus (HCV) genotype, tissue HCV antigens, hepatocellular expression of HLA-A,B,C, and intracellular adhesion-1 molecules. *Journal of Clinical Investigation* **95:** 2067–2075.

Benvegnù L, Pontisso P, Cavalletto D et al (1995) Hepatitis C virus (HCV) genotypes and clinical course of anti-HCV positive cirrhosis. *Hepatology* **22:** 343A.

Bhattacherjee V, Prescott LE, Pike I et al (1995) Use of NS-4 peptides to identify type-specific antibody to hepatitis C virus genotypes 1,2,3,4,5 and 6. *Journal of General Virology* **76:** 1737–1748.

Brown EA, Day SP, Jansen RW & Lemon SM (1991) The 5′ nontranslated region of hepatitis A virus RNA: secondary structure and elements required for translation in vitro. *Journal of Virology* **65:** 5825–5838.

Bukh J (1995) Genetic heterogeneity of hepatitis C virus: quasispecies and genotypes. *Seminars in Liver Disease* **15:** 41–36.

Chan SW, Simmonds P, McOmish F et al (1991). Serological reactivity of blood donors infected with three different types of hepatitis C virus. *Lancet* **338:** 1391.

Chan CY, Lee SD, Hwnang SJ et al (1995) Quantitative branched DNA assay and genotyping for hepatitis C virus RNA in Chinese patients with acute and chronic hepatitis C. *Journal of Infectious Diseases* **171:** 443–446.

Chemello L, Bonetti P, Cavalletto L et al (1995) Randomized trial comparing three different regimens of alpha-2a-interferon in chronic hepatitis C. *Hepatology* **22:** 700–706.

Chemello L, Cavalletto D, Casarin C et al (1996) Persistent hepatitis C viraemia predicts late relapse after sustained response to alpha-interferon in chronic hepatitis C. *Annals of Internal Medicine* (in press).

Choo QL, Kuo G, Ralston R et al (1994) Vaccination of chimpanzees against infection by the hepatitis C virus. *Proceedings of the National Academy of Science of the USA* **91:** 1294–1298.

Collins ML, Zayati C, Detmer JJ et al (1995) Preparation and characterization of RNA standards for use in quantitative branched DNA hybridization assays. *Analytical Biochemistry* **226:** 120–129.

Conjeevaram HS, Everhart JE & Hoofnagle JH (1995) Predictors of a sustained beneficial response to interferon alfa therapy in chronic hepatitis C. *Hepatology* **22:** 1326–1329.

Darwish MA, Raouf TA, Rushdy P et al (1993) Risk factors associated with a high seroprevalence of hepatitis C virus infection in Egyptian blood donors. *American Journal of Tropical Medicine and Hygiene* **49:** 440–447.

Davidson F, Simmonds P, Ferguson JC et al (1995) Survey of major genotypes and subtypes of hepatitis C virus using RFLP of sequences amplified from the 5′ non-coding region. *Journal of General Virology* **76:** 1197–1204.

De Mitri MS, Poussin K, Baccarini P et al (1995) HCV-associated liver cancer without cirrhosis. *Lancet* **345:** 413–415.

Dhaliwal SK, Munoz A, Ness PM et al (1996) Influence of viraemia and genotype upon serological reactivity in screening assays for antibody to hepatitis C virus. *Journal of Medical Virology* **48:** 184–190.

Donahue JG, Munoz A, Ness PM et al (1992) The declining risk of post-transfusion hepatitis C virus infection. *New England Journal of Medicine* **327:** 369–373.

Dusheiko G, Schmilovitz-Weiss H, Brown D et al (1994) Hepatitis C virus genotypes: an investigation of type-specific differences in geographic origin and disease. *Hepatology* **19:** 13–18.

Enotomo N, Sakuma, I, Asahina Y et al (1995a) Comparison of full-length sequences of interferon-sensitive and resistant hepatitis C virus 1b—sensitivity to interferon is conferred by amino acid substitutions in the NS5 region. *Journal of Clinical Investigation* **96:** 224–230.

Enotomo K, Sakuma I, Asahina Y et al (1995b). Mutations in the nonstructural protein 5A gene and response to interferon in patients with chronic hepatitis C virus 1b infection. *New England Journal of Medicine* **334:** 77–81.

Farci P, Shimoda A, Wong D et al (1995) Prevention of HCV infection in chimpanzees by hyperimmune serum against the hypervariable region I (HVR1): emergence of neutralization escape mutants in vivo. *Hepatology* **22:** 220A.

Féray C, Gigou M, Samuel D et al (1994) The course of hepatitis C infection after liver transplantation. *Hepatology* **20:** 1137–1143,

Féray C, Gigou M, Samuel D et al (1995) Influence of the genotypes of hepatitis C virus on the severity of recurrent liver disease after liver transplantation. *Gastroenterology* **108:** 1088–1096.

Hagiwara H, Hayashi N, Mita E et al (1993) Quantitative analysis of hepatitis C virus RNA in serum during interferon alfa therapy. *Gastroenterology* **104:** 877–883.

Hoofnagle JH, Mullen KD, Jones DB et al (1986) Treatment of chronic non-A, non-B hepatitis with recombinant human alpha interferon. *New England Journal of Medicine* **315:** 1575–1578.

Jarvis LM, Watson HG, McOmish F et al (1994) Frequent reinfection and reactivation of hepatitis C virus genotypes in multitransfused hemophiliacs. *Journal of Infectious Disease* **170:** 1018–1022.

Kiyosawa K, Akahane Y, Nagata A et al (1982) Significance of blood transfusion in non-A, non-B chronic liver disease in Japan. *Vox Sanguinis* **43:** 45–52.

Kleinman S, Alter H, Bush M et al (1992) Increased detection of hepatitis C virus (HCV)-infected blood donors by a multiple-antigen HCV enzyme immunoassay. *Transfusion* **32:** 805–813.

Kohara M, Tanaka T, Tsukiyama-Kohara K et al (1995) Hepatitis C virus genotypes 1 and 2 respond to interferon alfa with different virologic kinetics. *Journal of Infectious Diseases* **172:** 934–938.

Koziel JM, Dudley D, Wong JT et al (1992) Intrahepatic cytotoxic T lymphocytes specific for hepatitis C virus in persons with chronic hepatitis. *Journal of Immunology* **149:** 3339–3344.

Lai ME, Mazzoleni AP, Argiolu F et al (1994) Hepatitis C virus in multiple episodes of acute hepatitis in polytransfused thalassaemic children. *Lancet* **343:** 388–390.

Lau JYN, Simmonds P Urdea MS (1995a) Implications of variations of 'conserved' regions of hepatitis C virus genome. *Lancet* **346:** 425–426.

Lau JYN, Mizokami M, Kolberg JA et al (1995b) Application of six hepatitis C virus genotyping systems to sera from chronic hepatitis C patients in the United States. *Journal of Infectious Disease* **171:** 281–289.

Liaw YF, Lee CS, Tsai SL et al (1995) T-cell mediated autologous hepatocytotoxicity in patients with chronic hepatitis C virus infection. *Hepatology* **22:** 1368–1373.

Machida A, Ohnuma H, Tsuda F et al (1992) Two distinct subtypes of hepatitis C virus defined by antibodies directed to the putative core protein. *Hepatology* **16:** 886–891.

McOmish F, Chittivudikarn C, Miyajima H et al (1993) Detection of three types of hepatitis C virus in blood donors: investigation of type-specific differences in serological reactivity and rate of alanine aminotransferase abnormalities. *Transfusion* **33:** 7–13.

McOmish F, Yap PL, Dow BC et al (1994) Geographical distribution of hepatitis C virus genotypes in blood donors—an international collaborative survey. *Journal of Clinical Microbiology* **32:** 884–892.

Mahaney K, Tedeschi V, Maertens G et al (1994) Genotypic analysis of hepatitis C virus in American patients. *Hepatology* **20:** 1405–1411.

Martell M, Esteban JI, Quer J et al (1992) Hepatitis C virus (HCV) circulates as a population of different but closely related genomes: quasispecies nature of HCV genome distribution. *Journal of Virology* **66:** 3225–3229.

Martinot-Peignoux M, Marcellin P, Pouteau M et al (1995) Pretreatment serum hepatitis C virus RNA levels and hepatitis C virus genotype are the main and independent prognostic factors of sustained response to interferon alfa therapy in chronic hepatitis C. *Hepatology* **22:** 1050–1056.

Mathiesen UL, Karlsson E, Foberg U et al (1993) Also with a restrictive transfusion policy, screening with 2nd generation anti-hepatitis C virus enzyme-linked immunosorbent assay would have reduced post-transfusion hepatitis C after open-heart surgery. *Scandinavian Journal of Gastroenteorlogy* **28:** 581–584.

Mellor J, Holmes EC, Jarvis LM et al (1995) Investigation of the pattern of hepatitis C virus sequence diversity in different geographical regions: implications for virus classification. *Journal of General Virology* **76:** 2493–2507.

Mellor J, Walsh EA, Prescott LE et al (1996) Survey of type 6-group variants of hepatitis C virus in South-East Asia using a core-based genotyping assay. *Journal of Clinical Microbiology* **34:** 417–423.

Murakawa K, Esumi M, Kato T et al (1992) Heterogeneity within the nonstructural protein-5-encoding region of hepatitis C viruses from a single patient. *Gene* **117:** 229–232.

Murphy D, Williams B & Delage G (1994) Use of the 5′ non-coding region for genotyping hepatitis C virus. *Journal of Infectious Disease* **169:** 473–475.

Nakao T, Enotomo N, Takada N et al (1991) Typing of hepatitis C virus (HCV) genomes by restriction fragment length polymorphisms. *Journal of General Virology* **72:** 2105–2112.

Nousbaum JB, Pol S, Nalpas B et al (1995) Hepatitis C virus type 1b (II) infection in France and Italy. *Annals of Internal Medicine* **122:** 161–168.

Ogata N, Alter HJ, Miller RH & Purcell RH (1991) Nucleotide sequence and mutation rate of the H strain of hepatitis C virus. *Proceedings of the National Academy of Sciences of the USA* **88:** 3392–3396.

Ohba K, Mizokami M, Ohno T et al (1995) Classification of hepatitis C virus into major types and subtypes based on molecular evolutionary analysis. *Virus Research* **36:** 201–214.

Okamoto H, Kojima M, Okada SL et al (1992a) Genetic drift of hepatitis C virus during an 8.2 year infection in a chimpanzee: variability and stability. *Virology* **190:** 894–899.

Okamoto H, Sugiyama Y, Okada S et al (1992b) Typing hepatitis C virus by polymerase chain reaction with type-specific primers: application to clinical surveys and tracing infectious sources. *Journal of General Virology* **73:** 673–679.

Okamoto H, Tokita H, Sakamoto M et al (1993) Characterization of the genomic sequence of type V (or 3a) hepatitis C virus isolates and PCR primers for specific detection. *Journal of General Virology* **74:** 2385–2390.

Pontisso P, Gerotto M, Chemello L et al (1995a) Hepatitis C virus genotypes HCV-1a and HCV-1b: the clinical point of view. *Journal of Infectious Disease* **171:** 760.

Pontisso P, Ruvoletto MG, Gerotto M et al (1995b) Genomic characterization of HCV in viremic patients with normal ALT. *Hepatology* **22:** 342A.

Pontisso P, Ruvoletto MG, Nicoletti M et al (1995c) Distribution of three major hepatitis C virus genotypes in Italy: a multicentre study of 495 patients with chronic hepatitis. *Journal of Viral Hepatitis* **2:** 33–38.

Preston FE, Jarvis LM, Makris M et al (1995) Heterogeneity of hepatitis C virus genotypes in haemophilia: relationship with chronic liver disease. *Blood* **85:** 1259–1262.

Silini E, Bono F, Cividini A et al (1994) Differential distribution of hepatitis C virus genotypes in patients with and without liver function abnormalities. *Hepatology* **21:** 285–290.

Simmonds P, Holmes EC, Cha TA et al (1993a) Classification of hepatitis C virus into six major genotypes and a series of subtypes by phylogenetic analysis of the NS-5 region. *Journal of General Virology* **74:** 2391–2399.

Simmonds P, McOmish F, Yap PL et al (1993b) Sequence variability in the 5′ non coding region of hepatitis C virus: identification of a new virus type and restrictions on sequence diversity. *Journal of General Virology* **74:** 661–668.

Simmonds P, Rose KA, Graham S et al (1993c) Mapping of serotype-specific, immunodominant epitopes in the NS-4 region of hepatitis C virus (HCV)—use of type-specific peptides to serologically differentiate infections with HCV type 1, type 2 and type 3. *Journal of Clinical Microbiology* **31:** 1493–1503.

Simmonds P, Alberti A, Alter HJ et al (1994) A proposed system for the nomenclature of hepatitis C viral genotypes. *Hepatology* **19:** 1321–1324.

Simons JN, Leary TP, Dawson GJ et al (1995a) Isolation of novel virus-like sequences associated with human hepatitis. *Nature Medicine* **1:** 564–569.

Simons JN, Pilot-Matias TJ, Leary TP et al (1995b) Identification of two flavivirus-like genomes in the GB hepatitis agent. *Proceedings of the National Academy of Sciences of the USA* **92:** 3041–3405.

Smith DB, Mellor J, Jarvis LM et al (1995) Variation of hepatitis C virus 5′ non-coding region: implications for secondary structure, virus detection and typing. *Journal of General Virology* **76:** 1749–1761.

Smith DB, Davidson F, Yap PL et al (1996) Levels of hepatitis C virus in blood donors infected with different viral genotypes. *Journal of Infectious Disease* **173:** 727–730.

Stuyver L, Rossau R, Wyseur A et al (1993) Typing of hepatitis C virus isolates and characterization of new subtypes using a line probe assay. *Journal of General Virology* **74:** 1093–1102.

Stuyver L, Wyseur A, Vanarnhem W et al (1995) Hepatitis C virus genotyping by means of 5′-UR/core line probe assays and molecular analysis of untypeable samples. *Virus Research* **38:** 137–157.

Sugiyama K, Kato N, Nakazawa T et al (1995) Novel genotypes of hepatitis C virus in Thailand. *Journal of General Virology* **76:** 2323–2327.

Tagariello G, Pontisso P, Davoli PG et al (1995) Hepatitis C virus genotypes and severity of chronic liver disease in haemophiliacs. *British Journal of Haematology* **91:** 708–713.

Tanaka T, Tsukiyama-Koara K, Yamaguchi K et al (1994) Significance of specific antibody assay for genotyping of hepatitis C virus *Hepatology* **19**. 1347–1353.

Taniguchi S, Okamoto H, Sakamoto M et al (1993) A structurally flexible and antigenically variable n-terminal domain of the hepatitis C virus e2/NS1 protein- implications for an escape from antibody. *Virology* **195**: 297–301.

Tanji Y, Kaneko T & Shimotohno K (1995) Phosphorylation of hepatitis C virus-encoded nonstructural protein NS5A. *Journal of Virology* **69**: 3980–3986.

Tisminetzky SG, Gerotto M, Pontisso P et al (1994) Genotypes of hepatitis C virus in Italian patients with chronic hepatitis C. *International Hepatology Communications* **2**: 105–112.

Tisminetzky SG, Gerotto M, Pontisso P et al (1995) Comparison of genotyping and serotyping methods for the identification of hepatitis C virus types. *Journal of Virological Methods* **55**: 303–307.

Tokita H, Okamoto H, Tsuda F et al (1994) Hepatitis C variants from Vietnam are classifiable into the seventh, eighth and ninth major genetic groups. *Proceedings of the National Academy of Sciences of the USA* **91**: 11 022–11 026.

Tokita H, Okamoto H, Luengrojanakul P et al (1995) Hepatitis C virus variants from Thailand classifiable into five novel genotypes in the sixth (6b), seventh (7c, 7d) and ninth (9b, 9c) major genetic groups. *Journal of General Virology* **76**: 2329–2335.

Tokita H, Okamoto H, Iizuka H et al (1996) Hepatitis C variants from Jakarta, classifiable into novel genotypes in the second (2e and 2f), tenth (10a) and eleventh (11a) genetic groups. *Journal of General Virology* **77**: 293–301.

Tsukiyama-Kohara K, Iizuka N, Kohara M et al (1992) Internal ribosome entry site within hepatitis C virus RNA. *Journal of Virology* **66**: 1476–1483.

van der Poel C, Cuypers T & Reesink HK (1994) Hepatitis C virus six years on. *Lancet* **344**: 1475–1479.

van Doorn LJ, Kleter GEM, Stuyver L et al (1995) Sequence analysis of hepatitis C virus genotypes 1 to 5 reveals multiple novel subtypes in the Benelux countries. *Journal of General Virology* **76**: 1871–1876.

Viazov S, Zibert A, Ramakrishnan K et al (1994) Typing of hepatitis C virus isolates by DNA enzyme immunoassay. *Journal of Virological Methods* **48**: 81–91.

Wang C, Sarnow P & Siddiqui A (1993) Translation of human hepatitis C virus RNA in cultured cells is mediated by an internal ribosome-binding mechanism. *Journal of Virology* **67**: 3338–3344.

Wang JT, Wang TH, Lin JT et al (1995) Effect of hepatitis C antibody screening in blood donors on post-transfusion hepatitis in Taiwan. *Journal of Gastroenterology and Hepatology* **10**: 454–458.

Wiener AJ, Geysen HM, Christopherson C et al (1992) Evidence for immune selection of hepatitis C virus (HCV) putative envelope glycoprotein variants: potential role in chronic HCV infections. *Proceedings of the National Academy of Sciences of the USA* **89**: 3468–3472.

Wright TL, Donegan E, Hsu H et al (1992) Recurrent and acquired hepatitis C viral infection in liver transplant recipients. *Gastroenterology* **103**: 317–322.

Yamada G, Takatani M, Kishi F et al (1995) Efficacy of interferon alfa therapy in chronic hepatitis C patients depends primarily on hepatitis C virus RNA levels. *Hepatology* **22**: 1351–1354.

Yoshioka K, Kakamu S, Wakita T et al (1992) Detection of hepatitis C virus by polymerase chain reaction and response to interferon alpha therapy: relationship to genotypes of hepatitis C virus. *Hepatology* **16**: 293–299.

Zein NN, Rakela J & Persing DH (1995) Genotype-dependent serologic reactivities in patients infected with hepatitis C virus in the United States. *Mayo Clinic Proceedings* **70**: 449–452.

5

Pathogenesis of chronic hepatitis C and associated clinical manifestations

JONATHAN C. L. BOOTH
HOWARD C. THOMAS

Infection with the hepatitis C virus results in a variety of hepatic and extra-hepatic diseases. In a minority of patients, infection results in an acute hepatitis which is usually asymptomatic. In 80% of infected patients, infection persists for many years and results in a variable degree of hepatitis. In the majority of patients over the initial 10–20 years of infection, the degree of hepatitis is minimal, but as time goes on, fibrosis occurs, and up to 20% of patients followed for 20 years will develop cirrhosis, and 1% of these develop hepatocellular cancer each year. Thus, although initially a mild disease, eventually hepatitis C virus infection produces serious pathology. Extrahepatic diseases have also been seen with this infection. Type 2 cryoglobulinaemia, particularly in Southern Europe, is usually associated with this persistent viral infection. Initial reports that the virus might be aetiologically involved in autoimmune thyroiditis and diabetes mellitus have not been confirmed. A small proportion of the patients with persistent infection and chronic hepatitis have type 2 liver/kidney microsomal antibodies present in their serum. In this group of patients whether the liver damage is caused by the virus or by the auto-immune response remains to be established.

THE NATURAL HISTORY OF HCV INFECTION

Hepatitis C virus infection results in persistent infection in 80% of cases and, in a proportion of these, becomes a progressive disease (Alter, 1989). The factors influencing the natural history of HCV infection remain obscure.

Although serial transaminase levels have been used to assess HCV-related liver disease, the most accurate way is to examine the histological appearances by liver biopsy. There is general agreement that histological changes need to be divided into necro-inflammatory activity (grade) and level of fibrosis (stage). The Knodell scoring system (Knodell et al, 1981), the Scheuer (Scheuer et al, 1992) and modified histological activity index (HAI) (Ishak et al, 1995) have all been used. The more recent Scheuer and

Baillière's Clinical Gastroenterology—
Vol. 10, No. 2, July 1996
ISBN 0–7020–2094–X
0950–3528/96/020257 + 18 $12.00/00

Copyright © 1996, by Baillière Tindall
All rights of reproduction in any form reserved

modified HAI systems classify the histological changes according to a dissociated semiquantitative assessment of necro-inflammatory lesions (grade) and fibrosis (stage). These systems offer more reproducibility than the older Knodell system that used a global numerical index incorporating discontinuous numerical scores of both necro-inflammatory lesions and fibrosis.

Using these systems, HCV 1 shows an overall tendency to display more active histological disease (Booth et al, unpublished). In this analysis, patients infected with genotypes 2 and 3 were pooled together and compared to those patients infected with HCV 1, the genotype previously associated with more severe disease and a poorer response to interferon therapy. The comparisons between HCV 1-infected patients and those infected with either HCV 2 or 3 revealed significant differences in inflammatory activity, as scored by the modified HAI and the Scheuer scoring systems, that were not detected by the original Knodell system. Although the level of fibrosis (stage) did not differ significantly between the groups there was, again, a clear tendency for greater fibrosis scores in HCV 1 infections. This difference approached significance under the Scheuer scoring system.

The possibility that genetic heterogeneity of HCV infections might lead to variability in the severity of observed liver disease was further suggested by Pozzato et al who studied a group of Italian patients and found that 90% (9/10) patients infected with Japanese type HCV (Simmonds type 1b) had chronic active hepatitis with cirrhosis compared to 0% (0/9) patients infected with non-1b virus (Pozzato et al, 1991). The patients not infected with 1b virus had chronic persistent hepatitis in 66% (6/9) of cases and chronic active hepatitis without cirrhosis in 33% (3/9) of cases.

The finding of higher levels of necro-inflammatory activity could be explained by a longer duration of infection with HCV 1 so that the differences simply reflect a later stage in the disease process at the time of biopsy. In a French study, although infection with type 1b was more frequently associated with cirrhosis (59%) compared with 1a infections (23%), the patients with type 1b infections were older, suggesting a longer duration of infection in these patients (Qu et al, 1994). However, in a study of British patients the average age of HCV 1-infected patients was lower than in the other groups (HCV 1—41.75 ± 10.4 years, HCV 2—48 ± 8.9 years, HCV 3—45.1 ± 13.4 years), and in those patients with a definable date of infection, there was no trend towards longer duration of disease (Booth et al, 1996). Additionally, it remains unclear whether altering patterns of the relative prevalence of HCV genotypes exist over time. In an American study, there did not appear to be any change in the distribution of infecting strains of HCV over a 20-year period (Mahaney et al, 1994), but in France changing prevalences of hepatitis C virus genotypes were observed in a group of haemodialysis patients (Pol et al, 1995). In those patients haemodialysed before 1977 16/24 were infected with HCV type 1b, compared with 5/12 haemodialysed after 1985.

It has been suggested that the mode of transmission influences the histological severity of HCV-associated liver disease, with patients infected following blood transfusion tending to have more severe histological lesions compared with patients infected by other routes (Gordon et al, 1993). In particular, the post-transfusion group had more periportal necrosis, fibrosis and a higher total histological activity score, as assessed by the Knodell system. Bile duct damage was also found to be more common in the post-transfusion hepatitis (PTH) group. It has been suggested that the more severe histological lesions seen in this group of patients is related to the larger initial infecting innoculum, an idea supported by Lau et al who showed higher levels of viraemia in patients infected following blood transfusion (Lau et al, 1993b).

A further study assessed the influence of HCV genotype and viraemia on the rate of development of fibrotic liver disease (Booth et al, 1995). Roughly one-third of the patients (6/20) studied had developed histological evidence of cirrhosis within 10 years of infection with HCV. A further four patients had developed cirrhosis after intervals of more than 15, 18, 14 and 16 years, although these patients were excluded from the severity study as they had been infected for longer than 10 years. These findings indicate that a significant proportion of patients develop progressive liver disease leading to cirrhosis with the associated risks of liver failure and the development of hepatocellular carcinoma, underlining the clinical importance of persistent HCV infection. These figures are in agreement with a 1992 study where follow-up of 65 PTH patients revealed that 32% had developed cirrhosis after a mean follow-up of 7.5 years (Tremolada et al, 1992). A more recent study of 131 PTH patients reported that about 50% of patients developed cirrhosis after a mean follow-up of 20 years (Tong et al, 1995). However, it needs to be stressed that the patients studied in these trials have been referred to specialist centres, and so represent the severe end of the spectrum, and the true number of patients infected with HCV but who have no or only mild liver disease remains unknown. Results from follow-up studies of single-source outbreaks of HCV, such as the one reported by Meisal et al (Meisal et al, 1995) on a group of women infected with contaminated anti-D immunoglobulin, are eagerly awaited. Initial results presented in abstract form suggest that half of the women infected remain PCR-positive at 15 years and all had mild histological abnormalities described as chronic persistent hepatitis (Wiese, 1995). However, none of these infected women had histological evidence of chronic acute hepatitis (CAH) or cirrhosis.

Although genotype has been associated with the severity of liver histological lesions, little has been published on the contribution of genotype to the natural history of chronic HCV infection. We believe that the rate of progression to hepatic fibrosis is the most clinically relevant variable and have used this indicator as a marker of disease severity. Using this marker of disease severity, patients infected with HCV type 1 appeared to develop cirrhosis more rapidly when compared with patients infected with other genotypes (Booth et al, 1995). However, this difference was not statistically significant, and it should be noted that half of the patients infected with genotype 1 had mild disease. Hence, HCV genotype may play a minor role in determining the outcome of infection, but other factors are clearly involved. It is interesting that only 1/8 (12.5%) patients infected with HCV by IVDU had severe disease, compared with 6/11 (54.5%) patients infected by blood transfusion. As previously mentioned, it has been suggested that patients infected via blood transfusion tended to have more severe histological liver disease (Gordon et al, 1993). There were no major differences in mean age or sex ratio between the groups, although the proportion of females was higher in the mild disease group.

Fluctuating viraemia, as measured by RNA concentration in serum (Gunji et al, 1992) is also a feature of chronic HCV infection, and it has been suggested that the level of viraemia is related to the histological grade of liver disease. However, the relationship of HCV viraemia to stage of liver disease is unclear, with some studies showing a correlation between high-level viraemia and severe histology (Hagiwara et al, 1993; Kato et al, 1993b) and others showing lower levels in advanced disease (Magrin et al, 1994). In another study the level of viraemia was shown to be very high at a time when the patient's liver disease was progressing most rapidly (Gunji et al, 1992). It is also unclear whether level of viraemia correlates accurately with serum ALT (Magrin et al, 1994).

Since the level of viraemia varies in any individual, it seems unlikely that a single measurement will be able to predict disease outcome (Booth et al, 1995). In a further study, use was made of a PCR-based quantification method (Kumar et al, 1994) which has a sensitivity of 3.3×10^2 virus particles per millilitre compared with the lower limit of detection of the branched DNA (bDNA) assay of 3.5×10^5 virus particles per millilitre. Previous methods, involving either serial dilutions of cDNA or the use of a shortened cDNA template, make assumptions on the efficiency of the reverse transcription and PCR sensitivity and thus make inter-sample comparisons unreliable. Using a shortened RNA template in a competitive PCR assay (Kumar et al, 1994), the concentration of serum RNA can be estimated by identifying the point of equivalence of the PCR products. This comparison is not influenced by the efficiency of either reverse transcription or PCR. The results show a tendency towards severe disease in patients found to have high levels of viraemia, although this was not statistically significant. However, a relatively crude quantification assay (greater than or less than 3.3×10^5 genomes per millilitre) was used and it is possible that a more sensitive assay may have shown a significant difference.

It is possible that different genotypes may differ in replication efficiencies, thus giving rise to different levels of viraemia which might contribute to differing clinical outcomes and susceptibility to interferon (IFN). Using the semi-quantitative PCR technique, similar proportions of HCV 1-infected patients with high-level viraemia, compared with those patients infected with HCV 2 or 3, were found (Booth et al, 1995). Thus, any effect of genotype on the rate of disease progression did not seem to be related to a higher level of viraemia. These data agree with other studies showing no significant difference in the concentration of serum HCV between patients infected with different genotypes using competitive PCR (Tsubota et al, 1994). However, other studies using the branched DNA assay (Chiron HCV-RNA, Chiron Corporation, Emeryville, CA) have suggested that HCV 1 infections tend to have higher levels of viraemia compared with HCV 2 and 3 (Yuki et al, 1995). These results need to be carefully considered because the b-DNA assay, although incorporating oligonucleotide sequences from the major genotypes, is more sensitive for HCV 1 infections compared with HCV 2 and HCV 3 infections.

In conclusion, infection with HCV is associated with progression to cirrhosis in a significant proportion of patients. Although HCV 1 infections tend to display a more rapid course of disease, this is not always the case— indicating that other factors are involved in determining the natural history of HCV infection. The value of measuring viraemia in HCV remains to be established.

MECHANISMS OF VIRAL PERSISTENCE

The ability to establish persistent infection is an extremely important aspect of HCV infection. Many viruses, both human and animal, are known to establish persistent infection in their hosts and several principles have emerged about the mechanisms of viral persistence from studies of these viruses (for review see Oldstone, 1991). First, as viruses are obligate intra-cellular parasites, the virus needs to establish persistent non-cytopathic infection. Although vital cellular functions are not affected in this type of infection, certain 'luxury' functions may be altered. Second, the virus must evade the host's immune response, which involves both humoral and cellular mechanisms. Evidence is starting to emerge on the interaction of HCV and the immune system and how the virus is able to establish persist-ent infection. Evidence is available on the following aspects.

Infection of lymphoid cells

By analogy with Epstein–Barr virus (EBV) and hepatitis B virus (HBV) (Pontisso et al, 1984; Yoffe et al, 1986) infections, chronic hepatitis C infection might be due to lymphotropic characteristics of the virus. This concept was suggested by the observation that the inflammatory infiltrate in the liver of patients with non-A, non-B (NANB) hepatitis was similar to that seen in EBV where the infected mononuclear cells were lined up in the hepatic sinusoids and not juxtaposed to areas of hepatocyte necrosis (Bamber et al, 1981). Hellings et al (1985) showed that mononuclear cells, prepared by ficoll-paque gradient centrifugation from a haemophilia A patient with NANB hepatitis, could transmit NANB when infused into a susceptible chimpanzee. Further studies showed that T lymphocytes, rather than B cells, were responsible for the transmission (Hellings et al, 1988). The results of these experiments are consistent with the hypothesis that the putative NANB virus might reside in cells involved in the immune response and that this property might contribute to viral persistence.

Following the identification of HCV, generic analysis led to the obser-vation of similarity between HCV and flavi-/pestiviruses which are known to infect cells of the reticuloendothelial system (Moennig and Plagemann, 1992).

HCV is found in the peripheral blood mononuclear cells (PBMC) of the majority of patients chronically infected with HCV (Bouffard et al, 1992; Wang et al, 1992; Zignego et al, 1992; Muller et al, 1993; Yun et al, 1994; Booth et al, unpublished). It seems unlikely that detection of HCV RNA is an artefact due to adhesion of circulating serum virions to the cells, as the cells in one study (Booth et al, unpublished) were washed extensively and the final cell washes also underwent PCR and were always found to be negative. Bouffard et al (1992) confirmed that HCV was inside the cell, rather than adherent, by showing cytoplasmic staining of cells with a monoclonal antibody against HCV core. In another study, PBMCs were stimulated with pokeweed mitogen, and synthesis of HCV RNA was determined by incorporation of [^{3}H]-uridine into nascent viral RNA molecules (Muller et al, 1993).

Infection of cells involved in the immune response may alter their function and influence whether the infection is self-limited or persistent. At present it is not known whether patients with HCV infection of PBMCs have differing clinical outcomes compared to those that do not. However, there were no major differences in biochemical or histological assessment of the patients with or without HCV infection of total PBMC populations in one study (Booth et al, unpublished). In a study of 18 patients treated with interferon, five were considered as complete responders with no HCV detectable by PCR from liver tissue (Saleh et al, 1994). However, three of these five patients had HCV detectable in PBMCs, and of these three patients two subsequently relapsed, indicating that eradication of HCV from this site may be a better predictor of response to IFN than clearance of detectable RNA from the serum or, indeed, the liver. It is also possible that replication in this site may allow the evolution of viral variants capable of evading the host's immune response, as will be discussed in more detail later.

It is important to define the particular cell subset with which HCV is associated. HCV was not detected in enriched populations of CD4$^+$ T lymphocytes (Booth et al, unpublished). The inability of HCV to infect CD4 cells in patients with chronic HCV suggests that there are restrictions to the generalized tropism of the virus and that there may be specific mechanisms for viral penetration into lymphoid cells. The negative result with this population suggests that the washes were sufficient to remove any adherent virus. However, HCV RNA was detectable in CD8$^+$ T lymphocytes (6/17), adherent monocyte/macrophage cells (3/8) and CD19$^+$ B lymphocytes (4/6). There did not appear to be any clinical differences between those patients with cellular HCV RNA and those without. In four of six patients with HCV RNA detected in the CD8-enriched populations, these were the only cell populations that were positive, excluding the possibility of contamination of the CD8 cells by other types of cell as the cause of PCR positivity.

The finding of HCV associated with CD8 cells agrees with other studies showing infection of total T cell populations in HIV/HCV-infected patients (Zignego et al, 1992). The demonstration of infection of MOLT 4 cells (CD4$^+$) by HCV (Shimizu et al, 1992) is at odds with our failure to show infection of CD4 cells in patients (Booth et al, unpublished). Our own attempts to infect MOLT 4 cells have been unsuccessful (Kumar,

Monjardino and Thomas, personal communication). Another study failed to show a positive PCR signal from T cells, but the cells had been isolated from heparinized blood samples and it is therefore possible that the heparin may have affected the sensitivity of the PCR in these experiments (Muller et al, 1993). The detection of HCV RNA in CD8 cells, which are non-phagocytic, suggests that these sequences arise as a direct result of infection rather than by phagocytosis. In remains to be established whether HCV infection of cytotoxic T lymphocytes can influence the immune functions of these cells and therefore contribute to the persistence of the virus. In another latent viral infection, cytomegalovirus (CMV), infection of cytotoxic T-cells has been shown to suppress CMV-specific HLA-restricted cytotoxic T-lymphocyte activity (Schrier and Oldstone, 1986). Measles virus is also known to infect T-cells and has been shown to suppress lymphocyte proliferation (McChesney and Oldstone, 1987).

The HCV found in monocyte/macrophage populations could be due to phagocytosis of the virus but could also represent true infection of these cells. Infection of monocytes has also been suggested by others (Bouffard et al, 1992), and functional studies have suggested that monocytes from patients infected with HCV have decreased cytoskeletal vimentin inter-mediate filaments and HLA-DR antigens in addition to a reduced phago-cytic activity (Castilla et al, 1989). It remains to be seen whether these findings are reproducible and what effect they might have on the course of HCV infection. In another well studied virus, the arenavirus lymphocytic choriomeningitis virus (LCMV) of the mouse, the ability of the virus to cause persistent viral infections appears dependent on the ability of the virus to infect cells of the immune system, in particular monocyte/macrophages (Matloubian et al, 1993).

The presence of HCV in B lymphocytes has also been suggested by Muller et al (1993). Another flavivirus, hog cholera virus, is known to infect B lymphocytes and causes a dramatic depletion of these cells in the end stage of the host's disease. In contrast, in HCV no major lymphocyte alterations have been observed. In herpes simplex virus infection of mice, B lymphocytes have been identified that suppress the delayed cellular responses to the virus in a specific way (Nash and Gell, 1988). It is tempting to hypothesize along the same lines about the potential immuno-logical effect of infection of B cells by HCV. However, no specific B cell effects have been documented in HCV infection. Despite knowledge of antibody produced against HCV antigens, there is so far little evidence to suggest that this antibody is neutralizing.

In situ hybridization, using an antisense HCV-RNA probe, has been used to show the presence of HCV in hepatocytes (scattered distribution of infected cells) as well as in mononuclear cells within the inflammatory infiltrates in HIV/HCV co-infected individuals (Lamas et al, 1992). These findings were confirmed in patients with lone HCV infection by non-isotopic in situ hybridization using a digoxigenin-labelled probe to the NS5 region of HCV (Nouri Aria et al, 1993). A later study, using dual immunostaining of liver sections for lymphocyte differentiation markers and HCV antigens, revealed that most of the HCV staining cells were

CD20[+] B lymphocytes (62–64%) or CD8[+] T cells (47–50%) with only a small number of CD4[+] T cells (2–4%) staining positive (Blight et al, 1994).

Unfortunately there is no reliable in vitro culture system for HCV at present so there is no way of confirming the presence of infectious virus from these sites other than by chimpanzee transmission studies as previously described (Hellings et al, 1988). The genetic similarities of HCV to flavi-/pestiviruses suggested that the virus probably replicates via a full-length negative RNA strand via semiconservative RNA replication using the positive strand as template (Chambers et al, 1990). The positive strand is then amplified from the positive/negative double-strand template as has been demonstrated for type 2 dengue virus (Cleaves et al, 1981). Several authors have subsequently described techniques for the specific detection of HCV negative strand, using the sense primer specifically to generate positive-strand prior to cDNA synthesis, and have suggested that this confirms the presence of replicating virus in PBMCs (Artini et al, 1993) and liver (Fong et al, 1991; Takehara et al, 1992). However, a number of additional steps had to be included in these techniques to ensure specific detection of negative strand. One concern was that false-positive results for negative strand could occur due to insufficient inactivation of reverse transcriptase after cDNA synthesis or by reverse-transcriptase like properties of taq polymerase used for PCR. Another was that certain RNA secondary structures could lead to self priming. To avoid these problems the HCV RNA was heated prior to cDNA synthesis and was treated with RNAse and heat inactivation after cDNA synthesis. However, despite these precautions, 'false' negative strands could still be generated, suggesting that reliable detection of HCV-negative strand cannot be achieved by these methods (Willems et al, 1993; McGuiness et al, 1994). One explanation for these findings was that a thermostable hairpin loop existed in the 5′ end of HCV and led to false priming during cDNA synthesis (Han et al, 1991). The observation that, in some patients, a positive PCR signal could be produced in the absence of any cDNA primer supported the stable hairpin loop theory (Willems et al, 1994).

Lymphocytes have been cloned from liver biopsy specimens from patients infected with other hepatotrophic viruses such as HAV, with successful culture of CD4[+] and CD4/8[-] T lymphocyte clones. In recent experiments (Booth et al, unpublished) we have used similar culture methods to generate cell lines from liver infiltrating lymphocytes in HCV-infected patients. CD8[+] cell lines were generated and the PCR results indicated that HCV was present in these liver-infiltrating lymphoid cells for up to 6 months in culture. In addition, two PCR-positive cell lines were produced that were mostly CD4/8[-] cells. These results indicate latent infection or low-level persistent replication in these cells.

Few attempts to study in vitro infection of HCV have been published, although several reports of replication of HCV have been reported in T cell lines, fetal hepatocytes and a human-derived bone-marrow line. A more recent study used strand-specific PCR and in situ hybridization to demonstrate in vitro infection of cultured peripheral blood mononuclear cells by HCV from HCV-positive sera (Cribier et al, 1995). It was suggested that, although the presence of HCV RNA observed immediately after inoculation was due to absorption of the positive inoculum, the presence of detectable HCV RNA in 7 of 10 donors at days 10–15 were in favour of HCV infection of PBMC and replication. The fact that other cell lines inoculated in the same way lost all detectable HCV after 3–6 days indicated that the detection of HCV RNA after the second week of culture was not due to persistent adherence of the virus to the cells. These experiments reinforce the interpretation that the detection of HCV in cultured cells for 6 weeks does reflect replication of the virus in these cells.

Infection of lymphocytes is also thought important in well studied persistent animal virus infections such as lymphocytic choriomeningitis virus of the mouse (LCMV) (Matloubian et al, 1993) and bovine viral diarrhoea virus (BVDV) of cattle (Bielefeldt Ohmann et al, 1987). The case of BVDV, the aetiological agent of mucosal disease of cattle, is particularly interesting as this virus is classified as a flavivirus and therefore shares similarities with HCV. BVDV isolates are divided into two biotypes according to their cytopathic effect in cell culture. Infection with the non-cytopathic biotype during early gestation leads to the birth of persistently infected (PI) calves. PI animals are immunologically tolerant to the non-cytopathic BVDV strain, but if infection with a cytopathic biotype takes place, the animal will die of mucosal disease. It has been shown that mucosal disease develops only in cattle persistently infected with non-cytopathic BVDV, established by fetal infection with the virus, and that a state of virus-specific tolerance is established characterized by the absence of BVDV-specific neutralizing antibody. The virus has been shown to replicate in monocytes and T cells, both $CD4^+$ and $CD8^+$, but there is debate as to whether infection of B lymphocytes occurs (Bielefeldt Ohmann et al, 1987; Lopez et al, 1993). It has been shown that calves infected with BVDV exhibit an alteration of some immune functions, and this has been linked to the observation of enhancement of concurrent infections (Lopez et al, 1993). The mechanism leading to tolerance in PI with BVDV and the interactions between the virus and cells of the immune system are unknown. Possible explanations include an indirect effect on B cell functions caused by a defect of antigen presentation by macrophages or by the failure to produce some essential factor caused by infection of macrophages and/or T lymphocytes. Alternatively, infection of either T cells or monocyte/macrophages could include virus-specific suppressor cells in both of these types of cell. It is also possible that infection of B cells, perhaps in the bone marrow, may lead to a clonal deletion of the virus-specific precursor cells. It is possible that some of these mechanisms contribute to the persistence of HCV infection as the virus does seem to have a similar cellular tropism. The experiments with BVDV were able to show the presence of viral RNA, viral antigen and the replication of the virus in these cellular sites as an in vitro co-cultivation system revealed that infectious virus could be isolated from the enriched cell populations.

Lysis of infected hepatocytes

The mechanisms whereby HCV causes liver disease are poorly understood. It remains possible that both direct, virus cytopathic, and indirect, immune-mediated mechanisms are involved. The demonstration of a direct cyto-pathic effect of HCV has been hampered by the lack of a reliable tissue culture system. The proliferative responses of peripheral blood CD4[+] T lymphocytes suggested that core, NS4 and NS5 antigens are the most frequently recognized (Ferrari et al, 1994). A proliferative response to core protein has been linked to a benign course of HCV infection (Botarelli et al, 1993). A study of liver-infiltrating lymphocytes showed that NS4 antigen was able to stimulate CD4[+] T-cell lines in 3/19 liver biopsies, but all other antigens failed to establish T-cell lines (Minutello et al, 1993). All the liver-derived clones appeared identical, compared with the peripheral blood T-cell clones—which differed in their major histocompatibility complex restriction, as confirmed by sequence analysis of the variable and hypervariable regions of the T-cell receptor. None of the peripheral clones had the same T-cell receptor, suggesting preferential intrahepatic local-ization of these T cells. Interestingly, the liver-derived T cells provided help for polyclonal IgA production by B cells that was 10-fold more effective than that provided by the peripheral blood derived clones.

The first description of the CD8 cytotoxic response to HCV was given by Imawara et al (1989), prior to the discovery of HCV. A peripheral blood T-cell line was produced that recognized an NANB hepatitis-related antigen expressed on hepatocytes. Further studies have confirmed the presence of cytotoxic T cells in lymphocytes derived from the liver (Koziel et al, 1992, 1993), but not from the peripheral blood. HLA class-I-restricted cytotoxic T lymphocyte (CTL) epitopes from the core and envelope regions have been identified using liver-derived CD8[+] T-cell lines (Koziel et al, 1993). The lack of CTLs in the peripheral blood in these patients suggests that these cells may have been preferentially recruited to the liver, perhaps because they are HCV-infected and the peripheral CTL response is limited.

The importance of CD8[+] T cells in the liver pathology associated with HCV is suggested by the observation that some of these cells are in close contact with HCV-infected hepatocytes and apoptotic bodies (Ballardini et al, 1995). The correlation of ALT to numbers of lobular CD8[+] cells, as well as the lack of correlation between number of hepatocytes positive for HCV antigens and ALT levels, further supports the prominent role of CD8[+] cells in determining hepatocellular damage (Hayata et al, 1991).

If the cells mediating the immune response are infected by HCV non-cytopathically, as our results suggest, then the specific immune functions of these cells may be compromised contributing to the ability of HCV to establish chronic infection. Several viruses are thought to modulate the immune response by mechanisms including inhibition of interferon pathways, inhibition of complement pathways, interference with HLA expression, altered cytokine production and lymphocyte signal trans-duction (McChesney and Oldstone, 1987; Gooding, 1992). Although other viruses, such as HBV (Pignatelli et al, 1986), are able to down-regulate

HLA and the intracellular adhesion molecule expression (ICAM-1), the finding that HCV-infected hepatocytes express these antigens suggests that defective T-cell recognition due to a lack of cellular expression of these antigens is not important in HCV infection (Ballardini et al, 1995). The presence of HCV in both systemic and liver-derived CD8 cell populations is particularly interesting as these cells are thought to be important in the pathogenesis of HCV-associated liver disease. However, the elucidation of the effects of HCV on cellular immune function await the development of more reliable cell culture systems.

Antigenic variation of the envelope proteins

Comparative studies of HCV isolates suggest the existence of a hyper-variable region (HVR—27 amino acids) near the amino terminus of NS1/E2 proteins, which appears similar to the second envelope protein of pestiviruses (Weiner et al, 1991). Expression of the E2/NS1 protein domain in mammalian CHO cells suggests that this protein is not secreted, unlike the NS1 protein of flaviviruses, and is probably a membrane-associated glycoprotein with the C-terminus in and the N-terminus outside the membrane (Spaete et al, 1992). Thus, the N-terminus of the protein would be subject to immune surveillance with its attendant selective pressure in favour of antigenically altered variants. By using recombinant protein it has been shown that this region of the virus is recognized by circulating antibody from HCV-infected individuals (Spaete et al, 1992). It remains uncertain whether these antibodies are neutralizing, as they co-exist with HCV viraemia, but a recent study revealed that anti-HCV antibody could block the initiation of HCV replication in susceptible cells (Shimuzu et al, 1994). Although it is not known whether these antibodies were directed to viral envelope epitopes, the fact that they correlated with the detection of antibody bound to the surface of the virus, as well as knowledge that neutralizing antibody to most enveloped viruses is directed to envelope proteins, suggests that the envelope protein is the likely target of neutraliz-ing antibody in HCV. These antibodies were shown to be isolate-specific and to change over time (Shimuzu et al, 1994).

Genetic drift in HCV infections has been observed by sequence analysis of partial (Ogata et al, 1991) and full-length (Okamoto et al, 1992) viral genomes. Both studies confirmed the presence of a hypervariable region at the N-terminus of the envelope glycoprotein. Such observations suggest that genetic variation in the envelope proteins can lead to escape from the host immune response and contribute to the ability of HCV to establish persistent infection. Studies in both humans and chimpanzees have documented genetic variation in the HVR during chronic infection, and have demonstrated that these changes can lead to escape from antibody binding (Weiner et al, 1992; Taniguchi et al, 1993). The immune system was implicated by finding that the titres of anti-HVR antibody against a particular epitope reached maximum levels several months after that specific sequence of HVR was first isolated (Kato et al, 1993) and in the presence of a predominant viral species bearing a variant HVR sequence.

In a corroborative study of chimpanzees, two out of three animals showed sequence evolution of the HVR in association with varying but detectable levels of anti-HVR antibody (van Doorn et al, 1995). In the third animal the HVR remained conserved for 6 years in the presence of antibody and only after 7 years was anti-HVR first detected, in association with the presence of a variant virus with HVR amino acid alterations. Another study suggested that particularly high rates of HVR variation in acute HCV infection may be one of the mechanisms of establishing persistent infection (Yamaguchi et al, 1994). These findings indicate that the high rate of amino acid variation in HCV infections is driven by host immune pressure and that persistent infections develop with the emergence of variants capable of escaping the host's immune system.

A similar mechanism has been suggested to explain the persistence of HIV where sequence variation of the third variable domain (V3), the principal neutralization epitope of HIV, appears to be host dependent (Wolfs et al, 1990). The clinical outcome appears to depend on the ability of the host immune system to suppress the selected variants. Novak et al (1991) unpublished a mathematical model of the interaction of viral diversity and the cellular immune system and suggested the existence of an antigen diversity threshold below which the immune system can regulate the viral population but above which the virus is able to overcome the CD4$^+$ lymphocyte population.

We have recently shown that the rate of amino acid variation in the HVR of HCV is significantly lower in common variable immunodeficiency (CVID) patients compared with the rate observed in control subjects. These findings suggest that, in the absence of humoral immune selection, and in spite of active viral replication suggested by relatively high viraemias, the frequency of occurrence of genetic variation in the major viral species is reduced (Booth et al, unpublished). The mutations will still occur at a rate which is presumably determined by the rate of genomic replication, but in the absence of immune selection, will remain as minor species. The finding of single amino acid changes in the HVR in three of four hypogamma-globulinaemic patients suggests that there is some additional selection pressure on this region. Koziel et al (1993) have identified HCV-specific, HLA class I-restricted cytotoxic T lymphocytes that recognize epitopes in the HVR. It is possible that the observed changes in these hypogamma-globulinaemic patients is due to cellular, as opposed to humoral, selection pressure. Three of the four CVID patients received intravenous immunoglobulin up to 1992, and it is therefore possible that the anti-HCV antibody levels contained in these preparations was sufficient to drive the observed amino acid variation, albeit at a reduced rate compared with control subjects.

While a well-defined hypervariable region exists at the amino-terminus of E2/NS1, it is interesting to find three well conserved amino acids within this region. Out of the 60 clones sequenced in our studies, amino acid position 408 (glycine) and 411 (glutamine) were found in all clones sequenced. In a review of 55 published sequences glycine was found in 100% and glutamine in 98.2% of isolates in these same positions

(Lesniewski et al, 1993). More recent studies have found both amino acids in all sequenced isolates (Okada et al, 1992; Sakamoto et al, 1994). The threonine at amino acid 387 was found in 96.67% of clones sequenced in this study and has also been found in the vast majority of isolates sequenced so far. It is intriguing to speculate about the possible role of these conserved amino acids. They may help receptor recognition for all viral isolates or in some way contribute to the overall structure of the envelope protein.

The finding of relatively high levels of HCV RNA in CVID patients suggests that the low level of observed amino acid variation over time is not a result of a reduced replication rate in these patients. The lower rates of amino acid variation found during interferon treatment have been explained by the reduction in viral replication during therapy (Kumar et al, 1993). The finding of high levels of viral RNA in most of the renal transplant patients receiving high-dose immunosuppression again suggests that the host's immune system exerts some control over viral replication and has been observed in other studies of renal transplant recipients (Lau et al, 1993a).

All four hypogammaglobulinaemic patients demonstrated aggressive forms of HCV-related liver disease (Booth et al, unpublished). These clinical findings are in agreement with other studies documenting severe and rapid progression of liver disease in patients with defects of the humoral immune system (Bjoro et al, 1994).

Associated conditions

HCV infections have been associated with a number of immunological disorders, including autoimmune hepatitis (AIH), Sjögrens, lichen planus, thyroiditis, glomerulonephritis, cryoglobulinaemia and polyarteritis nodosa (Lunel, 1994). The role of HCV infection in the pathogenesis of most of these conditions remains obscure. Initial studies with first-generation diagnostic assays demonstrated prevalence rates of 40–80% in patients classified as autoimmune hepatitis (Esteban et al, 1989; McFarlane et al, 1990). More recently, second-generation assays have shown a 48% prevalence rate in patients with type 2 AIH, associated with anti-LKM antibody, and no association with type 1 AIH, associated with AMA and ANA antibodies (Michel et al, 1992). Michel described the presence of anti-GOR antibody in 11/14 patients with type 2 AIH and anti-HCV antibody and only 1/15 type 2 patients without evidence of HCV infection. The GOR protein is thought to be host-derived, but antibody to this protein is seen in the majority of patients with HCV infections (Mishiro et al, 1990). The finding of anti-GOR antibody in patients with AIF suggested that HCV may have induced autoimmunity to GOR and LKM. Indeed, the presence of anti-GOR identified a subgroup of type 2 patients (type 2b) who tended to be older, less likely to be female, to have less severe disease and to respond poorly to immunosuppressive therapy (Michel et al, 1992). Whether anti-GOR is a true marker of autoimmunity or simply a response to a cross-reactive core epitope remains unclear. Koskinas et al (1994) studied the humoral and cellular response to HCV core, GOR and to liver-specific asialo glycoprotein receptor (ASGP-R) and found a very close correlation in the responses to core and GOR, suggesting that the antibody is not a marker of autoimmunity. In a study of in vitro production of anti-HCV antibody, Lohr et al (1994) found the two antibodies to be independently regulated, suggesting that anti-GOR may indeed reflect HCV associated autoimmunity.

HCV has also been shown to be present in many patients with essential mixed cryoglobulinaemia (EMC) (Disdier et al, 1991; Marcellin et al, 1993; Bichard et al, 1994). Viral RNA has been shown to be concentrated in the cryoprecipitate (Chung et al, 1992), and in some cases interferon treatment will not only normalize LFTs but also lead to the disappearance of the cryoprecipitate (Marcellin et al, 1993). The demonstration of HCV in the cryoglobulin suggests that HCV is present in the circulating immune complexes and may be responsible for the vasculitis.

Recognition of HCV involvement in disorders such as cryoglobulin-aemia and idiopathic thrombocytopenic purpura (Silva et al, 1992) will allow consideration of interferon therapy for these non-hepatic as well as hepatic diseases.

SUMMARY

In 20% of patients exposed to hepatitis C virus, infection is transient but, after a few months, the patient remains susceptible to infection with the same strain. Protective immunity is short-lived. This suggests that recovery is related to the cellular immune response, which presumably lyses infected cells, and that the need during recovery for a virus-neutralizing anti-envelope response, is transient. In 80% of patients the infection is persistent, and it seems that antigenic variation of the envelope proteins allows the virus to escape neutralization by anti-envelope responses. The fact that this antigenic variation occurs at a much lower rate in agammaglobulin-aemic subjects suggests that the major immune pressure producing this variation is humoral. How the virus-infected cells avoid lysis by cytotoxic T cells, which can be demonstrated in small numbers in the infected liver, remains unclear. The recent observation, that HCV infects CD8 lymphocytes, raises the possibility that virus infection of CD8 cells may impair their function and contribute to persistent infection. The mechanisms of production of cryoglobulin and of autoantibody formation are both unclear.

REFERENCES

Alter H (1989) *Chronic Consequences of Non-A, Non-B Hepatitis*. New York: Plenum Medical Book.
Artini M, Natoli G, Avantaggiati M et al (1993) Detection of replicative intermediates of viral RNA in peripheral blood mononuclear cells from chronic hepatitis C virus carriers. *Archives of Virology* **(supplement 8):** 23–29.
Ballardini G, Groff P, Pontisso P et al (1995) Hepatitis C virus (HCV) genotype, tissue HCV antigens, hepatocellular expression of HLA-A, B, C and intercellular adhesion-1 molecules. *Journal of Clinical Investigation* **95:** 2067–2075.
Bamber M, Murray A, Arborgh B et al (1981) Short incubation NANB hepatitis transmitted by factor VIII concentrate in patients with congenital coagulation disorders. *Gut* **22:** 854–859.

Bichard P, Ounanian A, Girard M et al (1994) High prevalence of hepatitis C virus RNA in the supernatant and the cryoprecipitate of patients with essential and secondary type II mixed cryoglobulinaemia. *Journal of Hepatology* 21: 58–63.

Bielefeldt Ohmann H, Ronsholt L & Bloch B (1987) Demonstration of bovine viral diarrhoea virus in peripheral blood mononuclear cells of persistently infected, clinically normal cattle. *Journal of General Virology* 68: 1971–1982.

Bjoro K, Froland S, Yun Z et al (1994) Hepatitis C infection in patients with primary hypogammaglobulinaemia after treatment with contaminated immune globulin. *New England Journal of Medicine* 331: 1607–1611.

Blight K, Lesniewski R, LaBrooy J & Gowans E (1994) Detection and distribution of hepatitis C-specific antigens in naturally infected liver. *Hepatology* 20: 553–557.

Booth J, Foster G, Kumar U et al (1995) Chronic hepatitis C virus infections: predictive value of genotype and level of viraemia on disease progression and response to interferon α. *Gut* 36: 427–432.

Botarelli P, Brunetto MR, Minutello MA et al (1993) T-Lymphocyte response to hepatitis C virus in different clinical courses of infection. *Gastroenterology* 104: 580–587.

Bouffard P, Hayashi P, Acevedo R et al (1992) Hepatitis C virus is detected in a monocyte/macrophage subpopulation of peripheral blood mononuclear cells of infected patients. *Journal of Infectious Diseases* 166: 1276–1280.

Castilla A, Subira M, Civeira M & Prieto J (1989) Correlation between lymphocyte and monocyte function in patients with chronic non-A, non-B hepatitis. *American Journal of Gastroenterology* 84: 978.

Chambers T, Hahn C, Galler R & Rice C (1990) Flavivirus genome organization, expression and replication. *Annual Review of Microbiology* 44: 649–688.

Chung R, Agnello V, Weiner N et al (1992) A role for hepatitis C virus infection in the pathogenesis of essential mixed cryoglobulinaemia: selective concentrations of HCV antigen and RNA in cryoprecipitates. *Gastroenterology* 102: A794.

Cleaves G, Ryan T & Schlesinger R (1981) Identification and characterization of type 2 dengue virus replicative intermediate and replicative form RNAs. *Virology* 111: 73–83.

Cribier B, Schmitt C, Bingen A et al (1995) In vitro infection of peripheral blood mononuclear cells by hepatitis C virus. *Journal of General Virology* 76: 2485–2491.

Disdier P, Harle J-R & Weiller P-J (1991) Cryoglobulinaemia and hepatitis C infection. *Lancet* 338: 1151–1152.

Esteban J, Viladomiu L, Gonzalez A et al (1989) Hepatitis C virus antibodies among risk groups in Spain. *Lancet* 334: 294–297.

Ferrari C, Valli A, Galati L et al (1994) T-cell response to structural and nonstructural hepatitis C virus antigens in persistent and self-limited hepatitis C virus infections. *Hepatology* 19: 286–295.

Fong T-L, Shindo M, Feinstone SM et al (1991) Detection of replicative intermediates of hepatitis C. Viral RNA in liver and serum of patients with chronic hepatitis C. *Journal of Clinical Investigation* 88: 1058–1060.

Gooding L (1992) Virus proteins that counteract host immune defenses. *Cell* 71: 5–7.

Gordon S, Elloway R, Long J & Dmuchowski C (1993) The pathology of hepatitis C as a function of mode of transmission: blood transfusion vs intravenous drug use. *Hepatology* 18: 1338–1343.

Gunji T, Kato N, Mori S et al (1992) Correlation between serum level of hepatitis C virus RNA and disease activities in acute and chronic hepatitis C. *International Journal of Cancer* 52: 726–730.

Hagiwara H, Hayashi N, Mita E et al (1993) Quantitation of hepatitis C virus RNA in serum of asymptomatic blood donors and patients with type C chronic liver disease. *Hepatology* 17: 545–550.

Han J, Shyamala V, Richman K et al (1991) Characterization of the terminal regions of hepatitis C viral RNA: identification of conserved sequences in the 5' untranslated region and poly (A) tails at the 3' end. *Proceedings of the National Academy of Sciences of the USA* 88: 1711–1715.

Hayata T, Nakano Y, Yoshizawa T et al (1991) Effects of interferon on intrahepatic human leukocyte antigens and lymphocyte subsets in patients with chronic hepatitis B and C. *Hepatology* 13: 1022–1028.

Hellings J, van der Veen-du Prie J, Snelting-van Densen R & Stute R (1985) Preliminary results of transmission of non-A non-B hepatitis by mononuclear leucocytes from a chronic patient. *Journal of Virological Methods* 10: 321–326.

Hellings J, van der Veen-du Prie J & Boender P (1988) Transmission of non-A, non-B hepatitis by leucocyte preparations. *Viral Hepatitis and Liver Disease* 543–549.

Imawara M, Nomura M, Kaieda T et al (1989) Establishment of a human T-cell clone cytotoxic for both autologous and allogeneic hepatocytes from chronic hepatitis patients with type non-A, non-B virus. *Proceedings of the National Academy of Sciences of the USA* **86:** 2883–2887.

Ishak K, Baptista A, Bianchi L et al (1995) Histological grading and staging of chronic hepatitis. *Journal of Hepatology* **22:** 696–699.

Kato N, Sekiya H, Ootsuyama Y et al (1993a) Humoral immune response to hypervariable region 1 of the putative envelope glycoprotein (gp 70) of hepatitis C virus. *Journal of General Virology* **67:** 3923–3920.

Kato N, Yokosuka O, Hosoda K et al (1993b) Quantification of hepatitis C virus by competitive reverse transcription–polymerase chain reaction: increase of the virus in advanced disease. *Hepatology* **18:** 16–20.

Knodell R, Ishak K, Black W et al (1981) Formulation and application of a numerical scoring system for assessing histological activity in asymptomatic chronic active hepatitis. *Hepatology* **1:** 431–435.

Koskinas J, McFarlane B, Nouri-Aria K et al (1994) Cellular and humoral immune reactions against autoantigens and hepatitis C viral antigens in chronic hepatitis C. *Gastroenterology* **107:** 1436–1442.

Koziel M, Dudley D, Wong J et al (1992) Intrahepatic cytotoxic T lymphocytes specific for hepatitis C virus in persons with chronic hepatitis. *Journal of Immunology* **149:** 3339–3344.

Koziel M, Dudley D, Afdhal N et al (1993) Hepatitis C virus (HCV)-specific cytotoxic T lymphocytes recognize epitopes in the core and envelope proteins of HCV. *Journal of Virology* **67:** 7522–7532.

Kumar U, Brown J, Monjardino J & Thomas H (1993) Sequence variation in the large envelope glycoprotein (E2/NS1) of hepatitis C virus during chronic infection. *Journal of Infectious Diseases* **167:** 726–730.

Kumar U, Thomas H & Monjardino J (1994) Serum HCV RNA levels in chronic HCV hepatitis measured by quantitative PCR assay; correlation with serum AST. *Journal of Virological Methods* **47:** 95–102.

Lamas E, Baccarini P, Housset C et al (1992) Detection of hepatitis C virus (HCV) RNA sequences in liver tissue by in situ hybridization. *Journal of Hepatology* **16:** 219–223.

Lau JYN, Davis GL, Brunson ME et al (1993a) Hepatitis C virus infection in kidney transplant recipients. *Hepatology* **18:** 1027–1031.

Lau JYN, Davis GL, Kniffen J et al (1993b) Significance of serum hepatitis C virus RNA levels in chronic hepatitis C. *Lancet* **341:** 1501–1504.

Lesniewski R, Boardway K, Casey J et al (1993) Hypervariable 5′-terminus of hepatitis C virus E2/NS1 encodes antigenically distinct variants. *Journal of Medical Virology* **40:** 150–156.

Lohr H, Gerken G, Michel G et al (1994) In vitro secretion of anti-GOR protein and anti-hepatitis C virus antibodies in patients with chronic hepatitis C. *Gastroenterology* **107:** 1443–1448.

Lopez O, Osorio F, Kelling C & Donis R (1993) Presence of bovine viral diarrhoea virus in lymphoid cell populations of persistently infected cattle. *Journal of General Virology* **74:** 925–929.

Lunel F (1994) Hepatitis C virus and autoimmunity: fortuitous association or reality? *Gastroenterology* **107:** 1550–1555.

McChesney M & Oldstone M (1987) Viruses perturb lymphocyte functions: selected principles characterising virus-induced immunosuppression. *Annual Review of Immunology* **5:** 279–304.

McFarlane J, Smith H, Johnson P et al (1990) Hepatitis C virus antibodies in chronic active hepatitis: pathogenetic factor of false-positive results? *Lancet* **335:** 754–757.

McGuiness P, Bishop G, McCaughan G et al (1994) False detection of negative-strand hepatitis C virus RNA. *Lancet* **343:** 551–552.

Magrin S, Craxi A, Fabiano C et al (1994) Hepatitis C viremia in chronic liver disease: relationship to interferon-α or corticosteroid treatment. *Hepatology* **19:** 273–279.

Mahaney K, Tedeschi V, Maertens G et al (1994) Genotypic analysis of hepatitis C virus in American patients. *Hepatology* **20:** 1405–1411.

Marcellin P, Descamps V, Martinot-Peignoux M et al (1993) Cryoglobulinaemia with vasculitis associated with hepatitis c virus infection. *Gastroenterology* **104:** 272–277.

Matloubian M, Kolhekar S, Somasundaram T & Ahmed R (1993) Molecular determinants of macrophage tropism and viral persistence: importance of single amino acid changes in the polymerase and glycoprotein of lymphocytic choriomeningitis virus. *Journal of Virology* **67:** 7340–7349.

Meisal H, Reip A, Faltus B et al (1995) Transmission of hepatitis C virus to children and husbands by women infected with contaminated anti-D immunoglobulin. *Lancet* **345:** 1209–1211.

Michel G, Ritter A, Gerken G et al (1992) Anti-GOR and hepatitis C virus in autoimmune liver diseases. *Lancet* **339:** 267–269.

Minutello M, Pileri P, Unutmaz D et al (1993) Compartmentalisation of T lymphocytes to the site of disease: intrahepatic CD4⁺ T cells specific for the protein NS4 of hepatitis C virus in patients with chronic hepatitis C. *Journal of Experimental Medicine* **178:** 17–23.

Mishiro S, Hoshi Y, Takeda K et al (1990) Non-A, non-B hepatitis specific antibodies directed at host-derived epitope: implication for an autoimmune process. *Lancet* **336:** 1400–1403.

Moennig V & Plagemann P (1992) The pestiviruses. *Advances in Virus Research* **41:** 53–98.

Muller HM, Pfaff E, Goeser T et al (1993) Peripheral blood leukocytes serve as a possible extrahepatic site for hepatitis C virus replication. *Journal of General Virology* **74:** 669–676.

Nash A & Gell P (1988) Cell mediated immunity in herpes simplex virus-infected mice: suppression of delayed hypersensitivity by an antigen specific B-lymphocyte. *Journal of General Virology* **48:** 359–364.

Nouri Aria K, Sallie R, Sangar D et al (1993) Detection of genomic and intermediate replicative strands of hepatitis C virus in liver tissue by in situ hybridization. *Journal of Clinical Investigation* **91:** 2226–2234.

Novak M, Anderson R, Mclean A et al (1991) Antigenic diversity thresholds and the development of AIDS. *Science* **254:** 963–969.

Ogata N, Alter HJ, Miller RH & Purcell RH (1991) Nucleotide sequence and mutation rate of the H strain of hepatitis C virus. *Proceedings of the National Academy of Sciences of the USA* **88:** 3392–3396.

Okada S-I, Akahane Y, Suzuki H et al (1992) The degree of variability in the amino terminal region of the E2/NS1 protein of hepatitis C virus correlates with responsiveness to interferon therapy in viremic patients. *Hepatology* **16:** 619–624.

Okamoto H, Kojima M, Okada S-I et al (1992) Genetic drift of hepatitis C virus during an 8.2-year infection in a chimpanzee: variability and stability. *Virology* **190:** 894–899.

Oldstone M (1991) Molecular anatomy of viral persistence. *Journal of Virology* **65:** 6381–6386.

Pignatelli M, Waters J, Brown D et al (1986) HLA class I antigens on hepatocyte membrane during recovery from acute hepatitis B infection and during interferon therapy in chronic hepatitis B virus infection. *Hepatology* **6:** 349–353.

Pol S, Thiers V, Nousbaum J-P et al (1995) The changing relative prevalence of hepatitis C virus genotypes: evidence in haemodialysed patients and kidney recipients. *Gastroenterology* **108:** 581–583.

Pontisso P, Poon M, Tiollais P & Brechot C (1984) Detection of hepatitis B virus DNA in mononuclear blood cells. *British Medical Journal* **288:** 1563–1566.

Pozzato G, Moretti M, Franzin F et al (1991) Severity of liver disease with different HCV clones. *Lancet* **338:** 509.

Qu D, Li J, Vitviski L et al (1994) Hepatitis C virus genotypes in France: comparison of clinical features of patients infected with HCV type I and type II. *Journal of Hepatology* **21:** 70–75.

Sakamoto N, Enomoto N, Kurosaki M et al (1994) Sequential change of the hypervariable region of the hepatitis C virus genome in acute infection. *Journal of Medical Virology* **42:** 103–108.

Saleh M, Tibbs C, Koskinas J et al (1994) Hepatic and extrahepatic hepatitis C virus replication in relation to response to interferon therapy. *Hepatology* **20:** 1399–1404.

Scheuer PJ, Ashrafzadeh P, Sherlock S et al (1992) The pathology of hepatitis C. *Hepatology* **15:** 567–571.

Schrier R & Oldstone M (1986) Recent clinical isolates of cytomegalovirus suppress human cytomegalovirus-specific human leucocyte antigen-restricted cytotoxic T-lymphocyte activity. *Journal of Virology* **59:** 127–131.

Shimizu YK, Iwamoto A, Hijikata M et al (1992) Evidence for in vitro replication of hepatitis C virus genome in a human T-cell line. *Proceedings of the National Academy of Sciences of the USA* **89:** 5477–5481.

Shimuzu Y, Hijikata M, Iwamoto A et al (1994) Neutralizing antibodies against hepatitis C virus and the emergence of neutralization escape mutant viruses. *Journal of Virology* **68:** 1494–1500.

Silva M, Li X, Cheinquer H et al (1992) HCV-associated idiopathic thrombocytopenic purpura (ITP). *Gastroenterology* **102:** A889.

Spaete R, Alexander D, Rugroden M et al (1992) Characterization of the hepatitis C virus E2/NS1 gene product expressed in mammalian cells. *Virology* **188:** 819–830.

Takehara T, Hayashi M, Mita E et al (1992) Detection of the minus strand of hepatitis C virus RNA by reverse transcription and polymerase chain reaction: implications for hepatitis C virus replication in infected tissue. *Hepatology* **15:** 387–390.

Taniguchi S, Okamoto H, Sakamoto M et al (1993) A structurally flexible and antigenically variable N-terminal domain of the hepatitis C virus E2/NS1 protein: Implication for an escape from antibody. *Virology* **195:** 297–301.

Tong M, El-Farra N, Reikes A & Co R (1995) Clinical outcomes after transfusion-associated hepatitis C. *New England Journal of Medicine* **332:** 1463–1466.

Tremolada F, Casarin C, Alberti A et al (1992) Long-term follow-up of non-A, non-B (type C) post-transfusion hepatitis. *Journal of Hepatology* **16:** 273–281.

Tsubota A, Chayama K, Ikeda K et al (1994) Factors predictive of response to interferon-α therapy in hepatitis C virus infection. *Hepatology* **19:** 1088–1094.

van Doorn L-J, Capriles I, Maertens G et al (1995) Sequence evolution of the hypervariable region in the putative envelope region E2/NS1 of hepatitis C virus is correlated with specific humoral immune responses. *Journal of Virology* **69:** 773–778.

Wang J-T, Sheu J-C, Lin J-T et al (1992) Detection of replicative form of hepatitis c virus RNA in peripheral blood mononuclear cells. *Journal of Infectious Diseases* **166:** 1167–1169.

Weiner A, Brauer M, Rosenblatt J et al (1991) Variable and hypervariable domains are found in the regions of HCV corresponding to the flavivirus envelope and NS1 proteins and the pestivirus group glycoproteins. *Virology* **180:** 842–848.

Weiner AJ, Geysen M, Christopherson C et al (1992) Evidence for immune selection of hepatitis C virus (HCV) putative envelope glycoprotein variants: potential role in chronic HCV infections. *Proceedings of the National Academy of Sciences of the USA* **89:** 3468–3472.

Wiese M (1995) Natural course of hepatitis C: 15 year analysis in an unselected group with an identical parenteral infection. *Journal of Hepatology* **23 (supplement 1):** 89 (abst. P/C1/11).

Willems M, Moshage H & Yap S (1993) PCR and detection of negative HCV RNA strands. *Hepatology* **17:** 526.

Willems M, Peerlinck K, Moshage H et al (1994) Hepatitis C virus-RNAs in plasma and in peripheral blood mononuclear cells of haemophiliacs with chronic hepatitis C: evidence for viral replication in peripheral blood mononuclear cells. *Journal of Medical Virology* **42:** 272–278.

Wolfs T, de Jong J-J, van den Berg H et al (1990) Evolution of sequences encoding the principal neutralization epitope of human immunodeficiency virus 1 is host dependent, rapid and continuous. *Proceedings of the National Academy of Sciences of the USA* **87:** 9938–9942.

Yamaguchi K, Tanaka E, Higashi K et al (1994) Adaptation of hepatitis C virus for persistent infection in patients with acute hepatitis. *Gastroenterology* **106:** 1344–1348.

Yoffe B, Noonan A, Melnick J & Blaine Hollinger F (1986) Hepatitis B virus DNA in mononuclear cells and analysis of cell subsets for the presence of replicative intermediates of viral DNA. *Journal of Infectious Diseases* **153:** 471–477.

Yuki N, Hayashi N, Kasahara A et al (1995) Pretreatment viral load and response to prolonged interferon-α course for chronic hepatitis C. *Journal of Hepatology* **22:** 457–463.

Yun Z, Sonnerborg A & Weiland O (1994) Hepatitis C virus replication in liver and peripheral blood mononuclear cells of interferon α treated and untreated patients with chronic hepatitis C. *Scandinavian Journal of Gastroenterology* **29:** 82–86.

Zignego A, Macchia D, Monti M et al (1992) Infection of peripheral mononuclear cells by hepatitis C virus. *Journal of Hepatology* **15:** 382–386.

6

The natural history of hepatitis C

MASSIMO COLOMBO

Understanding the natural history of hepatitis C virus (HCV) infection is crucial for cost-effective monitoring of the patients and development of treatment strategies.

Unfortunately, our understanding of hepatitis C is unsatisfactory because of a number of 'black holes', the most important of which is early identification of patients who are prone to develop cirrhosis. Because of the lack of recognizable risk factors, prospective follow-up studies aimed at studying the natural history of HCV in the many patients with the so-called community-acquired hepatitis are difficult (Alter et al, 1992).

Like any communicable disease, both the transmission and the natural history of hepatitis C may have changed following improvements in community medicine and transfusion policies and changes in sexual activity. With decreasing numbers of 'ordinary' patients with newly acquired infections, the number of 'problematic' patients with hepatitis C and associated risks, in whom the natural history of HCV is even more obscure than in the former, is steadily increasing. This is frequently a consequence of co-infection with the human immunodeficiency virus (HIV1) acquired with self-injection of illicit drugs, altered immunity following cytotoxic treatment for cancer or prophylaxis of graft rejection or exposure to hepatotoxic environmental factors (Wright et al, 1994).

ACUTE HEPATITIS

In transfusion recipients the time-lag between the patient's exposure to HCV and development of hepatitis is 2–26 weeks, with a peak of onset between 6 and 12 weeks (Alter et al, 1989). Using second-generation ELISA assays that detect serum antibodies against both structural and non-structural components of HCV, the mean time between exposure and seroconversion is much shorter, i.e. approximately 2 weeks (Aach et al 1991; Mattsson et al, 1992). The time between exposure to HCV and onset of virus replication detected by serum HCV RNA may be as short as 1 week (Farci et al, 1991). Thus, a consistent feature of HCV infection is that viral replication can be detected very soon after exposure, and that the appearance of antibodies to multiple epitopes does not coincide with the first ALT peak.

Baillière's Clinical Gastroenterology—
Vol. 10, No. 2, July 1996
ISBN 0–7020–2094–X
0950–3528/96/020275 + 14 $12.00/00

Copyright © 1996, by Baillière Tindall
All rights of reproduction in any form reserved

In most patients the hepatitis is clinically mild during its acute phase, with ALT levels only occasionally exceeding 600 IU/l; 75% of the cases are anicteric and relatively asymptomatic (Aach et al, 1991; Alter et al, 1989). In contrast, it is more difficult to define the clinical profile of community-acquired hepatitis, which is more often a symptomatic disease (Alter et al, 1992). One possible explanation for the discrepancies is that the starting point of studies of community-acquired hepatitis is the enrolment of patients with clinically detectable disease. Thus, the occurrence, chronicity rate and severity of this form of hepatitis could have been wrongly evaluated because of the large number of subclinical cases that escaped detection.

The course of hepatitis C is variable, although its most characteristic feature is a fluctuating, polyphasic ALT pattern (Alter et al, 1989; Aach et al, 1991). Most patients have variations of several hundreds of IU/l within a 1-week period, and such variations are sometimes recurrent, with the magnitude of the ALT elevations diminishing with time. There are also patients with a single monophasic ALT peak proceeding to apparent full recovery or with a plateau-like mild elevation of ALT, which remained the same from the onset of the disease with little variation. The disturbing feature of hepatitis is that there sometimes occurs an apparent long-lasting normalization of ALT, suggesting full recovery, but this is followed later by symptom-less enzymatic exacerbations.

The antibody against the non-structural C-100$_3$ epitope of HCV (first-generation ELISA) persisted in patients with chronic hepatitis and disappeared from almost all patients who recovered clinically and biochemically (Alter et al, 1989; Alberti, 1991).

While the majority of acute hepatitis cases are clinically indolent, individual severe cases occur. Fulminant hepatic failure rarely occurred in patients infected parenterally, unless they also had immunodeficiency or pre-existing liver disease (Fagan, 1994). Based on serum HCV RNA, a marker for replicating HCV, HCV was the cause of hepatic failure in only 12% of American patients with fulminant non-A, non-B hepatitis referred for liver transplantation (Liang et al, 1993), as reported in other centres (Fagan, 1994). However, there may be geographical differences, because one study in Japan showed that HCV was a common (> 50%) cause of late-onset fulminant hepatitis (Yoshiba et al, 1994). The incubation period for hepatitis C cases was longer than for hepatitis B or non-A, non-B, non-C cases (25 days versus 2 and 12). The survival rate was 46% for hepatitis C, as compared to 86% for hepatitis B and 40% for non-A, non-B, non-C. In other studies, HCV was implicated as a co-factor of fulminant hepatitis in conjunction with hepatitis A or B, or with drugs (Fagan, 1994).

CHRONIC INFECTION

Chronic HCV infection is by far more common than previously thought. When longer than 6-month elevations of serum ALT were used as a marker of chronicity, 62–77% of the patients with transfusion-associated hepatitis and 62% of those with community-acquired infection were estimated to have chronic hepatitis. Using serum HCV-RNA to detect persistent infection, the rates of chronicity rose to 82–100% (Omata et al, 1991, Alter et al, 1992, Hwang et al, 1994, Lampertico et al, 1994, Barrera et al, 1995) (Table 1).

Table 1. Rates of chronic hepatitis in prospectively followed-up patients with acute hepatitis C.

Author	Type of hepatitis	Number of patients	Chronicity	
			ALT	HCV RNA
Barrera et al (1995)	Transfusion	41	77%	90%
Omata et al (1991)	Transfusion	14	78%	82%
Lampertico et al (1994)	Transfusion	16	63%	100%
Hwang et al (1994)	Transfusion	17	62%	87%
Alter et al (1992)	Community-acquired	106	62%	15/15

Although the mechanisms underlying persistence of virus in patients with hepatitis C are largely unknown, a faulty immune reaction to HCV is a likely candidate. Perhaps persistence of HCV is due to immune escape of neutralizing antibodies and/or lack of cytotoxic T-cell activity in situ, or to extrahepatic replication of the virus. Clearly, chronicity is not related to viral integration into the host genome because there are no DNA intermediates in the viral life cycle.

In chronic infection there is usually an indolent course, but there can be a variety of histological lesions. Existing data suggest that the bursts of inflammatory activity with HCV disease tend to occur more in the early phase of the disease and to diminish with time. It is important to note that HCV is not a progressive disease in all infected patients. The spectrum of histological lesions ranges from minimal hepatic inflammation to severe active cirrhosis and hepatocellular carcinoma (HCC). It is controversial whether or not there are HCV carriers with normal liver histology (Alberti et al, 1992).

The risk that HCV-infected patients will develop severe hepatic sequelae is difficult to assess, mainly because of methodological weaknesses of the available studies.

Two studies have depicted hepatitis as a severe condition, with a large number of patients developing cirrhosis or dying of liver-related causes. In a prospective cohort study, approximately 30% of Spanish patients developed cirrhosis, 2–7% developed HCC, and 4–9% died in an average time period of 10 years (Sanchez-Tapias, personal communication). In a tertiary referral centre in the USA, 50% of patients with transfusion-associated hepatitis C developed cirrhosis and 5% had hepatocellular carcinoma (Tong et al 1995). During a follow-up of 4 years (range 1–15), 15% of these patients died from complications of cirrhosis or HCC. However, the average interval between transfusion and cirrhosis was 20 years, with a standard deviation of ±10 years, suggesting that hepatitis C is indeed a potentially severe disease, but with a slowly progressive course.

The dismal prognosis of hepatitis C emerging from these two studies is mitigated by the results in other reports. In a long-term multicentre follow-up study of 568 patients who were transfused between 1967 and 1980, there was no increase in mortality from all causes 18 years after transfusion-associated hepatitis C, with 3.3% of the deaths being related to liver disease (Seeff et al, 1992). The Centers for Disease Control in Atlanta estimated that only 20% of acute cases of community-acquired infections progressed to chronic hepatitis, but cirrhosis and deaths were uncommon (Alter et al, 1992). In the NIH study, 92 patients had post-transfusion hepatitis, cirrhosis developed in 24% and the mortality rate after 23 years was only 3–6%, (Di Bisceglie et al, 1991). Similarly, 18% of 83 patients with transfusion-associated hepatitis followed up at UCLA (Los Angeles) developed cirrhosis within 16 years (Koretz et al, 1993). In a homogeneous group of 350 women infected with anti-D Ig, chronic hepatitis C developed in 50% of the cases within 15 years. Chronic persistent hepatitis was found in all of the 345 liver biopsies that were obtained (Wiese, 1995). It is possible that this cohort was too young or that women are less prone than men to have developed a significant incidence of progressive liver disease. However, existing data indicate that many carriers of serum HCV RNA who develop minimal liver damage or chronic persistent hepatitis remain unchanged over decades (Kiyosawa et al, 1990). Instead, in other studies, an apparently benign disease such as chronic persistent hepatitis did entail a risk of progression to cirrhosis (Hay et al, 1985).

Unlike hepatitis B, there is no clear-cut evidence that there are carriers with entirely normal liver histology. A few patients with serum anti-HCV and normal liver histology have been reported, but they were consistently serum-negative for HCV RNA (Alberti et al, 1992; Prieto et al, 1995; Shindo et al, 1995). By contrast, there also seem to be carriers with normal hepatic histology with detectable circulating levels of HCV RNA (Brillanti 1993, Zanella 1995).

HEPATOCELLULAR CARCINOMA

World-wide, the progression of hepatitis to cirrhosis was a clinically indolent process, with bleeding varices or hepatocellular carcinoma being common causes of death. In most patients, development of severe liver disease was heralded by persistent elevations of serum ALT activity for more than 6 months after the onset of acute hepatitis C. However, histo-logical features of chronic liver disease and cirrhosis have also been detected in seropositive, viraemic patients with persistently normal ALT (Alberti et al, 1992).

The sequential development of cirrhosis and liver cancer that has been observed in many patients with either community-acquired or transfusion-related hepatitis C first established a link between HCV and HCC (Table 2). The time lag between exposure to HCV and development of cancer varied greatly from patient to patient. However, it was an average of 29 years in one study (Kiyosawa et al 1990). In all cases, the tumour was a long-term sequela of HCV-related cirrhosis. However, there are cases of liver cancer that developed in non-cirrhotic livers (De Mitri et al, 1994). In Milan, the yearly rate of patients' transition from cirrhosis to liver cancer is approximately 2.5% (Colombo et al, 1991).

Table 2. Reports of progression from NANB(C) hepatitis to hepatocellular carcinoma.

Author	Year	Modality of infection	Histological follow-up	Incubation period (years)
Ayoola	1982	Sporadic	CAH→HCC	3
Resnick	1983	Transfusion	HCC	17
Gilliam	1984	Transfusion	CAH→CIRRH→HCC	9
Kiyosawa	1984	Transfusion	CPH→CAH→CIRRH→HCC	13
Cohen	1987	Sporadic	CAH→CIRRH→HCC	8

Modified from data reviewed by Tabor (1989).

The widespread use of abdominal ultrasound and the implementation of prospective studies of patients with cirrhosis have elucidated several important aspects of the natural history of this tumour (Okuda, 1992; Colombo, 1993). This tumour often has a subclinical incubation period, lasting 2 years or longer, during which it may grow as a solitary mass. However, in 8–36% of the patients, the tumour may be found as more than one nodule when it is first detected. In most Oriental and European patients the tumour presents as an expanding, encapsulated node rather than the more aggressive spreading form. However, many patients with apparently single encapsulated nodes of HCC may have ancillary tumours detectable only by highly sensitive imaging techniques or during surgery. There may be differences in the growth rates of HCV-related tumour even in a single patient with multiple nodes, which hinder correct prediction of patients' survival. Expressed as tumour volume doubling-time, the growth rate of liver cancer ranged from 1 to 19 months, with a median of 6 months. Because of this great diversity of the tumour growth rates, the predictive power of the number and size of tumour nodes is not absolute, and survival times were predicted better by the severity of liver impairment (Okuda, 1992).

PREDICTORS OF LIVER DISEASE SEVERITY

The epidemiological, clinical and virological covariates that influence the severity of liver damage in patients with HCV infection are poorly defined (Table 3). Among the many covariates that have been considered, modality of infection, patient age and duration of disease, type, serum load and degree of variation of HCV, host immunity and environmental co-factors (hepatitis B and alcohol) have been extensively investigated. In a 10-year study, the rate of apparent remission (6% versus 10%), development of cirrhosis (30% versus 39%) and overall mortality (4% versus 9%) were similar for 77 patients with transfusion-related hepatitis and 211 with community-acquired infection (Sanchez-Tapias, personal communication). The course of hepatitis was also similar for Spanish children with these two forms of hepatitis who were followed-up for 1–14 years (Bortolotti et al, 1994). Patient age and disease duration were correlated with an increased risk of severe hepatic lesions. Chronic active hepatitis and cirrhosis were detected more frequently among Spanish donors aged 40 years or older than in younger persons (66% versus 33%). Patients with histories of longer than 10 years' infection had chronic active hepatitis or cirrhosis more often than did patients who were infected for shorter times (70% versus 30%) (Esteban-Mur, 1990; Pontisso et al, 1993). Existing data would suggest that hepatitis C has a more favourable course in children than in adults. In a study of 73 Italian and Spanish children who were followed from 6 months to 14 years after diagnosis, 24 (33%) developed chronic active hepatitis and 2 (3%) developed cirrhosis, without any relation to the source of infection, i.e. transfusion or community-acquired (Bortolotti et al, 1994).

Table 3. Factors that may influence severity of hepatitis C.

• Epidemiology	Transfusion versus sporadic hepatitis
• Time	Patient age
	Duration of infection
• HCV	Type
	Load
	Degree of variation
• Host	Immunity
• Environment	Alcohol
	HBV

The identification of HCV as a genetically heterogeneous virus led to the concept that sequence variability of HCV could be a factor in the clinical heterogeneity of hepatitis C. With molecular evolutionary analysis techniques it has become possible to identify and quantify the major genetic groups (types) and more closely related subgroups (subtypes) of HCV, as well as to measure the dominant strains within the same infecting virus population (quasispecies).

Genotypes 1, 2 and 3 are the most frequently encountered genotypes in Europe, North America and Far East, with significant differences in subtype distribution. In many countries, genotype distribution has been found to vary with age, reflecting changes in HCV type prevalence within a given geographical area. As a general rule, genotype 1b of HCV was prevalent in patients with more severe liver diseases (Pozzato et al, 1994; Nousbaum et al, 1995; Silini et al, 1995). However, mitigating against virus genotypes as determinants of disease severity are studies in both Eastern and Western countries showing similar prevalences of genotype 1b in patients with cirrhosis and those without it (Yamada et al, 1994; Naito et al, 1995; Preston et al, 1995; Takano et al, 1995) (Table 4). A study in France and

Italy (Nousbaum et al, 1995) showed a low prevalence of HCV1b among young patients and those individuals more recently infected with cirrhosis, suggesting that the prevalence of this strain is decreasing in the general population. Data obtained for a homogeneous group of haemodialysed patients also showed a changing pattern of genotype prevalence with time (Pol et al, 1995). Altogether, these observations suggest that genotype 1b is found more often than other genotypes in long-lasting, old infections.

Table 4. Prevalence of HCV 1b genotype in patients with cirrhosis and patients with less advanced liver disease.

| | | Prevalence of HCV 1b | |
Author	Number of patients	Non-cirrhosis (%)	Cirrhosis (%)
Pozzato et al (1994)	54	64	100
Silini et al (1995)	207	38	54
Nousbaum et al (1995)	220	50	72
Naito et al (1995)	116	80	82
Preston et al (1995)	51	38	42
Yamada et al (1994)	251	65	73

The important bias of these studies, however, is that they were usually performed in referral centres, where most patients come with advanced liver disease. In fact, when HCV carriers with persistently normal or near-normal transaminase levels were investigated, the frequency of type 2 was significantly higher than in patients with liver disease in whom type 1 predominated (Silini et al, 1995).

The finding that there are million-fold differences in the copy numbers of HCV RNA among patients with chronic HCV infection led to the hypothesis that virus load could be a determinant of disease severity. The amounts of circulating HCV have been determined as infectivity titres by chimpanzee-transmission studies, by polymerase chain reaction (PCR) on serial dilutions of plasma, by competitive PCR using genetically mutated competitive templates, and by a signal amplification assay (branched DNA assay). The evidence suggesting that HCV viraemia might be a factor of disease severity is weakened by a number of methodological pitfalls. In fact, during chronic infections, the serum levels of HCV RNA fluctuate with time, although the magnitude of these fluctuations rarely exceeds 1 log (Brillanti 1991). As HCV RNA peaks usually precede ALT flares, identification of peak levels of viraemia is not possible in each patient. The lack of physiological standards for assessing sensitivity and specificity of the assays for HCV RNA makes it difficult to compare results from different studies. Finally, there is growing evidence that diagnostic accuracy of some assays is strain-dependent. With this as a background, it is not surprising that there are conflicting opinions about viraemia being a predictor of disease severity.

In both sporadic and transfusion-associated acute infection, the amounts of serum HCV RNA rose to a high level in the early phase of infection

(5–9.5 $\log_{10}$), and became exponentially larger as the interval after infection become longer (Kato et al, 1993; Naito et al, 1994, 1995). Using competitive PCR, two studies have shown that HCV RNA is higher in patients with advanced liver disease than in those with persistently normal liver chemistry (Hagiwara et al, 1993; Kato et al, 1993). Using different diagnostic tools (branched DNA assay), a correlation between serum HCV RNA levels and disease severity was not apparent (Nousbaum et al, 1995). In one study, high viraemia was more often detected in patients with lobular inflammation, lymphoid aggregates and bile duct lesions (Lau et al, 1993).

Severity of liver disease might also be related to predominance of selected virus strains within a single type of infection. Indeed, the mechanisms of persistence appear to reside in the ability of the virus to mutate under immune pressure and to survive as a series of related, but immunologically distinct variants (quasispecies). In newly infected persons, one HCV variant multiplies quickly and establishes a population that is initially almost homogeneous despite the heterogeneity of the donor population (Weiner et al, 1992). Once the hepatitis develops, the sequence diversity increased in the patients according to the severity of the liver disease (Honda et al, 1994). Studying the nucleotide sequences of HCV genome spanning the region from the core to envelope (hypervariable region), Honda and associates showed that the rate of nucleotide diversity was 0.85% in patients with chronic persistent hepatitis, 1.79% in patients with chronic active hepatitis and 3.05% in those with cirrhosis. However, no correlation between quasispecies and disease severity was found in other studies (Naito et al, 1995; Shindo et al, 1995), implying that in HCV infection the severity of liver disease depends upon a more complex interaction between virus and host immunity.

Indeed, immunological processes have been implicated as important determinants of hepatic injury during infection with HCV, although this virus may also have a (minor) direct cytotoxic effect on the liver. Liver disease in these patients seems to be influenced by cell-mediated immunity: CD8 cells isolated from infected livers show cytolytic activity against autologous or HLA-matched target cells that have HCV-encoded proteins via a recombinant vaccine vector (Koziel et al, 1992). In immuno-compromised patients, the course of hepatitis C seems to be exacerbated. As a result, HCV is a major cause of liver disease and mortality in renal-graft recipients (Chan et al, 1993; Hanafusa et al, 1995). High-titred recurrent HCV infection following liver transplantation is almost universal, with clinical hepatitis developing in 13–51% of the cases. In a 3-year period, 30% of these patients developed significant chronic liver disease, including cirrhosis and hepatocellular carcinoma, as compared with only 10% of the transplanted patients with de novo hepatitis C acquired via transfusion (Chazouilleres et al, 1994; Feray et al, 1994). In a multicentre study of the Italian Association for the Study of the Liver, the time lag between liver transplantation and development of HCV-related hepato-cellular carcinoma was as short as 5 years, on the average (G. Bellati, personal communication). Unlike immunocompetent individuals, only a few HCV carriers co-infected with the human immunodeficiency virus

(HIV-1) have serologically occult HCV viraemia (Wright et al, 1994). A large prospective study of haemophiliacs clearly suggests that HIV1 accelerates the clinical course of hepatitis C, especially in patients with low CD4 cell counts (Eyster et al, 1993). Other studies suggesting that immune dysfunction may influence the course of HCV infection have been those in patients with malignancies. Seventy-six percent of Japanese children with anti-HCV and malignant anaemia developed severe chronic liver disease, as compared with only 25% of carriers with benign anaemia. Hepatitis spontaneously remissed in 28% of the latter, but in none of the former (Inui et al, 1994). Another study reported the case of a patient who developed fulminant hepatitis C after bone marrow transplantation when cytotoxic treatment was terminated (Kanamori et al, 1992). Increased virus replication could have been the relevant factor, accounting for the increased severity of liver disease that has been observed in the immunocompromised patients.

Other data indicate that many environmental factors that adversely affect the liver might alter the natural history of hepatitis C. Combined HCV–HBV infection is quite frequent, being due to common sources of infection and similarities in the transmission modalities of both viruses in patients with parenteral exposure. In patients with replicating HCV, HBV replication is suppressed more often than vice versa (Pontisso et al, 1993). Concurrent HCV, HBV and HDV infections increase the risk of severe hepatitis and they can be associated with an increased risk of fulminant hepatic failure and HCC (Benvegnù et al, 1994; Fagan, 1994). In an endemic area for HBV, co-presence of HCV in HBsAg carriers increased progressively from patients with minimal liver lesions to patients with cirrhosis or HCC (Chen et al, 1990). The prevalence of anti-HCV was 5% in patients with chronic persistent hepatitis, but rose to 10% and 17% in patients with cirrhosis and liver cancer. A high prevalence of HCV markers has been described in patients with alcoholic liver disease and in chronic alcoholics with liver cancer (Mendenhall et al, 1991; Yamauchi et al, 1993). In the latter study, the risk of liver cancer was clearly increased in anti-HCV-positive alcoholics: the 10-year cumulative occurrence rate of HCC was 81% in anti-HCV-positive alcoholics, as compared with 18% for anti-HCV-negative alcoholics. The mechanisms of interaction between chronic alcohol abuse and liver cancer remain unclear.

EXTRAHEPATIC MANIFESTATIONS

In a recent study (Pawlotsky et al, 1994), the various immunological abnormalities that have been reported in patients with chronic hepatitis C were classified in four categories according to their putative mechanisms: (1) immune complex-mediated disease, mainly represented by mixed cryoglobulinaemia; (2) anti-tissue antibodies in serum and autoimmune thyroiditis; (3) salivary gland lesions characterized by lymphocytic capillaritis; (4) chronic liver disease associated with lichen planus.

Cryoglobulinaemia is detectable in 36–54% of patients with chronic hepatitis C, more likely for those with longer duration of HCV infection (Pawlotsky et al, 1995). Most patients with chronic hepatitis C and cryoglobulinaemia are asymptomatic. However, in 18% of the patients cryoglobulinaemia may cause arthralgias and pruritus, and in 2% purpura, neuropathy and glomerulonephritis.

HCV is implicated in 30–90% of type II cryoglobulinaemias, i.e. in a condition in which there is a mixture of a homogeneous immunoglobulin (mostly an IgM-Km component) with anti-IgG activity (rheumatoid factor) and heterogeneous IgG. Agnello et al detected HCV RNA in 16 of 19 such patients (two with chronic active hepatitis) and antibody to HCV in eight. In four patients, quantitative studies showed that almost all HCV RNA sequences were concentrated (1000-fold) in the cryoprecipitate. Moreover, anti-HCV, consisting of a mixture of heterogeneous IgM and heterogeneous IgG molecules, was found in five of 10 patients. Supporting evidence for the role of HCV in cryoglobulinaemia is the response of patients with cryoglobulinemia to alpha-interferon (Misiani et al, 1994).

Glomerulonephritis, with and without the presence of cryoglobulinaemia, is associated with HCV (Johnson et al, 1993). Eight patients with chronic hepatitis C developed proteinuria, and all had HCV RNA in the serum and membranoproliferative glomerulonephritis in the renal biopsy. A moderate proportion of patients with cryoglobulinaemia type II had a sicca-like syndrome resembling Sjogren syndrome, a condition thought to be another extrahepatic manifestation of HCV infection. In one study (Haddad et al, 1992), 29% of 28 patients with chronic hepatitis C had focal lymphocytic sialoadenitis and histological lesions of the labial salivary glands characteristic of Sjogren syndrome, compared with only 5% of controls with miscellaneous diseases. Although these studies demonstrated a striking association between HCV infection, cryoglobulinaemia and sialoadenitis, they do not prove a direct pathogenetic link.

Several observations are in favour of a direct role of HCV in immunity; for example, this virus was found to replicate within mononuclear cells (Qian et al, 1992), and many patients with hepatitis have been found to have smooth muscle, liver–kidney microsomal and thyroid antibodies and antibodies against host-derived epitopes (anti-GOR) (Nishiguchi et al, 1992; Pawlotsky et al, 1995). The possible link of HCV to such extrahepatic syndromes as polyarteritis nodosa and idiopathic pulmonary fibrosis is controversial. Anti-HCV was detected in 8% of 38 patients with polyarteritis nodosa and confirmed by a second-generation immunoblot assay (Deny et al, 1992). Anti-HCV was positive in 29% of 66 Japanese patients with idiopathic pulmonary fibrosis, whether or not they had chronic liver disease (Ueda et al, 1992). Lichen planus is often associated with immunological disease, and data suggest a link between lichen planus and chronic hepatitis C (Jubert 1994; Bellani et al, 1995). This association needs to be looked for in patients with chronic viral hepatitis who are candidates for interferon therapy because lichen planus can be exacerbated following interferon administration. HCV may contribute to the liver damage in patients with other diseases, such as porphyria cutanea tarda, autoimmune hepatitis type II and alcoholic liver diseases (Mendenhall et al, 1991; Herrero et al, 1993). HCV is responsible, in fact, for the portal and/or lobular hepatitis associated with these conditions. In patients with auto-immune hepatitis, the virus could also trigger the pathogenic process ab initio.

SUMMARY

The natural history of hepatitis C is complex and still poorly known. Hepatitis C virus (HCV) replication can be detected very soon after exposure and, at least in the transfusional setting, it persists indefinitely in up to 90% of the cases. While liver damage during the acute phase of hepatitis is almost invariably mild (fulminant cases are exceptions), chronic sequelae of HCV infection may be severe in the long run. Chronic hepatitis C, in fact, is a long-lasting indolent process which leads to cirrhosis in approximately 20% of all infected patients. Hepatocellular carcinoma is a well-recognized complication of old infections, as are a number of extra-hepatic manifestations, including type II cryoglobulinaemia. The determinants of the severity of the liver disease are still unclear. However, the risk of cirrhosis seems to be greater for patients with old infections, those infected with the genotype 1b and those with associated conditions. The latter are a heterogeneous and increasing group of 'problem' patients, including patients who are co-infected with the human immunodeficiency virus (HIV1), or who are being treated with cytotoxic or immunomodulating drugs. Data suggest that the natural history of hepatitis C is altered in patients with associated conditions, and this might have an impact on strategies of patient management and treatment.

REFERENCES

Aach RD, Stevens CE, Hollinger FB et al (1991) Hepatitis C virus infection in post-transfusion hepatitis. An analysis with first- and second-generation assays. New England Journal of Medicine 325: 1325–1329.

Agnello V, Chung RT & Kaplan LM (1992) A role for hepatitis C virus infection in type II cryoglobulinemia. New England Journal of Medicine 327: 1490–1495.

Alberti A (1991) Diagnosis of hepatitis C. Facts and perspectives. Journal of Hepatology 12: 279–282.

Alberti A, Morsica G, Chemello L et al (1992) Hepatitis C viremia and liver disease in symptom-free individuals with anti-HCV. Lancet 340: 697–698.

Alter HJ, Purcell RH, Shih JW et al (1989) Detection of antibody to hepatitis C virus in prospectively followed transfusion recipients with acute and chronic non-A, non-B hepatitis. New England Journal of Medicine 321: 1494–1500

Alter MJ, Margolis HS, Krawczynski K et al (1992) The natural history of community-acquired hepatitis C in the United States. New England Journal of Medicine 327: 1899–1905.

Barrera JM, Bruguera M, Ercilla MG et al (1995) Persistent hepatitis C viremia after acute self-limiting posttransfusion hepatitis C. Hepatology 21: 639–644.

Bellman B, Reddy KR & Falanga V (1995) Lichen planus associated with hepatitis C. Lancet 346: 1234.

Benvegnù L, Fattovich G, Noventa F et al (1994) Concurrent hepatitis B and C virus infection and risk of hepatocellular carcinoma in cirrhosis. A prospective study. Cancer 74: 2442–2448.

Bortolotti F, Jara P, Diaz C et al (1994) Posttransfusion and community-acquired hepatitis C in childhood. *Journal of Pediatric Gastroenterologic Nutrition* **18:** 279–283.

Brillanti S, Garson JA, Tuke PW et al (1991) Effect of interferon therapy on hepatitis C viraemia in community-acquired chronic non-A, non-B hepatitis: a quantitative polymerase chain reaction study. *Journal of Medical Virology* **34:** 136–141.

Brillanti S, Foli M, Gaiani S et al (1993) Persistent hepatitis C viraemia without liver disease. *Lancet* **341:** 464–465.

Chan TM, Lok ASF, Cheng IKP & Chan R (1993) A prospective study of hepatitis C virus infection among renal transplant recipients. *Gastroenterology* **104:** 862–868.

Chazouilleres O, Kim M, Combs C et al (1994) Quantitation of hepatitis C virus RNA in liver transplant recipients. *Gastroenterology* **106:** 994–999.

Chen DS, Kuo G, Sung JL et al (1990) Hepatitis C virus infection in an area hyperendemic for hepatitis B and chronic liver disease: the Taiwan experience. *Journal of Infectious Diseases* **162:** 817–822.

Colombo M (1993) Hepatocellular carcinoma in cirrhotics. *Seminars in Liver Disease* **13:** 374–383.

Colombo M, de Franchis R, Del Ninno E et al (1991) Hepatocellular carcinoma in Italian patients with cirrhosis. *New England Journal of Medicine* **325:** 675–680.

De Mitri MS, Poussin K, Baccarini P et al (1994) HCV-associated liver cancer without cirrhosis. *Lancet* **345:** 413–415.

Deny P, Bonacorsi S, Guillevin L & Quint L (1992) Association between hepatitis C virus and polyarteritis nodosa. *Clinical and Experimental Rheumatology* **10:** 319.

Di Bisceglie AM, Goodman WD, Ishak KG et al (1991) Long-term clinical and histopathological follow-up of chronic post-transfusion hepatitis. *Hepatology* **14:** 696–974.

Esteban-Mur JI (1990) Viral hepatitis C: progression to chronicity. *Second International Symposium of HCV*, p 30. Abstract.

Eyster ME, Diamondstone LS, Lien JM et al (1993) Natural history of hepatitis C virus infection in multitransfused hemophiliacs: effect of coinfection with human immunodeficiency virus. *Journal of Acquired Immune Deficiency Syndromes* **6:** 602–610.

Fagan AE (1994) Acute liver failure of unknown pathogenesis: the hidden agenda. *Hepatology* **19:** 1307–1312.

Farci P, Alter HJ, Wong D et al (1991) A long-term study of hepatitis C virus replication in non-A, non-B hepatitis. *New England Journal of Medicine* **325:** 98–104.

Feray C, Gigou M, Samuel D et al (1994) The course of hepatitis C virus infection after liver transplantation. *Hepatology* **20:** 1137–1143.

Haddad J, Deny P, Munz-Gotheil C et al (1992) Lymphocytic sialadenitis of Sjogren's syndrome associated with chronic hepatitis C virus liver disease. *Lancet* **339:** 321–323.

Hagiwara H, Hayashi N, Nita E et al (1993) Quantitation of hepatitis C virus RNA in serum of asymptomatic blood donors and patients with type C chronic liver disease. *Hepatology* **17:** 545–550.

Hanafusa T, Ichikawa Y, Kyo M et al (1995) Long-term impact of hepatitis virus infection on kidney transplantant recipient and a pilot study of the effects of interferon alpha on chronic hepatitis C. *Transplantation Proceedings* **27:** 956–957.

Hay CRM, Preston FE, Triger DR & Underwood JCE (1985) Progressive liver disease in haemophilia: an understated problem? *Lancet* **i:** 1495–1498.

Herrero C, Vicente A, Bruguera M et al (1993) Is hepatitis C virus infection a trigger of porphiria cutanea tarda? *Lancet* **341:** 788–789.

Honda M, Kaneko S, Sakai A et al (1994) Degree of diversity of hepatitis C virus quasispecies and progression of liver disease. *Hepatology* **20:** 1144–1151.

Hwang SJ, Lee SD, Chan CY et al (1994) A randomized controlled trial of recombinant interferon alpha-2b in the treatment of Chinese patients with acute post-transfusion hepatitis C. *Journal of Hepatology* **21:** 831–836.

Inui A, Fujisawa T, Miyagawa Y et al (1994) Histologic activity of the liver in children with transfusion-associated chronic hepatitis C. *Journal of Hepatology* **21:** 748–753.

Johnson RJ, Grecht DR, Yamabe H et al (1993) Membranoproliferative glomerulonephritis associated with hepatitis C virus infection. *New England Journal of Medicine* **328:** 465–470.

Jubert C, Pawlotsky JM, Ponget F et al (1994) Lichen planus and hepatitis C virus related chronic active hepatitis. *Archives of Dermatology* **130:** 73–76.

Kanamori H, Fukawa H, Maruta A et al (1992) Case report: fulminant hepatitis C viral infection after allogeneic bone marrow transplantation. *American Journal of the Medical Sciences* **303:** 109–111.

Kato N, Yokosuka O, Hosoda K et al (1993) Quantification of hepatitis C virus by competitive reverse transcription–polymerase chain reaction: increase of the virus in advanced liver disease. *Hepatology* **18:** 16–20.

Kiyosawa K, Sodeyama T, Tanaka E et al (1990) Interrelationship of blood transfusion, non-A, non-B hepatitis and hepatocellular carcinoma: analysis by detection of antibody to hepatitis C virus. *Hepatology* **12:** 671–675.

Koretz RL, Abber H, Coleman E & Gitnick G (1993) Non-A, non-B post-transfusion hepatitis. *Annals of Internal Medicine* **119:** 110–115.

Koziel MJ, Dudley D, Afdahl N et al (1992) Hepatitis C virus (HCV)-specific cytotoxic T lymphocytes recognize epitopes in the core and envelope proteins of HCV. *Journal of Virology* **67:** 7522–7532.

Lampertico P, Rumi MG, Romeo R et al (1994) A multicenter randomized controlled trial of recombinant interferon-alpha 2b in patients with acute transfusion-associated hepatitis C. *Hepatology* **19:** 19–22.

Lau JYN, Davis GL, Kniffen J et al (1993) Significance of serum hepatitis C virus RNA levels in chronic hepatitis C. *Lancet* **341:** 1501–1504.

Liang TJ, Jeffers L, Reddy RK et al (1993) Fulminant or subfulminant non-A, non-B viral hepatitis: the role of hepatitis C and E viruses. *Gastroenterology* **104:** 556–562.

Mattsson L, Grillner L & Weiland O (1992) Seroconversion to hepatitis C virus antibodies in patients with acute post-transfusion non-A, non-B hepatitis in Sweden with a second-generation test. *Scandinavian Journal of Infectious Diseases* **24:** 15–20.

Mendenhall CL, Seeff L, Diehl AM et al (1991) Antibodies to hepatitis B virus and hepatitis C virus in alcoholic hepatitis and cirrhosis: their prevalence and clinical relevance. *Hepatology* **14:** 581–589.

Misiani R, Bellavita P, Fenili D et al (1994) Interferon alfa-2a therapy in cryoglobulinemia associated with hepatitis C virus. *New England Journal of Medicine* **330:** 751–756.

Naito M, Hayashi N, Hagiwara H et al (1994) Serial quantitative analysis of serum hepatitis C virus RNA level in patients with acute and chronic hepatitis. *Journal of Hepatology* **20:** 755–759.

Naito M, Hayashi N, Moribe T et al (1995) Hepatitis C viral quasispecies in hepatitis C virus carriers with normal liver enzymes and patients with type C chronic liver disease. *Hepatology* **22:** 407–412.

Nishiguchi S, Kuroki T, Ueda T et al (1992) Detection of hepatitis C virus antibody in the absence of viral RNA in patients with autoimmune hepatitis. *Annals of Internal Medicine* **116:** 21–25.

Nousbaum JB, Pol S, Nalpas B et al (1995) Hepatitis C virus type 1b (II) infection in France and Italy. *Annals of Internal Medicine* **122:** 161–168.

Okuda K (1992) Hepatocellular carcinoma: recent progress. *Hepatology* **15:** 948–963.

Omata M, Yokosuka O, Takano S et al (1991) Resolution of acute hepatitis C alfter therapy with natural beta interferon. *Lancet* **338:** 914–915.

Pawlotsky JM, Yahia MB, Andre C et al (1994) Immunological disorders in C virus chronic active hepatitis: a prospective case–control study. *Hepatology* **19:** 841–848.

Pawlotsky JM, Roudot-Thorval F, Simmonds P et al (1995) Extrahepatic immunologic manifestation in chronic hepatitis C and hepatitis C virus serotypes. *Annals of Internal Medicine* **122:** 169–173.

Pol S, Thiers V, Nousbaum JB et al (1995) The changing relative prevalence of hepatitis C virus genotypes: evidence in hemodialyzed patients and kidney recipients. *Gastroenterology* **108:** 581–583.

Pontisso P, Ruvoletto MG, Fattovich G et al (1993) Clinical and virological profiles in patients with multiple hepatitis virus infections. *Gastroenterology* **105:** 1529–1533.

Pozzato G, Kaneko S, Moretti M et al (1994) Different genotypes of hepatitis C virus are associated with different severity of chronic liver disease. *Journal of Medical Virology* **43:** 291–296.

Preston FE, Jarvis LM, Makris M et al (1995) Heterogeneity of hepatitis C virus genotypes in hemophilia; relationship with chronic liver disease. *Blood* **85:** 1259–1262.

Prieto M, Olaso V, Verdu C et al (1995) Does the healthy hepatitis C virus carrier state really exist? An analysis using polymerase chain reaction. *Hepatology* **22:** 413–417.

Qian C, Camps J, Maluenda MD et al (1992) Replication of hepatitis C virus in peripheral blood mononuclear cells. Effects of alpha interferon therapy. *Journal of Hepatology* **16:** 380–383.

Seeff LB, Buskell-Bales Z, Wright EC et al (1992) Long-term mortality after transfusion-associated non-A, non-B hepatitis. *New England Journal of Medicine* **327:** 1905–1911.

Shindo M, Arai K, Sokawa Y & Okuno T (1995) The virological and histological states of anti-hepatitis C virus-positive subjects with normal liver biochemical values. *Hepatology* **22:** 418–425.

Silini E, Bono F, Cividini A et al (1995) Differential distribution of hepatitis C virus genotypes in patients with and without liver function abnormalities. *Hepatology* **21:** 285–290.

Tabor E (1989) Hepatocellular carcinoma: possible etiology in patients without serologic evidence of hepatitis B virus infection. *Journal of Medical Virology* **27:** 1–6.

Takano S, Yokosuka O, Imazeki F et al (1995) Incidence of hepatocellular carcinoma in chronic hepatitis B and C: a prospective study of 251 patients. *Hepatology* **21:** 650–655.

Tong MJ, El-Farra NS, Reikes R & Co RL (1995) Clinical outcomes after transfusion-associated hepatitis C. *New England Journal of Medicine* **332:** 1463–1466.

Ueda T, Ohta K, Suzuki N et al (1992) Idiopathic pulmonary fibrosis and high prevalence of serum antibodies to hepatitis C virus. *American Review of Respiratory Disease* **146:** 266–268.

Weiner AJ, Geysen HM, Christopherson C et al (1992) Evidence of immune selection of hepatitis C virus (HCV) putative envelope glycoprotein variants: potential role in chronic HCV infections. *Proceeding of the National Academy of Sciences of the USA* **89:** 3468–3472.

Wiese M (1995) Natural course of hepatitis C: 15-year-analysis in an unselected group with an identical parenteral infection. *Journal of Hepatology* **23:** 89.

Wright TL, Hollander H, Pu X et al (1994) Hepatitis C in HIV-infected patients with and without AIDS: prevalence and relationship to patient survival. *Hepatology* **20:** 1152–1155.

Yamada M, Kakumu S, Yoshioka K et al (1994) Hepatitis C virus genotypes are not responsible for development of serious liver disease. *Digestive Disease and Science* **39:** 234–239.

Yamauchi M, Nakahara M, Maexawa Y et al (1993) Prevalence of hepatocellular carcinoma in patients with alcoholic cirrhosis and prior exposure to hepatitis C. *American Journal of Gastro-enterology* **88:** 39–43.

Yoshiba M, Dehara K, Inoue K et al (1994) Contribution of hepatitis C virus to non-A, non-B fulminant hepatitis in Japan. *Hepatology* **19:** 829–835.

Zanella A, Conte D, Prati D et al (1995) Hepatitis C virus RNA and liver histology in blood donors reactive to a single antigen by second-generation recombinant immunoblot assay. *Hepatology* **21:** 913–917.

Zeldis JB & Jensen P (1994) Hepatitis C virus pathogenicity: the corner pieces of the jigsaw puzzle are found. *Gastroenterology* **106:** 1118–1120.

7

Interferon therapy for chronic hepatitis C

GARY L. DAVIS

Hepatitis C virus (HCV) infection is extremely common, with an estimated world-wide prevalence of chronic hepatitis ranging from 22 to 90 million (0.5–2%) (Alter and Sampliner, 1989; Kuo et al, 1989; Alter, 1995). In the United States, hepatitis C is the most common cause of chronic liver disease and affects about 3 500 000 individuals. It is estimated that more than 150 000 individuals are acutely infected with HCV annually (Alter and Sampliner, 1989). Of these, the majority (70–80%) develop chronic infection which is usually insidiously progressive, with cirrhosis develop-ing in 20–50% of patients over a 10–20 year period (Seeff et al, 1992)

HCV is thought to cause liver injury by either a direct cytopathic effect or through an immunological mechanism mediated by cytotoxic T-lymphocytes (CTL), (Gonzalez-Peralta et al, 1994). Although the former mechanism was originally favoured because of the rapid parallel fall in both virus levels and ALT after initiation of treatment, evidence supporting this route of cell injury for most cases of chronic hepatitis C is otherwise lacking. However, direct cytotoxicity may be responsible for cell injury in some immunosuppressed patients with extremely high levels of viraemia (Lim et al, 1994). Currently, evidence is building to support CTL as the major mechanism of cell injury (Gonzalez-Peralta et al, 1994; Nelson et al, 1995; Chapter 5). Thus, therapeutic intervention in patients with chronic hepatitis C must be either directly antiviral or modulate the immune response to the virus.

INTERFERON TREATMENT

Type 1, or alpha, interferons are the only agents thus far proven to be effective in the treatment of chronic hepatitis C (Davis, 1990). Alpha interferons are natural glycoproteins produced by cells in response to infection by viruses, including HCV (Davis and Hoofnagle, 1986; Peters et al, 1986; Kato et al, 1992). Interferons have many biological effects which might explain their activity in this disease (Davis and Hoofnagle, 1986; Peters et al, 1986). Interferon has been shown to inhibit the replication of a wide spectrum of RNA and DNA viruses, including hepatitis viruses. This occurs via a variety of mechanisms, including inhibition of virus attach-ment and uncoating, induction of intracellular proteins and ribonucleases

Baillière's Clinical Gastroenterology—
Vol. 10, No. 2, July 1996
ISBN 0–7020–2094–X
0950–3528/96/020289 + 10 $12.00/00

Copyright © 1996, by Baillière Tindall
All rights of reproduction in any form reserved

which convey antiviral properties to the cell, and amplification of both specific (cytotoxic T-lymphocyte) and non-specific (natural killer cell) immune response to viral proteins (Davis and Hoofnagle, 1986; Peters et al, 1986). The mechanism of interferon's effect in chronic hepatitis C infection remains poorly understood.

Because of its known antiviral properties and the experience with interferon (IFN) in the treatment of other forms of viral hepatitis, it was evaluated as a potential treatment for patients with non-A, non-B hepatitis (NANB) before the hepatitis C virus was even identified. The first efforts with alpha IFN in patients with this disease were conducted by Hoofnagle and colleagues at the National Institutes of Health (NIH) (Hoofnagle et al, 1986). Several subsequent reports have now confirmed that low doses of alpha IFN are useful in the treatment of patients with chronic hepatitis (Tiné et al, 1991). A large multicentre, randomized controlled study conducted in the United States demonstrated that treatment of patients with chronic NANB with alpha IFN resulted in normalization of serum ALT levels in 38% of patients treated for 6 months with a dose of three million units (MU) of recombinant IFN alfa-2b subcutaneously three times per week (t.i.w.) (Davis et al, 1989). The likelihood of response was only 4% in untreated controls (Davis et al, 1989). In retrospect, patients who responded to treatment could not be identified by any pretreatment clinical, biochemical or histological features (Davis et al, 1989). Significant reduction in inflammation on liver biopsy was seen in treated patients and was not confined only to the patients who had a biochemical response to treatment. In contrast to control patients, no patient in this treated group showed evidence of histological progression, regardless of the serum ALT response (Davis et al, 1989). These results were soon duplicated in several studies in Europe and Japan (Davis et al, 1989; Di Bisceglie et al, 1989; Jacyna et al, 1989; Gomez-Rubio et al, 1990; Realdi et al, 1990; Saracco et al, 1990; Weiland et al, 1990; Causse et al, 1991; Cimino et al, 1991; Gindici-Cipriani et al, 1991; Makris et al, 1991; Marcellin et al, 1991; Omata et al, 1991; Schvarcz et al, 1991a; Tiné et al, 1991). Despite considerable difference in the form of IFN, dose, duration of treatment and severity of illness, the results of these trials were remarkably similar. The proportion of patients normalizing serum ALT levels by the end of treatment was 2.6% (7/265; range, 0–6.6%) in the untreated control groups and 41.5% (76/183; range, 35–73%) in those treated with 3 MU thrice weekly for 6 months.

A response during interferon therapy can be anticipated in approximately 40% of patients, and it occurs quickly (Davis et al, 1989). HCV RNA levels fall dramatically and become undetectable within 4–8 weeks in the majority of patients who subsequently normalize their serum aminotransferases (Brillanti et al, 1991; Chayama et al, 1991; Shindo et al, 1991; Bresters et al, 1992; Hagiwara et al, 1992). The fall in the serum ALT level follows the virological response and normalizes between 4 and 12 weeks following initiation of treatment (Davis et al, 1989; Brillanti et al, 1991; Chayama et al, 1991; Shindo et al, 1991). These biochemical and virological changes are accompanied by histological improvement (Davis et al,

1989; Marcellin et al, 1991; Schvarcz et al, 1991b), restoration of hepatic functional impairment as measured by antipyrine clearance (Farrell et al, 1991), and normalization of markers of fibrinogenesis, including TGF-β1 mRNA and pro-collagen III mRNA expression and serum pro-collagen III peptide (Castilla et al, 1991).

Despite the prompt antiviral and biochemical response to treatment and the inability to detect residual HCV in either liver or serum in the responding patient (Roddenberry et al, 1991), biochemical normalization and absence of detectable viraemia in serum is maintained in only a minority of patients, ranging from 8 to 35%. Relapse, characterized by a rebound in serum ALT out of the normal range, occurs in 50–90% of successfully treated patients following the discontinuation of IFN treatment (Davis et al, 1989; Davis, 1990). Relapse is more common in patients with fibrosis on liver biopsy, high pre-treatment viraemia levels, and genotype 1 (Davis et al, 1990; Lau et al, 1993; Martinot-Peignoux et al, 1995). Re-institution of IFN treatment appears to be almost universally effective in re-inducing remission of disease (Davis et al, 1989; Davis, 1990). There are currently no available clinical data on how best to retreat patients who relapse, but it is apparent that IFN therapy serves only to reduce the HCV burden below levels which are overtly hepatotoxic, and therefore treatment regimens which maintain long-term response will be required if treatment is to alter the course of the disease.

At least half of patients with chronic NANBH who are treated with IFN fail to respond (Davis et al, 1989; Davis, 1990). Non-response is evident early in the treatment course because patients who fail to normalize the serum ALT level within 12 weeks are unlikely to do so with continuation of therapy (Davis et al, 1989, 1990). Escalation of the IFN dose does not appear significantly to enhance response in these patients, but is associated with greater side-effects (Feinman et al, 1991; Métreau et al, 1991; Marcellin et al, 1995). Thus, therapy can be discontinued after 12 weeks in these patients. Some patients who initially appear to respond to IFN by normalizing serum ALT levels will demonstrate a progressive rise in the serum ALT levels despite continuation of IFN (Di Bisceglie et al, 1989). Although the cause of this phenomenon is not yet clear, some of these cases may be due to selection of IFN-insensitive strains of HCV (Okada et al, 1992). The less likely possibilities of neutralizing antibodies or IFN-induced autoimmune hepatitis should also be considered under these circumstances.

Efforts to increase the response rate have concentrated on using higher doses and a longer duration of IFN therapy. In most studies, doses higher than 3 MU have not increased the response rate (Cimino et al, 1991; Schvarcz et al, 1991a). Although initial studies seemed to show a lack of benefit of longer durations of treatment (Gomez-Rubio et al, 1990; Realdi et al, 1990; Weiland et al, 1990; Sàez-Royuela et al, 1991), there is now no question that treatment for 12–24 months reduces relapse and thereby increases the longevity of response (Jouet et al, 1994; Benhamou et al, 1995; Kasahara et al, 1995; Poynard et al, 1995). There is growing evidence that different forms of alpha IFN are not necessarily dose equivalent.

Recombinant IFN alfa-2b and natural lymphoblastoid IFN appear to be similar (Tiné et al, 1991; Bacon et al, 1995); however, recombinant IFN alfa-2a and consensus IFN appear to require doses 2–5 times higher for equivalent response rates (Rakela et al, 1993; Tong et al, 1993). Of interest, one IFN preparation which was prepared from pooled donor buffy coats appears to have a biochemical (ALT) response rate similar to recombinant IFN alfa-2b or natural IFN, but there is virtually no antiviral response (loss of HCV RNA) at lower doses (Simon et al, 1995). Only recombinant IFN alfa-2b is approved for use in hepatitis in the United States, but several other forms of the drug are approved in other parts of the world.

SELECTION OF PATIENTS

Since chronic HCV infection is an insidiously progressive disease, all patients with HCV-induced hepatitis should at least be considered for possible IFN treatment. At the present time, a liver biopsy is critical in determining the degree of underlying liver injury, since the level of serum ALT may be misleading (Bodenheimer et al, 1990; Schoeman et al, 1990; Takahashi et al, 1993). Liver biopsy provides an estimation of prognosis as well as a reliable indicator of the likelihood of response to treatment. Until recently, most investigators confined treatment to patients with moderate-to-severe chronic hepatitis (formerly called chronic active hepatitis) in whom the risk of developing cirrhosis or subsequent hepatic failure was considered to be relatively high. A few groups have excluded cirrhotic patients from treatment because the sustained response to a short course of treatment is only about 30% and most of these responders relapse when the drug is stopped. However, the high risk of progression to hepatic failure in cirrhotic patients, estimated to be 25%, makes an attempt at treatment imperative in these patients (Dienstag, 1983; Davis, 1994; Tong et al, 1995). Furthermore, patients who repond to their initial treatment should either be left on treatment or retreated when relapse occurs. The group of patients with very mild histological disease, e.g. mild hepatitis or portal hepatitis (CPH), is the most controversial. These individuals have usually been excluded from treatment because the natural rate of progression to cirrhosis is usually slow (Takahashi et al, 1993). However, recent data are beginning to suggest that patients with histologically mild liver injury respond better to IFN with a 60–70% initial response rate and a >30% chance of eradicating infection (Bennett et al, 1995). Furthermore, decision modelling techniques have now demonstrated that treatment of mild chronic hepatitis C significantly extends life expectancy at minimal cost, at least in patients less than 60 years of age (older patients presumably die of natural causes before experiencing complication of HCV infection, thereby making treatment unnecessary) (Bennett et al, 1995). If it is confirmed that treatment is of benefit in all infected patients regardless of histology, liver biopsy may be less critical in our evaluation of these patients in the future. Regardless, if one does use the biopsy for selection of patients for treatment, it is important to realize that areas of portal hepatitis (CPH) and periportal hepatitis (chronic active hepatitis (CAH)) may co-exist within the same biopsy specimen (Jeffers et al, 1991). The decision to treat, where both patterns co-exist in the same specimen, is based upon the presence of the more severe lesion. Thus, the pathologist must be careful to examine all areas of the histological specimen. Additionally, the presence of portal inflammation (CPH) in chronic hepatitis C may not predict the same benign and non-progressive histological prognosis as the portal inflammation described in autoimmune hepatitis (Iwarson et al, 1979; Kiyosawa et al, 1982). It is therefore prudent to follow such patients closely if they are not treated. Liver biopsy may be the only means of detecting progressive liver disease in this largely asymptomatic population and this must be repeated every few years.

Numerous parameters, including younger age, female gender, low body mass, low pre-treatment HCV RNA level, loss of detectable HCV RNA during the initial month of treatment, non-type 1 viral genotype, absence of fibrosis or cirrhosis, higher or longer doses of IFN, and low serum ferritin or hepatic iron levels have been associated with a greater likelihood of response to IFN, and yet none of these has been able accurately and consistently to predict the patients who respond to IFN (Davis et al, 1989; Gomez-Rubio et al, 1990; Readi et al, 1990; Saracco et al, 1990; Weiland et al, 1990; Causse et al, 1991; Marcellin et al, 1991; Davis et al, 1994b; Olynyk et al, 1995; Orito et al, 1995). The most important pre-treatment factors which correlate with response are hepatic histology, pre-treatment viral levels, and viral genotype. The presence of mild chronic hepatitis is associated with a high response rate (Di Bisceglie et al, 1989; Weiland et al, 1990; Causse et al, 1991; Davis et al, 1994b). Initial response to IFN ranges from 30% in genotype 1 to as high as 60–70% in genotypes 2 and 3 (Chemello et al, 1995; Martinot-Peignoux et al, 1995; Nousbaum et al, 1995). Sustained response also varies considerably, with an 8–10% rate in genotype 1 and approximately 30% in genotypes 2 and 3 (Chemello et al, 1995; Martinot-Peignoux et al, 1995; Nousbaum et al, 1995). There have also been reports that minor genomic variability, known as quasispecies, influences IFN responsiveness. Patients with more than two predominant quasispecies tend to respond poorly to IFN (Enomoto et al, 1994). Low pre-treatment HCV RNA levels are associated with a lower relapse rate, but the initial response to IFN does not appear to be influenced by the level of viraemia (Lau et al, 1993). However, the most helpful clinical predictor of response to IFN is a decrease in the serum ALT level to normal during the first 12 weeks of therapy (Davis et al, 1990).

INTERFERON IN COMBINATION WITH OTHER AGENTS

Several agents or manoeuvres, including ursodeoxycholic acid, indomethacin, n-acetylcysteine, silymarin, and phlebotomy, have been reported to be useful adjuncts to interferon treatment. However, so far none of these has been shown consistently to be effective in controlled trials (Alter et al,

1989; Andreone et al, 1994; Angelico et al, 1995; Boucher et al, 1995). On the other hand, the combination of ribavirin and interferon shows promise.

Ribavirin is an unusual guanosine nucleoside analogue because its structural modification is limited to the base of the molecule. Ribavirin has a broad spectrum of in vitro activity against both DNA and RNA viruses, including flaviviridae. Although pilot studies demonstrated reduction of both serum ALT and HCV RNA levels in patients with chronic HCV infection (Reichard et al, 1991; Di Bisceglie et al, 1992), the antiviral effect of ribavirin could not be confirmed in a subsequent randomized controlled trial (Bodenheimer et al, 1994).

Kakumu first demonstrated the synergistic effect of ribavirin and IFN in patients with hepatitis C infection (Kakumu et al, 1993). In a small controlled trial, six of nine patients treated with the combination of ribavirin and β-IFN normalized serum ALT levels, while only 2/9 and 5/9 treated with ribavirin or IFN alone respectively, did so (Kakumu et al, 1993). These findings have also been confirmed in others studies which both demonstrated increased initial and sustained response in patients receiving the combination of ribavirin and IFN (Brillanti et al, 1994; Schvarcz et al, 1995). Several large randomized controlled studies of ribavirin/interferon combination therapy are underway in Europe and the United States.

Future options for combination therapy are likely to include a variety of antiviral agents directed at the replicative machinery of the hepatitis C virus. These regimens are likely to include viral enzyme inhibitors such as protease, helicase or polymerase inhibitors.

SUMMARY

Interferon alone is currently the treatment of choice for chronic hepatitis C. The optimal treatment regimen continues to be defined and refined by clinical studies. The variability of the response to interferon seems to be influenced by several factors, including liver histology, viral genotype, level of viraemia, number of predominant quasispecies, and perhaps the type of interferon and treatment regimen. It is therefore quite likely that, in the future, treatment regimens will be tailored to the individual patient in order to maximize the likelihood of a beneficial outcome. It is also likely that the increasing availability of sensitive, quantitative, and affordable assays of hepatitis C viral levels will allow physicians to assess treatment response quite differently from the way we do so today. This will change our philosophy such that we will begin to view and treat chronic hepatitis C as an infection, instead of simply as a liver disease.

REFERENCES

Alter MJ (1995) Epidemiology of hepatitis C in the West. *Seminars in Liver Disease* **15**: 5–14.
Alter MJ & Sampliner RE (1989) Hepatitis C and miles to go before we sleep. *New England Journal of Medicine* **321**: 1538–1540.

Andreone P, Cursaro C, Gramenzi A et al (1994) Indomethacin enhances serum 2'5'-oligoadenylate synthetase in patients with hepatitis B and C virus chronic active hepatitis. *Journal of Hepatology* 21: 984–988.

Angelico M, Gandin C, Pescarmona E et al (1995) Recombinant interferon alpha and ursodeoxycholic acid versus interferon alpha alone in the treatment of chronic hepatitis C: a randomized clinical trial with long-term follow-up. *American Journal of Gastroenterology* 90: 263–269.

Bacon BR, Farrell G, Benhamou JP et al (1995) Lymphoblastoid interferon improves long-term response to a six month course of treatment when compared with recombinant interferon alfa 2b: results of an international trial (abstract). *Hepatology* 22: 152A.

Benhamou JP, Hopf U, Rizzetto M et al (1995) Long-term lymphoblastoid interferon enhances sustained responses and improves histological activity up to 12 months post-treatment (abstract). *Hepatology* 22: 151A.

Bennett WG, Inoue Y, Beck JR et al (1995) Justification of a single 6-month course of interferon for histologically mild chronic hepatitis C (abstract). *Hepatology* 22: 290A.

Bodenheimer HC, Lefkowitch J, Lindsay K et al (1990) Histological and clinical correlation in chronic hepatitis C (abstract). *Hepatology* 12: 844.

Bodenheimer HC, Lindsay K, Davis GL et al (1994) Tolerance and safety of oral ribavirin treatment of chronic hepatitis C: a multicenter trial. *Hepatology* 20: 207A.

Boucher E, Jouanolle H, Andre et al (1995) Interferon and ursodeoxycholic acid combined therapy in the treatment of chronic viral C hepatitis: results from a controlled randomized trial of 80 patients. *Hepatology* 21: 322–327.

Bresters D, Mauser-Bunschoten EP, Cuypers HT et al (1992) Disappearance of hepatitis C virus RNA in plasma during interferon alpha-2b treatment in hemophilia patients. *Scandinavian Journal of Gastroenterology* 27: 166–168.

Brillanti S, Garson JA, Tuke PW et al (1991) Effect of alpha-interferon therapy on hepatitis C viremia in community-acquired chronic non-A, non-B hepatitis: a quantitative polymerase chain reaction study. *Journal of Medical Virology* 34: 136–141.

Brillanti S, Garson J, Foli M et al (1994) A pilot study of combination therapy with ribavirin plus interferon alfa for interferon alfa-resistant chronic hepatitis C. *Gastroenterology* 107: 812–817.

Castilla A, Prieto J & Fausto N (1991) Transforming growth factor beta 1 and alpha in chronic liver disease. Effects of interferon alfa therapy. *New England Journal of Medicine* 324: 933–940.

Causse X, Godinot H, Ouzan D et al (1991) Comparison of 1 or 3 MU of interferon alfa-2b and placebo in patients with chronic non-A non-B hepatitis. *Gastroenterology* 101: 497–502.

Chayama K, Saitoh S, Arase Y et al (1991) Effect of interferon administration on serum hepatitis C virus RNA in patients with chronic hepatitis C. *Hepatology* 13: 1040–1043.

Chemello L, Cavalletto L, Noventa F et al (1995) Predictors of sustained response, relapse and no response in patients with chronic hepatitis C treated with interferon alfa. *Journal of Viral Hepatitis* 2: 91–96.

Cimino L, Nardone G, Citarella C et al (1991) Treatment of chronic hepatitis C with recombinant interferon alfa. *Italian Journal of Gastroenterology* 23: 399–402.

Davis GL (1990) Recombinant alpha interferon treatment of non-A, non-B (type C) hepatitis: review of studies and recommendations. *Journal of Hepatology* 11 (**supplement 2**): 72–77.

Davis GL (1994) Interferon treatment of cirrhotic patients with chronic hepatitis C: a logical intervention. *American Journal of Gastroenterology* 89: 658–660.

Davis GL & Hoofnagle JH (1986) Interferon in viral hepatitis: role in pathogenesis and treatment. *Hepatology* 6: 1038–1041.

Davis GL, Balart LA, Schiff ER et al (1989) Treatment of chronic hepatitis C with recombinant interferon alfa: a multicenter randomized, controlled trial. *New England Journal of Medicine* 321: 1501–1506.

Davis GL, Lindsay K, Albrecht J et al (1990) Predictors of response to recombinant alpha interferon treatment in patients with chronic hepatitis C. *Hepatology* 12: 905.

Davis GL, Lau JYN & Lim HL (1994a) Therapy for chronic hepatitis C. *Gastroenterology Clinics of North America* 23: 603–613.

Davis GL, Lindsay K, Albrecht J et al (1994b) Clinical predictors of response to recombinant alpha interferon treatment in patients with chronic non-A, non-B hepatitis (hepatitis C). *Journal of Viral Hepatitis* 1: 55–63.

Di Bisceglie AM, Martin P, Kassianides C et al (1989) Recombinant interferon alfa therapy for chronic hepatitis C. A randomized, double-bind, placebo-controlled trial. *New England Journal of Medicine* 321: 1506–1510.

Di Bisceglie AM, Shindo M, Fong TL et al (1992) A pilot study of ribavirin therapy for chronic hepatitis C. *Hepatology* **16:** 649–654.

Dienstag JL (1983) Non-A, non-B hepatitis. I. Recognition, epidemiology, and clinical features. *Gastroenterology* **85:** 439–462.

Enomoto N, Kurosaki M, Tanaka Y et al (1994) Fluctuation of hepatitis C virus quasispecies in persistent infection and interferon treatment revealed by single-strand conformational polymorphism analysis. *Journal of General Virology* **75:** 1361–1369.

Farrell GC, Lin R & Coverdale S (1991) Prediction of response to interferon in patients with chronic active hepatitis C and evidence that this improves hepatic metabolic function. *Gastroenterologia Japonica* **26 (supplement 3):** 243–246.

Feinman SV, Willems B, Minuk G et al (1991) Treatment of chronic non-A, non-B hepatitis blood related and sporadic with recombinant interferon A (abstract). *Hepatology* **14:** 71A.

Giudici-Cipriani A, Rainisio C, Ponassi I et al (1991) Therapy of cheonic non-A, non-B hepatitis with interferon alfa-2b. A controlled clinical study and long-term follow-up. *Minerva Gastroenterologica Dietologica* **37:** 85–90.

Gomez-Rubio M, Porres JC, Castillo I et al (1990) Prolonged treatment (18 months) of chronic hepatitis C with recombinant alpha-interferon in comparison with a control group. *Journal of Hepatology* **11 (supplement 1):** S63–S67.

Gonzalez-Peralta RP, Davis GL & Lau JYN (1994) Pathogenetic mechanisms on hepatocellular damage in chronic hepatitis C virus infection. *Journal of Hepatology* **21:** 255–259.

Hagiwara H, Hayashi N, Mita E et al (1992) Detection of hepatitis C virus RNA in serum of patients with chronic hepatitis C treated with interferon-alpa. *Hepatology* **15:** 37–41.

Hoofnagle JH, Mullen KD, Jones DB et al (1986) Treatment of chronic non-A, non-B hepatitis with recombinant human alpha interferon: a preliminary report. *New England and Journal of Medicine* **315:** 1575–1578.

Iwarson S, Lindberg J & Lundin P (1979) Progression of hepatitis non-A, non-B to chronic active hepatitis: a histologic follow-up of two cases. *Journal of Clinical Pathology* **32:** 351–355.

Jacyna MR, Brooks MG, Loke RHT et al (1989) Randomized controlled trial of interferon alfa (lymphoblastoid interferon) in chronic non-A non-B hepatitis. *British Medical Journal* **298:** 80–82.

Jeffers L, Findor A, Thung SN et al (1991) Minimizing sampling error with laparoscopic guided liver biopsy of right and left lobes (abstract). *Gastrointestinal Endoscopy* **37:** 266.

Jouet P, Roudot-Thoraval F, Dhumeaux D et al (1994) Comparative efficacy of interferon alfa in cirrhotic and noncirrhotic patients with non-A, non-B C hepatitis. *Gastroenterology* **106:** 686–690.

Kakumu S, Yoshioka K, Wakita T et al (1993) A pilot study of ribavirin and interferon beta for the treatment for chronic hepatitis C. *Gastroenterology* **105:** 507–512.

Kasahara A, Hayashi N, Hiramatsu N et al (1995) Ability of prolonged interferon treatment to suppress relapse after cessation of therapy in patients with chronic hepatitis C: a multicenter randomized controlled trial. *Hepatology* **21:** 291–297.

Kato T, Esumi M, Yamashita S et al (1992) Interferon-inducible gene expression in chimpanzee liver infected with hepatitis C. *Virology* **190:** 856–860.

Kiyosawa K, Akahane Y, Nogata A et al (1982) Significance of blood transfusion in non-A, non-B chronic liver disease in Japan. *Vox Sanguis* **43:** 45–52.

Kuo G, Choo QL, Alter GL et al (1989) An assay for circulating antibodies to a major etiologic virus of human non-A, non-B hepatitis. *Science* **244:** 362–364.

Lau JYN, Davis GL, Kniffen J et al (1993) Significance of serum hepatitis C virus RNA levels in chronic hepatitis. *Lancet* **341:** 1501–1504.

Lim HL, Davis GL, Dolson DJ & Lau JYN (1994) Progressive cholestatic hepatitis leading to subfuminant hepatic failure in an immunosuppressed patient with organ transmitted hepatitis C virus infection. *Gastroenterology* **106:** 248–251.

Makris M, Preston FE, Triger DR et al (1991) A randomized controlled trial of recombinant interferon-alpha in chronic hepatitis C in hemophiliacs. *Blood* **78:** 1672–1677.

Marcellin P, Boyer N, Giostra E et al (1991) Recombinant human alpha-interferon in patients with chronic non-A non-B hepatitis: a multicenter randomized controlled trial from France. *Hepatology* **13:** 393–397.

Marcellin P, Pouteau M, Martinot-Peignoux M et al (1995) Lack of benefit of escalating dosage of interferon alfa in patients with chronic hepatitis C. *Gastroenterology* **109:** 156–165.

Martinot-Peignoux M, Marcellin P, Pouteau M et al (1995) Pretreatment serum hepatitis C virus RNA levels and hepatitis C virus genotype are the main and independent prognostic factors of sustained response to interferon alfa therapy in chronic hepatitis C. *Hepatology* **22**: 1050–1056.

Métreau JM, Calmus Y, Poupon R, et al (1991) Twelve-month treatment compared to 6-month treatment does not improve the efficacy of alpha-interferon in NANB chronic active hepatitis (abstract). *Hepatology* **14**: 72A.

Nelson DR, Marousis CG, Davis GL & Lau JYN (1995) Defining the role of intrahepatic HCV-specific cytotoxic T-lymphocytes in chronic hepatitis C (abstract). *Hepatology* **22**: 287A.

Nousbaum JB, Pol S, Nalpuas B et al (1995) Hepatitis C virus 1b (II) infection I France and Italy. *Annals of Internal Medicine* **122**: 161–173.

Okada S, Akahane Y, Suzuki H et al (1992) The degree of variability in the amino terminal region of the E2/NS1 protein of hepatitis C virus correlates with responsiveness to interferon therapy in viremic patients. *Hepatology* **16**: 619–624.

Olynyk JK, Reddy KR, Di Bisceglie AM et al (1995) Hepatic iron concentration as a predictor of response to interferon alfa therapy in chronic hepatitis C. *Gastroenterology* **108**: 1104–1109.

Omata M, Ito Y, Yokosuka O et al (1991) Randomized, double-blind, placebo-controlled trial of eight-week course of recombinant alpha-interferon for chronic non-A, non-B hepatitis. *Digestive Diseases and Sciences* **36**: 1217–1222.

Orito E, Mizokami M, Suzuki K et al (1995) Loss of serum HCV RNA at week 4 of interferon alpha therapy is associated with more favorable long-term response in patients with chronic hepatitis C. *Journal of Medical Virology* **46**: 109–115.

Peters M, Davis GL, Dooley JS & Hoofnagle JH (1986) The interferon system in acute and chronic viral hepatitis. In Popper H & Schaffner F (eds) *Progress in Liver Diseases*, vol 8, pp 453–467. New York: Grune and Stratton.

Poynard T, Bedossa P, Chevallier M et al (1995) A comparison of three interferon alfa-2b regimens for the long term treatment of chronic non-A, non-B hepatitis. *New England Journal of Medicine* **332**: 1457–1462.

Rakela J, Tong M, Shiffman M, et al (1993) An open-label, randomized parallel evaluation of one, three and six million units of interferon alfa-2a in the sixth-month treatment of patients with chronic non-A, non-B hepatitis (abstract). *Gastroenterology* **104**: A976.

Realdi G, Diodati G, Bonetti P et al (1990) Recombinant human interferon alfa-2a in community-acquired non-A, non-B chronic active hepatitis. Preliminary results of a randomized controlled trial. *Journal of Hepatology* **11 (supplement 1)**: S68–S71.

Reichard O, Andersson J, Schvarcz R & Weiland O (1991) Ribavirin treatment for chronic hepatitis C. *Lancet* **337**: 1058–1061.

Roddenberry JD, Balart LA, Regenstein FG et al (1991) Detection of hepatitis C viral RNA in liver tissue of chronic hepatitis C patients before and after treatment with interferon α-2b (abstract). *Hepatology* **14**: 75A.

Sàez-Royuela F, Porres JC, Moreno A et al (1991) High doses of recombinant alpha-interferon or gamma interferon for chronic hepatitis C: a randomized controlled trial. *Hepatology* **13**: 327–331.

Saracco G, Rosina F, Torrani Cerenzia MR et al (1990) A randomized controlled trial of interferon alfa-2b as therapy for chronic non-A, non-B hepatitis. *Journal of Hepatology* **11 (supplement 2)**: 43–49.

Schoeman MN, Liddle C, Bilous M et al (1990) Chronic non-A, non-B hepatitis: lack of correlation between biochemical and morphological activity, and effects of immunosuppressive therapy on disease progression. *Australian and New Zealand Journal of Medicine* **20**: 56–62.

Schvarcz R, Glaumann H, Weiland O et al (1991a) *Scandinavian Journal of Infectious Diseases* **23**: 413–420.

Schvarcz R, Glaumann H, Weiland O et al (1991b) Histological outcome in interferon alpha-2b treated patients with chronic posttransfusion non-A, non-B hepatitis. *Liver* **11**: 30–38.

Schvarcz R, Yun ZB, Sonnerborg A & Weiland O (1995) Combined treatment with interferon alpha-2b and ribavirin for chronic hepatitis C in patients with a previous non-response or non-sustained response to interferon alone. *Journal of Medical Virology* **46**: 43–47.

Seeff LB, Buskell-Bales Z, Wright EC et al (1992) Longterm mortality after transfusion-associated non-A, non-B hepatitis. *New England Journal of Medicine* **327**: 1906–1911.

Shindo M, Di Bisceglie AM, Cheung L et al (1991) Decrease in serum hepatitis C viral RNA during alpha-interferon therapy for chronic hepatitis C. *Annals of Internal Medicine* **115**: 700–704.

Simon DM, Gordon SC, Kaplan MM et al (1995) Natural alfa interferon (Alferon) treatment of chronic hepatitis C in previously untreated patients (abstract). *Hepatology* **22**: 151A.

Takahashi M, Yamada G, Miyamoto R et al (1993) Natural history of chronic hepatitis C. *American Journal of Gastroenterology* **88:** 240–243.

Tiné F, Magrin S, Craxi A & Pagliaro L (1991) Interferon for non-A, non-B chronic hepatitis: a meta-analysis of randomised clinical trials. *Journal of Hepatology* **13:** 192–199.

Tong MJ, Blatt LM, Resser K et al (1993) Treatment of patients with chronic HCV infection with a novel type-a interferon, concensus interferon (abstract). *Hepatology* **18:** 150A.

Tong MJ, El-Farra NS, Reikes AR & Co RL (1995) Clinical outcomes after transfusion-associated hepatitis C. *New England Journal of Medicine* **332:** 1463–1466.

Weiland O, Schvarcz R, Wejstal R et al (1990) Therapy of chronic post-transfusion non-A, non-B hepatitis with interferon alfa-2b: Swedish experience. *Journal of Hepatology* **11 (supplement 2):** 57–62.

8

New treatments for chronic viral hepatitis B and C

GEOFFREY M. DUSHEIKO

There are now six major viral hepatitides for which viruses have been isolated. These viruses have been given the nomenclature A, B, C, D, E and G /GBV-C. Hepatitis F has been tentatively reserved for a non-A to E virus associated with fulminant hepatitis. There are almost certainly other as yet unidentified viruses which may cause post-transfusion and fulminant hepatitis and perhaps chronic hepatitis and cirrhosis.

Hepatitis A virus and hepatitis E virus may lead to acute hepatitis. Although severe or prolonged illness can result from these viruses, hepatitis A and E generally cause a self-limited illness, and do not cause chronic hepatitis or cirrhosis. Effective antiviral therapy could be appropriate for severe and prolonged acute hepatitis A and E, but there are no agents of proven efficacy. Fulminant hepatitis A and E currently require liver transplantation. Similarly, fulminant hepatitis B and D require liver transplantation.

In contrast, chronic viral hepatitis caused by hepatitis B, C or D, and perhaps G/GBV-C, may lead to cirrhosis, hepatocellular failure and hepatocellular carcinoma. The morbidity of these diseases has necessitated an active and pro-longed search for effective therapy. Although a substantial number of antiviral compounds have been evaluated for the treatment of chronic viral hepatitis, few have achieved clinical applicability. Interferon-alpha has been widely studied, and remains the only licensed treatment. A number of other cytokines, and biological response modifiers, including thymosin, are being evaluated. Nucleoside analogues, alone or in combination with alpha interferon, may prove to be useful agents for the treatment of chronic hepatitis B and C.

Better animal and experimental models are required for test systems for the preliminary investigation of antiviral compounds in hepatitis B and C. The morbidity of hepatitis G (GBV-C) is not yet certain, but chronic viraemia can occur and the virus may be susceptible to interferon-alpha.

HEPATITIS B

Hepatitis B is caused by the hepatitis B virus (HBV), a large (42 nm) enveloped DNA virus that infects the liver, causing hepatocellular necrosis

Baillière's Clinical Gastroenterology—
Vol. 10, No. 2, July 1996
ISBN 0–7020–2094–X
0950–3528/96/020299 + 35 $12.00/00

299

Copyright © 1996, by Baillière Tindall
All rights of reproduction in any form reserved

and inflammation. The infection can be either acute or chronic, and can range from being an asymptomatic infection that resolves completely, to a severe, symptomatic infection with progressive and even fatal illness. Some patients with chronic hepatitis B have a spontaneous remission in disease, marked by disappearance of HBV DNA and HBeAg from serum with improvement in serum aminotransferases despite persistence of HBsAg. Measurement of serum HBV DNA in patients with chronic hepatitis B by polymerase chain reaction (PCR) demonstrates that the loss of HBeAg is associated with a decrease rather than complete clearance of HBV DNA in the serum (Kaneko et al, 1990). Other patients lose HBeAg, or are anti-HBe positive, yet continue to have active liver disease and HBV DNA detectable in serum by dot or blot hybridization techniques. These patients have been shown to be infected with replication competent HBV variants, and the absence of HBeAg expression is because of nucleotide substitution(s) in the pre-core region of the genome (Carman et al, 1989; Brunetto et al, 1990).

Most cases of acute symptomatic hepatitis B resolve with clearance of HBsAg and complete healing of the hepatic injury. Although non-specific symptoms may be improved, there is no evidence that antiviral therapy accelerates this healing or clearance of virus or that early treatment with interferon prevents the development of chronic disease.

Low levels of viral replication are found in patients with fulminant hepatitis B, suggesting that the pathogenesis of the disease is due to an exaggerated immune response to HBV (Figure 1). Interferon-alpha has not been found to be beneficial in fulminant hepatitis (Levin et al, 1989). Currently the optimal, albeit drastic therapy of fulminant hepatitis B is orthotopic liver transplantation, once prognostic factors indicate that survival is unlikely.

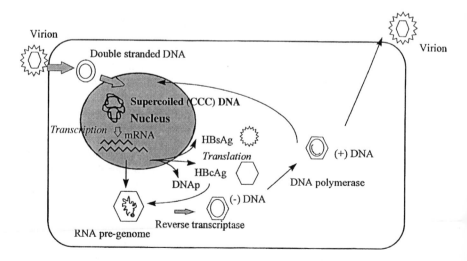

Figure 1. Replicative cycle of hepatitis B virus.

Interventional treatment of chronic hepatitis B is targeted at patients with active disease and viral replication, preferably at a stage before signs and symptoms of cirrhosis or significant injury have occurred. Eradication of the infection is possible in only a minority of patients. Permanent loss of HBV DNA and HBeAg is considered a response to antiviral treatment, as this result is associated with an improvement in necro-inflammatory damage, and reduced infectivity. It is possible, but unproven, that the accompanying reduction in histological chronic active hepatitis lessens the risk of cirrhosis and hepatocellular carcinoma. HBV DNA may still be detectable in serum and liver after loss of HBeAg and HBsAg induced by antiviral therapy, but this is often not associated with progressive disease (Marcellin et al, 1990b).

Therapeutic use of interferon-alpha in chronic hepatitis B

Alpha, beta and gamma interferons were recombinantly cloned and became available for therapeutic use after 1981, facilitating studies of treatment. Recombinant interferon-alpha has since been licensed for treatment of chronic hepatitis B in many countries. Response rates tend to be higher in carriers with higher base-line serum aminotransferase levels. The subclinical exacerbation of the hepatitis frequently seen in responders suggests that interferon acts by augmenting the immune response to HBV, perhaps triggered by the inhibition of viral replication as well as the effects of interferon on cytotoxic T cells. Although 35% of HBeAg-positive patients are effectively treated by this agent, interferon therapy has several drawbacks: the treatment is effective in less than half of cases of chronic hepatitis B, is relatively expensive, requires administration by injection, is often unpredictable in its effects, and is not without side-effects. Sustained loss of HBeAg is generally associated with histological reduction in inflammation (Brook et al, 1989b; Hope et al, 1995).

Although parameters that predict responsive patients are difficult to characterize fully, those carriers with elevated pre-treatment serum amino-transferase levels, with chronic active hepatitis, lower serum HBV DNA, females, those negative for anti-HIV, those with a history of hepatitis, Caucasians with more recent onset of this disease, with IgM anti-HBc may respond more favourably (Quiroga et al, 1988; Brook et al, 1989a). Although these factors provide some predictive information, none of these criteria is absolute. Specific mutations in the core protein that could interfere with T cell recognition may also preclude responsiveness to interferon (Fattovich et al, 1995; Naoumov et al, 1995). However, interferon may improve the long-term prognosis of chronic hepatitis B (Reichen et al, 1994).

Patients with anti-HBe-positive chronic hepatitis

Patients who are anti-HBe-positive but who have hepatitis B core antigen in hepatocytes and histological chronic active hepatitis due to infection with HBV pre-core mutants affecting the expression of HBeAg may have severe disease. In parts of Europe, and elsewhere, disease caused by this variant of hepatitis B is more common than disease caused by 'wild type' of HBeAg-positive chronic hepatitis. Approximately 10–25% of patients have long-term responses, as relapse rates tend to be high in these patients (Brunetto et al, 1989, 1995).

Children

Children who are infected perinatally, and have mild disease activity, respond poorly to interferon treatment (Lok et al, 1989; Milich et al, 1990). Children with active disease and high serum aminotransferases respond to interferon therapy similarly to adults and usually accept treatment reasonably well (Ruiz-Moreno et al, 1990; Kato et al, 1991). The appropriate dose of interferon in children is $5 \, MU/m^2$ s.c. three times weekly for 4 months.

Other groups with chronic hepatitis B

Patients with cirrhosis and ascites, encephalopathy or persistent jaundice from chronic hepatitis B have a dire prognosis without treatment, but are prone to developing multiple, serious side effects from higher (2–10 MU) of interferon-alpha, particularly bone marrow suppression, neutropenia and an increased incidence of serious bacterial infections (Liaw et al, 1991). Low doses of interferon (1–3 MU t.i.w.) could be considered in these patients (Rakela et al, 1990). The safety and efficacy of low dose, titratable interferon-alpha has been assessed in a recent trial (Perrillo et al, 1995).

Chronic hepatitis B is relatively common among patients on renal dialysis, patients with malignancies receiving chemotherapy and patients who have kidney, heart or liver transplants. Anecdotal experience suggests that interferon has little effect in patients with major immune deficiencies (Davis, 1989). Glomerulonephritis caused by chronic hepatitis B virus has been treated with recombinant interferon-alpha 2b (Lisker-Melman et al, 1989). In patients in whom HBeAg disappears and aminotransferases fall into the normal range, urine protein excretion also decreases and resolution of the glomerulonephritis occurs (Lin, 1995).

Patients who do not respond to therapy with interferon-alpha represent a difficult management problem. The prescription of interferon-alpha is also limited by the relatively high costs, but an economic evaluation of the costs of interferon-alpha for chronic hepatitis B suggests that some benefit can be obtained (Garcia de Ancos et al, 1990; Wong et al, 1995).

Other antiviral agents

Other antiviral therapies of chronic hepatitis B have been attempted, using a variety of agents. These agents, which have not proven useful, include the following:

Acyclovir (an acyclic analogue of deoxyguanosine, ACV), is a synthetic nucleoside analogue in which a linear side chain has been substituted for the cyclic sugar of the naturally occurring guanosine molecule. Acyclovir is converted intracellularly, and is phosphorylated to the active compound acyclovir triphosphate. Its antiviral activity is particularly effective against herpes simplex, because herpes viruses accelerate the phosphorylation of ACV in infected cells. The initial step in this conversion is facilitated by a virus-encoded thymidine kinase. ACV acts as a subtrate for, and is a modest inhibitor of, HBV DNA polymerase; however, HBV does not encode a thymidine kinase. Indeed, in two controlled studies, using ACV at a high dose, the drug appeared to have little effect. A pro-drug, 6-dexoxyacyclovir is completely absorbed by mouth, but appears to have little efficacy.

Foscarnet (trisodium phosphonoformate) is an inhibitor of DNA polymerase which has been shown to have activity against hepatitis B in vitro. Patients with fulminant and chronic hepatitis B have been treated intravenously with this drug, but the results do not suggest an important role for this agent in these diseases (Bain et al, 1989). Renal dysfunction may occur with continuous intravenous infusion, and the blood levels achieved are disappointing (Schvarcz et al, 1994).

Phyllanthus amarus. In a preliminary study, a high proportion of hepatitis B carriers (59%) treated with this plant extract lost HBsAg. Extracts of *Phyllanthus amarus* and species of the genus *Phyllanthus* (Euphorbiaceae) have since been tested for their efficacy as antivirals, and although these species have been shown to inhibit the DNA polymerase of HBV virus and hepatitis virus in vitro, the first striking results have not been confirmed (Blumberg et al, 1990; Unander et al, 1995). Although several species in China had a demonstrable antiviral effect (Wang et al, 1995), five species of an Australian *Phyllanthus* species, while able to inhibit endogenous HBV DNA polymerase activity, were unable to prevent or eliminate duck hepatitis B infection.

Adenine arabinoside is an analogue of adenine, and a potent inhibitor of hepatitis B virus DNA polymerase. Adenine arabinoside 5′-mono-phosphate, (ara-AMP) a water-soluble congener, can be administered intramuscularly. Suppression of HBV DNA has been demonstrated and clearance of HBeAg in 33% has been found in recent controlled trials. Usually 8 weeks of treatment is required to effect loss of HBeAg and HBV DNA, but, in many cases, serious neurotoxicity is seen after 4 weeks. A 28-day course suppresses HBV replication in patients with lower levels of replication (Marcellin et al, 1995). Although this drug is a potent inhibitor of hepatitis B virus, its future place as a single-agent therapy for chronic hepatitis B is uncertain. This drug may be effective in suppressing the disease activity and improving survival in patients with polyarteritis (Marcellin et al, 1989a).

Ara-AMP conjugated with lactosaminated albumin, a galactosyl terminating neoglycoprotein which selectively penetrates into hepatocytes by receptor mediated endocytosis, inhibits virus replication in patients with HBV infection, and in woodchucks with chronic WHV infection. Free and conjugated ara-AMP are active at doses of 10 and 0.75 mg/kg respectively Newer experiments in woodchucks using intramuscular injection resulted in marked inhibition of viraemia. Clinical trials with the intramuscular conjugate are now in progress (Fiume et al, 1995). This strategy may reduce the dose-related side effects. Ara -AMP coupled to high-molecular-mass lactosaminated poly-L-lysine and injected intramuscularly has a high molar ratio of drug to conjugate and is selectively taken up by the liver in mice after intramuscular administration (Fiume et al, 1994; Di Stefano et al, 1995).

Currently used antivirals and nucleoside analogues

Anti-retroviral therapies used in HIV infection have been attempted in chronic hepatitis B. Both of these viruses contain a reverse transcriptase. The functions of the viral polymerase include RNA-dependent DNA synthesis, and DNA-dependent DNA synthesis. This enzyme is a potential target for antiviral inhibition.

Initial experiments in hepatoblastoma cells transfected with hepatitis B (hepG2) suggested that $2',3'$-dideoxyguanosine (ddG), $2',3'$-dideoxy-inosine (ddI) and $3'$-azido-$2'$dideoxythymidine (AZT) diminished HBV replication by suppressing reverse transcription in the replicative cycle (Aoki-Sei et al, 1991). $2',3'$ dideoxycytidine (ddC) and $2',3'$-dideoxy-inosine (ddI) have also been investigated in animal and avian models of hepatitis B infection, and in pilot human studies. Inhibition of duck hepatitis B virus DNA in serum and liver has been demonstrated (Kassianides et al, 1989). However, the usefulness of all the 'first generation' nucleoside analogues in patients is limited. Zidovudine inhibits in vitro HBV DNA polymerase activity and reduces serum HBV DNA polymerase in patients with chronic hepatitis B at doses of 100–300 mg four times daily (Berk et al, 1992b). However, in a controlled trial of lymphoblastoid interferon (up to 5 MU daily plus zidovudine (1000 mg/day) only 8% of combination treatment patients versus 17% of interferon recipients lost HBeAg. Side-effects necessitating dose reductions were common in the recipients of both drugs. Other investigators have also failed to find an effect (Marcellin et al, 1989b). Phase I clinical trials of ddI using escalating doses of 3, 6 and 9 mg/kg/day for 3 months have not been encouraging (Fried et al, 1992). There was no appreciable change in HBV DNA levels during ddI therapy in five patients with both human immunodeficiency virus (HIV) and hepatitis B infection (Catterall et al, 1992).

Ganciclovir [9-[2-hydroxy-1-hydroxymethyl)ethoxymethyl]guanine] has been used to treat recurrence of hepatitis B after transplantation. This drug inhibits hepatitis B DNA but needs to be given intravenously, and replication re-ensues when treatment is stopped.

New nucleoside analogues

Fialuridine

Research development of this drug suffered a recent setback with reports of an unanticipated lethal toxicity with fialuridine (1-(2-deoxy-2-fluoro-beta-D-arabinofuranosyl)-5-iodouracil, or FIAU) at the NIH (a phase II study), using 0.1 mg/kg/day and 0.25 mg/kg/day. The trial was stopped in June, 1993, after 15 patients had been enrolled. Seven of the 15 patients developed severe liver toxicity, including hepatic failure with lactic acidosis, pancreatitis, myopathy and neuropathy. Of the seven patients with severe hepatotoxicity, five died and two survived after liver transplantation. Histological analysis of liver tissue revealed marked accumulation of microvesicular and macrovesicular fat, with minimal necrosis of hepatocytes or architectural changes. The lethal toxicity of the drug may be related to its incorporation into mitochondrial DNA (McKenzie et al, 1995).

The clinical course in the affected patients has been described. (McKenzie et al, 1995; Stevenson et al, 1995)

Famciclovir

Recent research efforts have resulted in the development of famciclovir (Figure 2), the oral precursor of penciclovir, a purine nucleoside (9-(4-hydroxy-3-hydroxymethylbut-1-yl)guanine; BRL 39123). Penciclovir is poorly absorbed orally, but famciclovir is readily absorbed and rapidly converted into the active molecule penciclovir by enzyme hydrolyisis; this conversion occurs partly in the intestinal wall. The residual ester group is removed in the liver, where oxidation of the purine at position 6 also occurs. Phosphorylation leads to the triphosphate compound and interference with synthesis of viral DNA; penciclovir triphosphate reduces varicella zoster

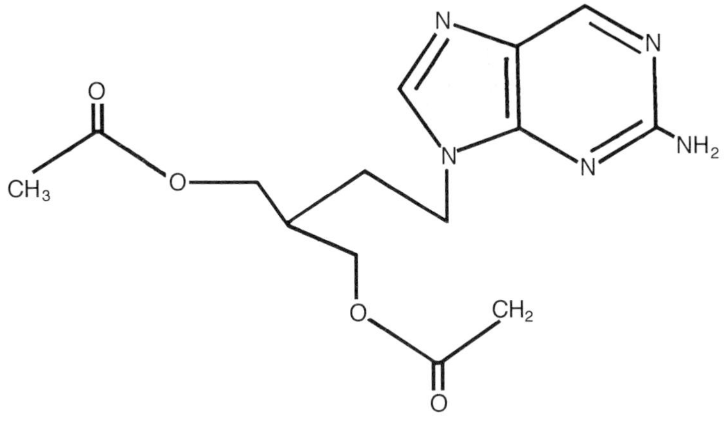

Figure 2. Structure of famciclovir.

and herpes simplex concentrations in cells, and oral famciclovir is an effective treatment of shingles.

The duck model was first used to assess this new agent for hepatitis B. Day-old ducklings hatched from eggs were administered famciclovir (25 mg/kg/b.d.) orally for periods of 1 to 12 days. Plasma levels of DHBV DNA were significantly reduced compared to levels in samples collected before treatment. DHBV DNA replicative intermediates in all the tissues examined were also reduced (Tsiquaye et al, 1994).

The effect of penciclovir been also been examined in primary duck hepatocyte cultures congenitally infected with DHBV. Penciclovir was more active than ganciclovir both during longer-term continuous treatment (50% inhibitory concentrations: penciclovir, 0.7 ± 0.1 μM: ganciclovir, 4.0 ± 0.2 μM) and in washout experiments (Shaw et al, 1994).

It is uncertain to what degree the drug is transformed to active metabolites in different infected tissues, including hepatocytes or bile duct cells. Famciclovir has been tested in a phase II trial in over 300 HBeAg and HBV DNA patients with chronic hepatitis B, using dosing schedules of 125, 250 and 500 mg three times daily for 16 weeks. The trial has been completed and the results will be published in 1996.

Lamivudine

$2',3'$-Dideoxy-$3'$-thiacytidine $((+)(-)$-SddC$)$ (3TC, lamivudine, Figure 3) is a potent inhibitor of human hepatitis B virus as well as human immuno-deficiency virus. The drug acts by inhibition of DNA synthesis through chain termination of the nascent pro-viral DNA.

The $(-)$ form $((-)$-SddC$)$, which is resistant to deoxycytidine deaminase, is more active as an antiviral stereoisomer than is the $(+)$-form. Unlike $2',3'$-dideoxycytidine, which is a potent inhibitor of mitochondrial DNA synthesis and results in delayed toxicity such as peripheral neuropathy with long-term usage, $(-)$-SddC does not appear to affect mitochondrial DNA synthesis. Metabolic studies have shown that the drug is converted to the monophosphate, diphosphate and triphosphate form. The $(-)$-form is phos-phorylated to $(-)$-SddCMP and is subsequently converted to $(-)$-SddCDP and $(-)$-SddCTP (Chang et al, 1992a).

The enzyme responsible for the formation of monophosphates has been identified as cytoplasmic deoxycytidine kinase. The selective inhibition of DNA synthesis in isolated mitochondria by $(+)$- and $(-)$- SddCTP suggests a stereospecificity on the mitochondrial uptake of deoxynucleoside tri-phosphates (Chang et al, 1992b). The drug is rapidly absorbed after oral administration, with a bioavailability of >80%. The majority of drug is excreted unchanged in the urine.

Since 1990, lamivudine has been used in trials of treatment of HIV infection, and this compound has recently been licensed for this disease in the USA. Better efficacy has been observed in combination therapy. Lamivudine is active in vitro against human hepatitis B transfected cell lines and in ducklings affected with duck hepatitis B virus, as well as in chimpanzees infected with hepatitis B virus.

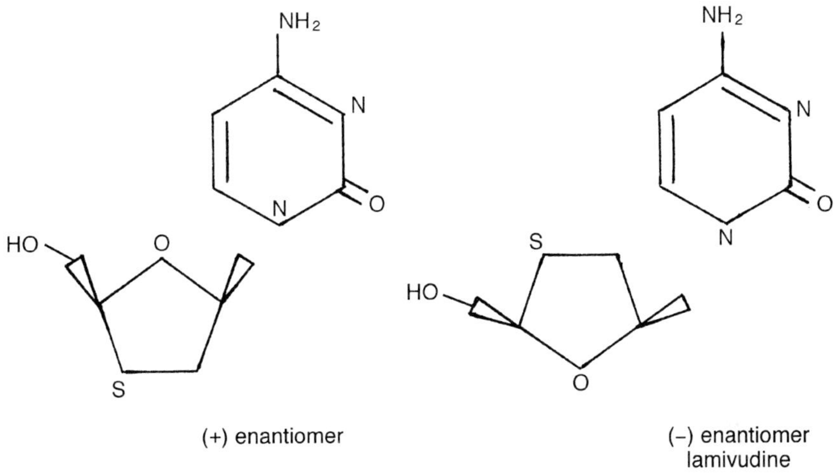

(+) enantiomer

(–) enantiomer
lamivudine

Figure 3. Structure of lamivudine.

Phase II and III studies in patients with chronic hepatitis B are in progress. In a preliminary trial, 75 patients with chronic hepatitis B were treated for 28 days with doses ranging from 5 to 600 mg/day. Doses above 5 mg reproducibly decreased HBV DNA levels in serum. Treatment has been extended to 12 weeks and 6 months, and over 200 patients have now been treated with lamivudine in dose-ranging studies with 5, 20, 100, 300 or 600 mg per day for 28 days, 12 weeks, 6, and now 12, months. The results of a randomized controlled trial have recently been published. Thirty-two patients were treated for 12 weeks. Levels of HBV DNA became undetectable (by Abbott liquid hybridization assay) in 70% of patients who received 25 mg, and 100% of those treated with 100 or 300 mg. In most patients, HBV DNA re-appeared after therapy was completed. Six patients (19%), including five who had not responded to interferon, had sustained suppression of HBV DNA, and HBeAg disappeared in four (12%). Sustained responses were more likely in patients with lower levels of HBV DNA or higher serum ALT levels. Only minor non-specific adverse events were seen that were not related to dose. Similar results have been observed after 6 months of treatment; a degree of histological improvement has been noted. HBV DNA has been undetectable at the end of treatment in approximately a quarter of patients treated for 6 months in a European study.

Patients with chronic hepatitis B are currently being treated for 1 year with combinations of lamivudine and interferon-alpha, or lamivudine only, in controlled trials.

The drug appears to be well tolerated, and relatively few serious side-effects have been reported. Serious side-effects have been observed in about 5% of patients; these include anaemia, neutropenia, an increase in liver enzymes, nausea and neuropathy. Increased lipases may occur, but uncommonly, and serious lactic acidosis has not been observed. More HIV-positive patients have been treated for longer than 6 months. The maximum duration of treatment has been 24 months. To date, over 170 paediatric patients (with HIV infection) have been treated.

Severe exacerbations of hepatitis accompanied by jaundice have been reported in patients whose HBV DNA became positive after stopping treatment (Honkoop et al, 1995). The preliminary results of treatment of patients to prevent recurrence of hepatitis B after liver transplantation are discussed below.

These data suggest that the most promising nucleoside analogues being assessed in clinical trials for hepatitis B are lamivudine and famciclovir. However, it is likely that in the absence of immune clearance to accelerate elimination of infected hepatocytes, inhibitors of virus replication would have to be administered for a long period to reduce substantially the burden of infected hepatocytes in the liver, and prevent relapse; at this time their long-term efficacy and safety is unproven: chronic type B hepatitis disease will require relatively long courses of treatment, often in asymptomatic carriers, including children, and viral resistance may emerge (as has been observed in immunosuppressed patients). The end points of treatment will require careful evaluation. There are several methods for testing HBV DNA, including hybridization and PCR methods and the sensitivity, analytical detection limits, dynamic range and standardization for determining antiviral effect need to be clarified (Hendricks et al, 1995).

Biological response modifiers

Gamma interferon

The pharmacokinetics, tolerance and anti-viral effect of human recombinant interferon-gamma have been studied in patients with chronic active hepatitis B, but most studies suggest that the antiviral effect of interferon-gamma is less than that of interferon-alpha (Di Bisceglie et al, 1990; Marcellin et al, 1990a; Lau et al, 1991).

Interferon-beta

Trials are in progress with this agent.

Levamizole

Levamizole, an anti-helminthic, has been claimed to inhibit HBV replication in up to 60% of patients (Fattovich et al, 1986). However, the initial good results have not proved reproducible. A combined trial of lympho-blastoid interferon (5 MU/m² plus levamizole (150 mg three times per week) revealed a higher response rate (38%) in patients treated with interferon alone compared to those treated with the combination (10%). Thus, levamizole has no added benefit when combined with interferon-alpha (Fattovich et al, 1992).

Isoprinosine (a molecular complex of inosine: 2-hydroxypropyldimethyl-ammonium 4-acetamidobenzoate 1:3), a compound with antiviral and immunoregulatory activity, has been reported to induce seroconversion in 43% of HBeAg-positive patients in a relatively small trial (Par et al, 1989).

Interleukin-2

Patients have been treated with 28 days with 15 fg of recombinant IL-2 intravenously. Some transient inhibition of HBV DNA polymerase was observed. The usefulness of IL-2 may be further explored, as the compound increases lymphocyte counts and CD4 cells (Onji et al, 1987; Minuk and LaFreniere, 1988; Yamaguchi et al, 1988; Bach et al, 1989).

Interleukin-12

Interleukin-12 is a 75 kDa heterodimeric protein and a member of the TNF receptor superfamily. This cytokine is a product of macrophages and dendritic cells, i.e. antigen-presenting cells. Interleukin (IL)-12 promotes Th-1 and suppresses Th-2 cell development, suggesting that IL-12 may be useful therapeutically to promote a cellular immune response. The compound induces secretion of interferon-gamma from T and natural killer cells, and increases the lytic activity of NK cells and facilitates specific CTL responses. In experimental mouse virus models of acute viral infections, IL-12 reduces morbidity and prevents re-infection to HSV-2 and CMV. The effect of systemic IL-12 treatment on in vivo autoantibody synthesis in hepatitis B e antigen (HBeAg)-expressing transgenic mice has been tested. Low-dose IL-12 significantly inhibited autoantibody (anti-HBe) production by shifting the Th-2-mediated response toward Th-1 predominance.

Additionally, previous studies suggest that a predominance of HBeAg-specific Th-2-type cells may contribute to chronicity in hepatitis B virus infection. Therefore, IL-12 may also prove beneficial in modulating the antibody and cellular immune response in hepatitis B to improve clearance of hepatitis B (Milich et al, 1995). It has been shown that suppression of intrahepatic replication of HBV DNA in transgenic mice is mediated through cytokines such as interferon-gamma and TNF. Pilot studies in humans with hepatitis B infection have begun. In experimental animals, fever, lethargy, anorexia, anaemia, thrombocytopenia, stomatitis, pulmonary oedema and increased serum ALT have been observed. IL-12 can also aggravate autoimmune processes, and deaths in patients with renal carcinoma have been observed.

Thymopentin

A randomized, controlled trial has been performed to to assess the safety and efficacy of thymopentin therapy in 30 patients with chronic hepatitis B.

At the conclusion of the study (1 year), HBV DNA was negative and alanine aminotransferase had normalized in 13 and 20% of treated cases and in 20 and 27% of controls. None of the ten treated and one of the nine control patients who were initially HBeAg positive subsequently cleared HBeAg. The results are not encouraging (Fattovich et al, 1994).

Thymosin

This is an immune stimulant which is known to enhance suppressor T cell activity and in vitro B cell synthesis of IgG. Peptide preparations of thymosin have been evaluated in small controlled trials, and HBV DNA has been noted to become negative in some of these patients in chimpanzees with chronic hepatitis B (Mutchnick et al, 1991). It is given parenterally by subcutaneous injection. This interesting agent's possible therapeutic role has been evaluated in a larger controlled trial in which HBeAg sero-conversion rates were not significantly different from those of placebo recipients. The place of this drug is still being appraised as few side-effects are observed with thymosin injected subcutaneously.

Polyadenylic polyuridylic acid [poly(A) × poly(U)]

In a small trial, this compound normalized elevated ALT levels and induced loss of HBeAg in 11/19 patients (57.9%) and loss of HBV DNA in 12 out of 19 patients (63.1%) (Hahm et al, 1994).

GM-CSF

Recombinant human granulocyte–macrophage colony-stimulating factor therapy reduced serum hepatitis B virus DNA levels in nine patients with chronic hepatitis B. The effect of this compound may be to alter immune function and enhance cytokine production (Martín et al, 1994).

Colchicine

Colchicine does not improve the cumulative survival rates in patients with chronic hepatitis B (Wang et al, 1994).

Combination therapies

Pulsed corticosteroid treatment and interferon

A multi-centre trial comparing the efficacy of prednisolone withdrawal plus interferon (alpha 2b) to interferon alone (5 MU daily to 16 weeks) has not shown an added benefit of corticosteroids plus interferon: 38% of patients in both groups lost HBeAg, and 12% and 10%, respectively, lost HBsAg (Perrillo et al, 1990). However, the response rates with combined treatment were better than for IFN alone in those patients with pre-treatment serum ALT less than 100 IU/l (44 versus 18%). These data could mean that 'unprimed' carriers, with inactive disease, are poorly responsive. Carriers with lower concentrations of HBV DNA (< 100 pg/ml) were also more likely to respond to treatment.

Treatment with prednisolone followed by interferon-alpha appeared safe and effective in inducing stable clearance of HBeAg and, in some cases, HBsAg in *children* with chronic hepatitis B with a low level of viral replication (Krogsgaard, 1994; Utili et al, 1994). It is also suggested that prednisolone withdrawal followed by interferon therapy is effective and safe in Chinese patients with chronic hepatitis B, particularly those with lower pre-treatment serum ALT and hepatitis B DNA levels (Liaw et al, 1994).

The treatment is still used, and a meta-analysis of this form of treatment indicates the potential benefit of prednisolone interferon combination (Cohard et al, 1994). A disadvantage of this treatment is the increase in production of HBsAg associated with corticosteroid treatment (Mabit et al, 1994). This treatment regimen should be used with decompensated hepatitis B because of the risk of inducing severe hepatic necrosis.

Interferon-gamma and interferon-alpha

In eight patients treated with a combination of interferon-gamma and -alpha, interferon-gamma alone had minimal inhibitory effects upon serum levels of hepatitis B virus DNA. Troublesome side-effects were also encountered. In contrast, a more potent antiviral effect was found with interferon-alpha, which had fewer side-effects. When combined, the two interferons showed little synergistic effect in inhibiting HBV DNA (Di Bisceglie et al, 1990).

Interferon-gamma and interferon-beta

Interferon-gamma has a greater immune modulating effect, but a less potent antiviral effect. A recent study of interferon-gamma and -beta treatment of 20 patients with chronic hepatitis B was successful in reducing viraemia in 5 of 10 patients treated for 23 days. The interferon-beta was given intravenously, and the interferon-gamma subcutaneously (Caselmann et al, 1989).

Acyclovir and interferon-alpha

An initial pilot study showed that this combination was efficacious in eradicating HBV DNA. In a subsequent controlled study, clearance of HBeAg in patients treated with acyclovir and lymphoblastoid interferon was not greater than that observed with interferon alone (Berk et al, 1992a).

Steroid withdrawal and acyclovir

A relatively high HBeAg seroconversion rate has been observed in patients treated with this regimen (Minuk et al, 1992).

Indomethacin and interferon

In 1991 Hannigan and Williams (Heinrich and Maier, 1995) described a synergistic signal transduction effect in human fibroblasts after exposure to interferon. Inhibition of the arachidonic acid (AA) oxidation pathways by addition of inhibitors of the enzymes involved, for example indomethacin, results in marked amplification of the interferon signal. This could theoretically improve the efficacy of interferon therapy (acetyl salicylic acid, a cyclo-oxygenase inhibitor, does not improve hepatitis C) (Heinrich and Maier, 1995).

Interferon and thymus humoral factor gamma 2

A small trial of this combination indicated that HBV DNA levels were reduced compared to previous treatment with interferon alone. The agent has functional effects upon T lymphocytes. Few side-effects were observed (Farhat et al, 1995).

Experimental systems for studying new antivirals

Human hepatitis B virus is a member of the family of hepadnaviridiae, affecting woodchucks, duck, ground squirrels and humans. These viruses share a similar hepatotropism, propensity to chronic infection and genome organization and replication strategy. It has become possible to study the effect of a variety of antiviral compounds in ducks and woodchucks affected with duck hepatitis B (DHBV) and woodchuck hepatitis B (WHV) respectively, and to develop experimental systems for drug screening. Using these models, a number of new compounds, particularly new nucleoside analogues, have been tested and formulated. Some of these compounds appear to inhibit HBV and may prove useful clinically (Dusheiko and Zuckerman, 1991).

Inhibition of duck HBV replication in vivo

The effect of nucleoside analogues, acting as reverse transcriptase inhibitors or chain terminators, has been studied, particularly in ducks. Ganciclovir [9-[2-hydroxy-1-(hydroxymethyl)ethoxymethyl]guanine] and nalidixic acid, either alone or in combination, have an effect on duck hepatitis B virus DNA replication in vivo in ducks; viral supercoiled DNA and RNA are suppressed (Wang et al, 1995). However, of the viral replicative forms, supercoiled DNA is the most resistant to treatment and returns to base-line levels within days of stopping treatment (Dean et al, 1995).

Primary duck hepatocyte cultures

Primary duck hepatocyte cultures from ducks congenitally infected with duck hepatitis B virus have proven a useful in vitro system for detecting compounds with recognized or potential anti-viral activity (Bishop et al, 1990). Compounds with potential antiviral activity have included agents with reverse transcriptase inhibitory activity and activity against super-coiled DNA, and DNA-binding agents. Conventional antivirals which inhibit duck HBV DNA replication include ganciclovir, acyclovir, riba-virin, phosphonoformate and dideoxyadenosine. These do not generally significantly inhibit DHBsAg production. Novobiocin and nalidixic acid act at the level of supercoiled DNA and significantly inhibit the production of duck HBsAg (Civitico et al, 1990a). Because supercoiled DNA may be the template from which re-activation of hepatitis B virus occurs after transient inhibition by antiviral agents, these compounds may merit further study in humans (Civitico et al, 1990b).

The carbocyclic analogue of 2'-deoxyguanosine (2'-CDG) is a strong inhibitor of hepatitis B virus (HBV) DNA synthesis in primary cultures of duck hepatocytes and experimentally infected ducks. The compound failed to inhibit the DNA repair reaction that occurs during the initiation of infection which converts virion relaxed circular DNA to covalently closed circular DNA (the template for viral mRNA transcription). The drug can be orally administered to ducklings (Fourel et al, 1994b; Mason et al, 1994).

A cell culture system for the evaluation of compounds which inhibit HBV replication has been developed into a standardized assay in which toxicity of test compounds can be assessed by the uptake of neutral red dye under culture and treatment conditions identical to those used for the anti-viral assays. Activities of several 2'-substituted and 3'-substituted deoxy-nucleoside analogues against HBV replication have been compared using this standardized assay. Several 2'-fluorinated pyrimidine arabinosyl furanosides, reported to be potent (but toxic) inhibitors of hepadnaviruses in vivo, demonstrated relatively low selective antiviral activities in 2.2.15 cells (Korba and Gerin, 1992).

Transient expression systems

Transient expression systems achieved by transfection of human hepato-blastoma (Hep G2 cells) with HBV DNA have been used. HBV has been inhibited by co-transfection with poly(I):poly(C). This effect may be achieved by intracellular induction of interferon-alpha in Hep G2 cells and selective inhibition of HBV gene expression. Interferon inhibition of hepatitis B replication has been found by analysing the effect of interferons on the transcription of a chloramphenicol acetyltransferase reporter gene under the control of HBV regulatory sequences in permanently HBV transfected Hep G2 cells (Tur-Kaspa et al, 1990). Other investigators have suggested that interferon inhibits HBV replication in transfected cells by blocking a step in the pre-genome RNA primed assembly of core particles.

Inhibition in vitro

The inhibitory effects of selected compounds on the RNA polymerase (reverse transcriptase) and DNA-dependent DNA polymerase activity of duck hepatitis B virus have been investigated (Lofgren et al, 1989; Yokota et al, 1990). HBV from serum has been used as a source of the polymerase activity in these experiments. Marked inhibition has been obtained with 3-fluoro-2′,3′-dideoxythymidine-5′-triphosphate, 2′,3′-dideoxyguanosine-5′-triphosphate and 2′,3′-dideoxythymidine-5′-triphosphate. Among tested pyrophosphate analogues only phosphonoformate was inhibitory.

New experimental nucleoside analogues with activity against hepatitis B virus

The in vitro and in vivo antiviral effects of new purine and pyrimidine 2′,3′-dideoxynucleosides on duck hepatitis B virus have been compared. Several purine 2′,3′-dideoxynucleosides are potent inhibitors of HBV, and rapid clearance of hepadnavirus DNA has been observed with 2,6-diamino-purine-2′,3′-dideoxyriboside at a dose of 10 mg/kg i.m. twice daily (Lee et al, 1989).

Several other analogues have been tested for their potential antiviral activity in vitro using the human hepatoblastoma cell line, Hep G2 2.2.15, transfected with a vector containing hepatitis B virus (HBV). 2′,3′-Dideoxy-3′-fluorothymidine (FddThd), 2′,3′-dideoxy-3′-fluoro-5-methyl-cytidine (FddMeCyt), 2′,3′-dideoxy-3′-fluoro-5-ethylcytidine (FddEtCyt) and other analogues display cytostatic activity at concentrations (CD50 values) between 0.54 (FddMeCyt) and 3.93 µM (FddEtCyt). Of these, FddThd is the most effective antiviral agent: at a concentration of 0.03 µM a more than 90% reduction of HBV DNA synthesis was measured. The most powerful antiviral agents in a group of cytidine analogues tested in vitro were FddMeCyt (more than 90% reduction of HBV DNA synthesis at 0.10 µM) and ClddMeCyt (0.10 µM); FddThd and FddMeCyt were also effective against duck HBV in vivo. Administration of FddThd and FddMeCyt to ducks infected with DHBV for 12 days blocked virus pro-duction. Termination of treatment with FddThd of infected animals led to the re-appearance of the virus in the serum though at lower levels (Matthes et al, 1992).

Synthesis of enantiomerically pure (2′R,5′S)-(−)-1-[2-(hydroxymethyl) oxathiolan-5-yl]cytosine has been accomplished. This isomer exhibits potent anti-HIV and anti-HBV activities (Beach et al, 1992). The anti-hepatitis B (anti-HBV) activities of the (−) and (+) enantiomers of cis-5-fluoro-1-[2-(hydroxy-methyl)-1,3-oxathiolan-5-yl]cytosine (2′-deoxy-3′-thia-5-fluorocytosine [FTC]) have been studied using HepG2 derivative cells. The (−) isomer was found to be a potent inhibitor of viral replication, with an apparent 50% inhibitory concentration of 10 nM, while the (+) isomer was found to be considerably less active. Both isomers showed minimal toxicity to Hep G2 cells and showed minimal toxicity in the human bone marrow progenitor cell assay. The 5′-triphosphate of (−)-FTC also inhibited viral DNA synthesis in an endogenous HBV DNA polymerase assay, while the 5′-triphosphate of the (+) isomer was inactive. Both (−)- and (+)-FTC are anabolized to the corresponding 5′-triphosphates in chronically HBV-infected Hep G2 cells. (−)-FTC is not a substrate for cytidine deaminase and, therefore, is not subject to deamination and conversion to an inactive uridine analogue. The (+) isomer is, however, a good substrate for cytidine deaminase (Furman et al, 1992). The super-coiled form of liver viral DNA was found to be less affected by the therapy (Fourel et al, 1992).

The nucleoside analogue 2,4-diamino-7-(2-deoxy-2-fluoro-beta-D-arabinofuranosyl)pyrrolo[2,3-d]pyrimidine (T70080) and several related compounds have been assessed in cultured 2.2.15 cells. T70080 reduced episomal viral replication in these cells by 50% (Ojwang et al, 1995).

Accelerated hepatocyte turnover enhances the rapid clearance of infected hepatocytes in ducks induced by by 2'-deoxycarbocyclic guanosine (2'-CDG). The same effect on viral clearance was not seen with 5-fluoro-2',3'-dideoxy-3'-thiacytidine (524W), which did not accelerate hepatocyte turnover in ducks. Thus, liver injury is correlated with hepatocyte turnover and clearance of infected hepatocytes (Fourel et al, 1994a).

Other agents

The effects on duck hepatitis B virus (DHBV) replication of specific analogues of two classes of chemical compound not previously tested against hepadnaviruses have been described: erythromycin A-9-methyl-oxime (EMO) and other oxime derivatives of erythromycin A, and purine nucleoside analogues (cyclobut A and cyclobut G) with cyclobutane rings.

Immunotherapy

There has been a resurgence of interest in the possibility of successfully immunizing chronically infected hepatitis B-positive patients to activate an immune response and eradicate viraemia (Figure 4). A recent pilot study to immunize 32 patients with HBeAg-positive, HBV DNA-positive chronic hepatitis B with three standard doses of *GenHevac vaccine* at monthly intervals. Six months after the first injection, 37% had undetectable DNA. Eight responders were given interferon-alpha to maintain viral inhibition (Pol et al, 1994; Pol, 1995). These results require explanation, as earlier

- *Interferon alpha*
- *Steroid priming and interferon alpha*
- Thymosin
- GM-CSF
- Interleukins: IL-2, IL-12
- TNF
- Tucaresol
- *HBIg (prophylaxis post transplantation)*
- Hepatitis B vaccination: HBsAg, HBcAg
- Bone marrow transplantation
- Activated autologous lymphocytes

Figure 4. Immunotherapies: hepatitis B.

trials of HBsAg vaccination had no demonstrable efficacy. The effects may be the result of altered antigen presentation. A larger controlled trial is currently in progress.

There is considerable interest in the possibility of provoking a cytotoxic immune response to HBV core epitopes, as the CTL response contributes to viral clearance in acute hepatitis B. A strong cytotoxic T cell response has been observed in HLA A2.1 individuals with acute hepatitis B against an epitope (FLPSDFFPSV) that contains an HLA A2-binding motif located between residues 18 and 27 of the hepatitis B nucleocapsid protein (Bertoletti et al, 1993). This identification has led to development of a therapeutic vaccine (*Theradigm HBV*®) which is now undergoing assessment (Bertoletti et al, 1993).

Recently, DNA-based immunization, using purified plasmid DNA, containing protein coding sequences and the necessary regulatory elements to express them, has been tested. The DNA is introduced into tissues of the organism by means of a parenteral injection; the number of cells transfected and the amount of protein produced is sufficient to produce a broad-based immune response to a wide variety of foreign proteins. A response to HBsAg has been achieved using this form of antigen presentation. A CD8⁺ CTL response has been induced in BALB/c mice, suggesting a pathway for exogenous presentation of hepatitis B envelope protein for class I expression (Davis et al, 1995). If the safety of DNA-mediated immunization can be assured, then this form of vaccination may also have therapeutic potential (Whalen and Davis, 1995).

Solid matrix–antigen–antibody complexes were able to clear viraemia in persistent duck infection. In these experiments rabbit anti-duck HBs complexed to a solid matrix (*Staphylococcus aureus*) with purified duck HBsAg bound to this matrix was used as an immunogen (Wen et al, 1994).

Intravenous immunoglobulin has been reported to benefit a patient with polyarteritis nodosa associated with hepatitis B (Boman et al, 1995). Hepatitis B immune globulin (HBIg) has been effective in post-exposure prophylaxis; the treatment of ongoing disease is more problematical, as hepatitis B infection is characterized by high levels of circulating HBsAg, requiring large amounts of antibody for neutralization. *Monoclonal antibodies* with specificity to *a* determin*ants* are being assessed. Small pilot studies have indicated that extrahepatic HBsAg can decline and that HBV DNA levels decrease as hepatocytes are not re-infected. The acute and chronic immunological effects of immune complexes will need careful monitoring.

Variants can appear during monoclonal antibody prophylaxis of hepatitis B following liver transplantation.

Bone marrow transplantation

Adoptive transfer of immunity to hepatitis B has been observed in recipients of bone marrow from immune or immunized HBV donors. Clearance of replicating virus has been observed, and immunity has been induced after i.v. injection of peripheral blood lymphocytes from immunized donors. The duration of this effect is uncertain however, as HBsAg may re-appear after recurrence of leukaemia (Ilan et al, 1993, 1994).

Molecular therapy, hormonal and targeted therapies

Molecular approaches to the therapy of hepatitis B are possible means of inhibiting hepatitis B. These experimental approaches have included the use of a synthetic oligodeoxynucleotide coding for three ribozyme motifs directed against three adjacent sites within the pre-genomic RNA (Figure 5). Experiments utilizing 5′ and 3′ end labelling of RNA have demonstrated that these three ribozymes accurately cleaved hepatitis B virus substrate RNA (von Weizsäcker et al, 1992).

Antisense oligodeoxyribonucleotides may inhibit the expression of the gene for hepatitis B virus surface antigen (Goodarzi et al, 1990), and experiments in ducks and HBV infected cell lines have been completed.

M13 bacteriophage DNA, *E. coli* DNA or PhIX 174 phage DNA injected intravenously causes a significant decrease in serum duck hepatitis B virus DNA. The efficacy has been reported to be twice that reported with antisense DNA. On treatment with M13 DNA serum 25A oligoadenylate synthetase levels were increased, suggesting that the antiviral effect of M13 DNA is at least in part due to induction of endogenous interferon (Iizuka et al, 1994). Our own experiments indicate that liposomes may target antisense oligonucleotides to hepatocytes, but that the inhibition of duck hepatitis B is not antisense-specific.

Chylomicrons transport dietary lipids to hepatocytes via apolipoprotein E specific receptors; recombinant chylomicrons have been used, too, for selective targeting of a nucleoside antiviral agent to achieve effective intracellular concentrations (Rensen et al, 1995).

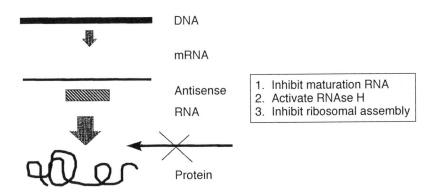

DNA

mRNA

Antisense
RNA

1. Inhibit maturation RNA
2. Activate RNAse H
3. Inhibit ribosomal assembly

Protein

Figure 5. Anti-sense oligonucleotides: interference with viral replication.

Antiviral therapy in liver transplantation for hepatitis B

The major shortcoming of liver transplantation as a treatment of chronic hepatitis is that re-infection of the engrafted liver and subsequent development of chronic hepatitis B commonly occurs. In HBsAg- and HBV DNA-positive carriers, HBsAg may initially disappear from the serum, only to almost invariably re-appear at 1 to 6 months after transplantation. The recurrent hepatitis can be severe and is almost invariably chronic. A proportion of patients who lack HBV DNA in serum (especially those with delta hepatitis) do not become re-infected. Immunosuppression, particularly with the drugs prednisolone and azathioprine, increase concentrations of HBsAg after transplantation (McMillan et al, 1995).

The most commonly used method for preventing re-infection has been the use of high doses of hepatitis B immune globulin (HBIg). This strategy may be effective in up to 40%. Unfortunately, most evidence indicates that HBIg delays but does not prevent recurrence (Kos et al, 1991; Lake and Wright, 1991; Martin et al, 1991). Furthermore, HBIg is expensive, and the duration of treatment has not been established. A human monoclonal anti-HBs has been reported to be more effective in HBIg in preventing recurrent hepatitis B in a small number of patients but such preparations are not widely available. The emergence of an antibody escape mutant of HBV lacking the a determinant of HBsAg has also been observed in such patients. Treatment with interferon-alpha has also been used at or around the time of transplantation to prevent recurrence of hepatitis B, but again without significant success, except perhaps in those who become PCR-negative prior to transplantation. It is unlikely that interferon-alpha will prove useful for immunosuppressed patients (Marcellin et al, 1994).

Pre- and post-transplant treatment with lamivudine results in rapid suppression of HBV DNA prior to transplant, and clearance of HBsAg following treatment in a high proportion of patients. We have observed loss of HBsAg in 90% to date of 10 surviving patients after liver transplantation, in whom lamivudine was given for at least 1 month prior to transplant, and for a year afterwards. The drug may prevent re-infection of the liver, but it is not yet certain whether hepatitis B re-activation will occur after treatment is stopped. Depression and suicide occurred in one patient, and a neuropathy occurred in a diabetic patient. We have also observed re-activation of hepatitis B in two immunosuppressed patients who developed a methionine-to-valine or isoleucine substitution in the YMDD motif of the HBV polymerase (Ling et al, unpublished). The initial results are encouraging.

Post-transplant recurrence

Famciclovir has been shown to reduce levels of HBV DNA in patients with hepatitis B recurrence after transplant, and to improve hepatic histology in responsive patients (Kruger et al, 1995). Ganciclovir (10 mg/kg/day) intravenously has been used for a 21-day period in patients in whom HBV recurred post-transplant. After 21 days of treatment, HBV DNA levels were significantly reduced in patients. The drug has been quite well tolerated with no significant adverse events. However, 3 months post-treatment, HBV DNA concentrations were again raised in patients (Gish et al, 1996).

HEPATITIS C

A viral agent responsible for most cases of post-transfusion hepatitis was recognized after serological tests for hepatitis A and hepatitis B viruses became available in 1974 (Feinstone et al, 1975). Several isolates of hepatitis C have been cloned. The sequence divergence of these isolates indicates that that are several major genotypes (serotypes) of hepatitis C, and component subtypes (Chan et al, 1991; McOmish et al, 1993). Geographical localization of these types has been reported. A standardized typing system or nomenclature has not been accepted at the time of writing.

The natural history of the disease is uncertain; the virus has a disturbing propensity to cause chronic infection, and it is believed that 10–20% of patients with chronic hepatitis C infections will progress to cirrhosis within a decade. The risk of further progression is probably cumulative, but is influenced by other cofactors which include viral genotype, level of viraemia, other viral infection, immunosuppression, age of acquisition, alcohol and perhaps parasitic disease. The infection causes systemic disease, and may be associated with a number of systemic complications, including a form of autoimmune hepatitis, cryoglobulinaemia, porphyria cutanea tarda, lymphocytic sialadinitis and membranous glomerulonephritis.

Interferons

Large therapeutic trials of interferon-alpha have been undertaken (discussed elsewhere in this volume). Preliminary therapeutic trials of interferon-alpha indicated that a proportion of patients may respond to treatment with this agent. Larger, placebo-controlled studies have indicated that approximately 50% of patients will have normal serum aminotransferases after treatment courses of interferon-alpha of approximately 3 million units three times a week for six months (Davis et al, 1989; Di Bisceglie et al, 1989).

However, after stopping treatment after 6 months, one-half of the responsive patients will promptly relapse. Our studies at the Royal Free Hospital indicate that 20% of patients have a prolonged response to therapy and do not again develop elevated serum aminotransferases (Varagona et al, 1992). Unfortunately, responsiveness to interferon-alpha remains somewhat unpredictable. Some differences in response rates have been observed in patients with different genotypes and levels of viraemia, emphasizing that there are a number of factors which appear to predict response. These have been well studied but suggested that selection of patients will be important for outcome.

Ribavirin

Ribavirin is a synthetic guanosine nucleotide analogue which possesses a broad spectrum of activity against both DNA and RNA viruses in vitro and in vivo (Fernandez et al, 1986). Efficacy has been demonstrated in several viral diseases. The drug exerts its action after intracellular phosphorylation to mono-, di- and triphosphate nucleotides. The precise mode of action probably includes perturbation of intracellular nucleoside triphosphate pools; interference with the formation of the 5′ cap structure of viral mRNA by competitive inhibition of both guanyltransferase and methyltransferase capping enzymes, direct inhibition of the viral mRNA polymerase complex, and possibly enhancement of macrophage inhibition of viral replication.

The pharmacokinetics of ribavirin have been studied. The bioavailability of oral formulations has been calculated at 19–65% (compared with i.v. administration). The distribution half-life is 1–3 hours, but the terminal half-life is prolonged (27–52 hours) perhaps due to sequestration within red cells and other tissues. Ribavirin is concentrated by a factor of 10–50 in red blood cells, and crosses the blood–brain barrier. Peak plasma levels range from 5 to 13 μM after single oral doses of 600–2400 mg. The excretion of the drug is predominantly renal.

The major side-effects of the drug that have been reported include anaemia, a metallic taste, dry mouth, flatulence, dyspepsia, nausea, headaches, irritability, emotional lability, fatigue, insomnia, skin rashes and myalgia. Mild reversible anaemia is common. Modest increases in uric acid have been reported.

Tong treated 22 patients with chronic hepatitis NANB with ribavirin 1200 mg daily for 4 weeks; although the details are not published, ALT and AST declined from a median of 145 to 78 and 86 to 52 IU respectively. After 4–8 weeks follow up, median levels of both ALT and AST had increased to pre-treatment levels. In an open-label study in Sweden, in which ribavirin was prescribed to 10 patients with chronic hepatitis C (1000–1200 mg/day) for 12 weeks, the median serum AST levels declined, but rose to pre-treatment levels upon completion (Reichard et al, 1991). A small study, using escalating doses of ribavirin (600–1200 mg) showed a somewhat slower fall in serum aminotransferases, perhaps reflecting the lower starting dose of ribavirin (Di Bisceglie et al, 1992). There was a significant decrease in geometric mean titres of HCV RNA. Several placebo-controlled trials have indicated that, despite the significant improvement in serum ALT, a marked decline in serum HCV concentrations does not occur. Most patients relapse when therapy is stopped.

Serum aminotransferases can be remain normal if therapy is prolonged and histological improvement has been observed in these patients. Thus, although ribavirin does not eradicate virus from the liver or peripheral blood mononuclear cells, it may be possible to use the drug in a selected group of patients for whom interferon is contraindicated. The effect on survival or disease progression with this strategy has not been proven however. Some patients may actually worsen on treatment with interferon, and develop increased serum aminotransferases. It is possible that such patients have an underlying autoimmune status associated with hepatitis C and exacerbated by interferon treatment. For such patients, and for patients who do not respond to treatment, ribavirin may be an alternative (Reichard et al, 1991).

Ursodeoxycolic acid (UCDA)

The affect of ursodeoxycolic acid on ALT has been investigated in multi-centre randomized controlled trials in patients with chronic hepatitis C. Doses have ranged from 150 to 900 mg/day. ALT values tend to decrease along with the change in composition of the bile. Serum aminotransferases decreased in those cases in which the hydrophobicity index decreased during treatment (Takano et al, 1994).

Combination therapy

Ribavirin and interferon

Relatively small pilot studies have been undertaken to assess the effect of ribavirin and interferon-alpha versus interferon-alpha alone. For example, in one study, interferon-alpha 2b given subcutaneously at a dose of 3 MU thrice weekly, together with ribavirin orally at a dose of 1–1.2 g/day, indicated that four patients with a prior non-sustained response to interferon had normal ALT levels at the end of treatment as well as during follow-up and that all these patients lost serum HCV RNA at the end of treatment. Thus, a substantial number of former transient responders and a smaller proportion of non-responder patients show a sustained biochemical response with eradication of HCV RNA (Schvarcz et al, 1995).

Other studies have included a combination study of interferon-alpha and ribavirin for 24 weeks (Braconier et al, 1995). Sixty percent of evaluable patients had complete clearance of HCV RNA as measured by PCR. HCV genotype did not seem to be correlated with response, but patients with sustained response to treatment had a significantly reduced number of HCV RNA copies per millilitre at the start of treatment (Braconier et al, 1995).

Combination therapy with interferon-alpha and ribavirin offers a chance of improving biochemical responses in patients who have not had sustained responses, and this is now being extensively investigated in a world-wide programme of controlled clinical trials (Brillanti et al, 1994; Schvarcz et al, 1995). It is not yet clear, however, whether relapse rates are reduced in responsive patients, or whether poor responders, particularly older patients with type 1b infection, cirrhosis and high levels of viraemia, are responsive to combination therapy.

Other combinations

Agents currently under investigation include thymic peptides, such as *thymosin alpha-1*, an important immunomodulator (Mutchnick et al, 1994) used in combination with interferon-alpha.

Recombinant interferon-alpha and ursodeoxycolic acid have been assessed against interferon-alpha alone for the treatment of chronic hepatitis C. The probability of a biochemical response was similar in both groups. The probability of relapse was also similar in both groups once treatment was stopped, but relapse occurred significantly later in the combination compared to the monotherapy group (Heinrich and Maier, 1995). Lobular necrosis improved in both groups, whereas portal inflammation improved only in the combination group. Virtually all patients remained HCV RNA-positive after treatment cessation. Thus, although UCDA appears to improve serum transaminases or prolong the period for which serum ALT remain within normal range after discontinuing interferon, there is no virological effect or significant histological improvement attributable to the addition of UCDA to interferon treatment. (Angelico et al, 1995; Boucher et al, 1995).

In an attempt to prove response rates, a pilot study using recombinant human *granulocyte colony stimulating factor* (GCSF), either alone or in combination with interferon-alpha, has been carried out in 15 cirrhotic patients. After 4 weeks of treatment with GCSF alone, no changes in ALT were observed. Three of 10 patients who completed GCSF-plus-interferon treatment had normal ALT values. This combination is being explored further (Pardo et al, 1995).

n-Acetyl cystein

Increased intracellular glutathione (GSH) levels may improve tissue injury and inhibit viral replication; n-acetyl cystein, a precursor of GSH is effective in increasing GSH levels. In patients with chronic hepatitis C, administration of n-acetyl cystein with interferon resulted in marked inhibition of HCV replication in lymphocytes and a decrease in serum ALT values (Beloqui et al, 1993).

Iron depletion

A number of authors have suggested that iron overload modifies the response to interferon therapy. The mean hepatic iron concentration has been found to be significantly higher in non-responders to interferon than in responders to interferon ($860 \pm 100 \, \mu g/g$ versus $548 \pm 85 \, \mu g/g$). The overwhelming majority of patients with a hepatic iron concentration greater than $1100 \, \mu g/g$ and 87% of patients with an elevated serum ferritin concentration did not respond to interferon-alpha therapy (Olynyk et al, 1995).

In a controlled trial of recombinant interferon-alpha in patients with thalassaemia major, the response to interferon-alpha therapy was inversely related to liver iron burden assessed by atomic absorption spectrometry, histological semiquantification or both methods (Clemente et al, 1994).

Serum transaminases may improve after phlebotomy in patients with chronic hepatitis C, although histological abnormalities of the liver are generally unchanged except for the disappearance of iron deposits (Hayashi et al, 1994, 1995).

Molecular treatments

Inhibition of hepatitis C antisense by oligonucleotides

Oligonucleotides complementary to the sequences containing the initiating codon AUG of the core region of positive-strand hepatitis C virus have been tested for the effects on viral translation in a cell-free protein synthesis system and on viral replication in the human T lymphotrophic virus type I infected cell line MT-2C. Treatment of HCV infection in two 2T cells with 10 μM antisense oligonucleotide had a dramatic inhibitory effect on viral replication and suggests that antisense oligonucleotides complementary to sequences close to the initiation codon of the core might be useful (Mizutani et al, 1995).

Others studies in vitro test systems and in cell cultures have supported the concept of an inhibitory effect of antisense phosphorothioate oligonucleotides on hepatitis C viral gene expression. Oligonucleotides directed against different stem root structures in the 5′ non-coding region of the hepatitis C virus and against a nucleotide stretch, including the start codon of the polyprotein precursor, appear inhibitory. The inhibitory effect of these has been quantified employing a viral RNA consisting of the first 407 nucleotides of HCV fused to the coding sequence of the fire-fly luciferase gene. This RNA were generated by in vitro transcription and used as a template in a rabbit reticulocyte lysate in vitro translation system. The production of active luciferase in the absence or presence of oligonucleotides suggests that the best results are obtained with oligonucleotides directed against oligonucleotides 326–348, comprising the start AUG of the polyprotein coding sequence. In cell culture experiments the hepatoblastoma cell line hep G2 was infected with a plasmid expressing the HCV luciferase fusion RNA.

In this assay oligonucleotides complementary to nucleotides 264–282 were most efficient and reduced viral translation. The inhibition was found to be specific because expression of the HCV luciferase fusion RNA was not significantly impaired by the control oligonucleotides and because an expression of an unrelated message RNA was not or only slightly down-regulated (Alt et al, 1995). Antisense mRNA constructs spanning the 5′ UTR and core ligated in adenovirus vectors express oligonucleotides that inhibit HCV replication in hepatocytes expressing HCV RNA genomes. Ribosymes may be used to check RNA and interfere with protein translation (Figure 6).

Plasmid-based DNA vaccination, using HCV core constructs, also generates a cytoxic T cell response in nude mice with tumour cell lines used to assay in vivo cytotoxicity. These vaccines will be going into phase I clinical trials shortly.

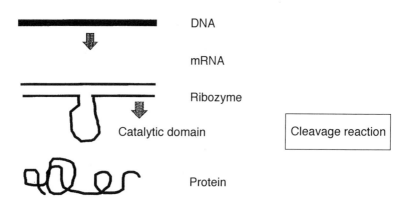

Figure 6. Ribozymes: interference with viral replication.

Antiviral treatment and liver transplantation for hepatitis C

Cirrhosis due to hepatitis C is becoming an important indication for liver transplantation, and the number of patients being transplanted for decompensated hepatic disease has increased in the past 5 years. It has become apparent that recurrence of hepatitis C virus infection is common, and that 90% or more of patients transplanted will again be HCV RNA-positive. The recurrence is rapid, and HCV RNA can be found in the engrafted liver within 2 weeks of the transplant. A number of studies have investigated the biochemical, virological and histological outcome of the transplantation (Read et al, 1991; Feray et al, 1992; Ferrell et al, 1992; Poterucha et al, 1992; Wright et al, 1992; Zignego et al, 1993). Episodes of biochemical hepatitis are more common in patients with recurrence of HCV than in control groups of patients transplanted for cirrhosis not due to chronic hepatitis.

Histological hepatitis is also more common, and chronic hepatititis is seen in approximately 60% of patients at 3 years. Cirrhosis occurs in about 10% of patients after 2–3 years.

Thus, although the recurrence is associated with relatively mild disease, follow-up of these patients has been short, and severe sequelae, including cirrhosis and even possibly hepatocellular carcinoma, may become more common with the passage of time. This provides the rationale for consideration of treatment. There is as yet little information in these patients. Preliminary studies have indicated that, in some interferon and ribavirin treated patients, levels of ALT may improve, along with a decline in concentrations of HCV RNA. As with chronic hepatitis, many patients are unresponsive, and biochemical deterioration may occur. Moreover, interferon is a powerful modulating agent, and there is concern that rejection may be increased with this treatment. Relapse rates are likely to be high. Carefully considered controlled trials are therefore indicated. The timing and dose of treatment will require assessment.

Treatment of cirrhosis due to chronic hepatitis B or C

There is some interest in inducing histological change, i.e. improving hepatic fibrosis using interferon-alpha. In studies in which patients with chronic hepatitis C have been treated with interferon, end-of-treatment biopsies for HCV RNA-negative groups have shown a significant alleviation of necrosis and inflammation. At the end of treatment, serum pro-collagen type III peptide levels and serum type IV collagen may also decrease significantly in HCV RNA-negative patients (Hiramatsu et al, 1995).

Serum pre-treatment levels of N-terminal pro-peptide of type III pro-collagen have been higher in non-responders than in transient or long-term responders. Serum pro-peptide levels decrease significantly during and after interferon-alpha therapy in treated groups, not only in responders but also in non-responders. These results suggest that interferon-alpha treatment induces long-term suppression of active fibrogenesis in chronic hepatitis C independent of the antiviral and necro-inflammatory effects observed and may help to prevent fibrosis or progression of fibrosis (Suou et al, 1995).

There may be a beneficial effect of interferon on markers of hepatic connective tissue turnover (suppression of serum pro-collagen III pro-peptide and laminin-P1 peptide) independent of its effect on viral repli-cation (Teran et al, 1994). It will be important to develop other measures of hepatic fibrosis and fibrogenesis, for example, amino terminal pro-peptide of type 3 pro-collagen and hyaluronan serum levels. These could prove to be important indicators of the extent of fibrosis and could be assayed to monitor the response to treatment in controlled clinical trials (Guéchot et al, 1994).

Histological outcome in patients with chronic hepatitis C who have been treated with interferon-alpha without sustained response may improve using numerical scoring systems to assess differences. These changes are generally not marked however. Whether such changes are beneficial requires further validation (Reichard et al, 1994).

Patients with chronic hepatitis and cirrhosis are at risk of developing hepatocellular carcinoma. In general, these patients have poor antiviral responses to interferon-alpha, but recent trials have suggested that patients with compensated chronic hepatitis with cirrhosis could be treated by interferon to prevent primary liver cancer. Oon (1995) has conducted a large trial of prevention of HCC in patients with resected HCC, and in at-risk patients, including approximately 600 patients with hepatitis B cirrhosis, as well as relatives of patients with HCC. The first group of patients included HBsAg-positive patients with resected HCC who were randomized to receive chemotherapy and interferon alpha$_n$ (Wellferon), or chemotherapy alone. Survival was improved in the chemotherapy and Wellferon group. In the second study, at-risk patients with cirrhosis due to hepatitis B were given intermittent interferon therapy or were monitoring only. A total of 162 patients were monitored, and 518 patients received 3 MU Wellferon daily for 10 days every 3 months. Most (85%) of the patients had cirrhosis. None of the patients in the Wellferon treatment arm has developed HCC, whereas 10/162 (6%) of the untreated patients have developed HCC. It is difficult to interpret this study, and a number of questions can be asked about the randomization of the patients. There were no virological measurements. The monitoring protocol was not detailed; there was little information regarding toxicity of interferon-alpha in a group of patients with advanced liver disease. Thus, there are some reservations about the conclusions drawn from this experience.

In another small study of 90 patients with chronic hepatitis C and cirrhosis, 45 patients were allocated to receive interferon-alpha 6 MU three times a week for 12–24 weeks, and 45 received symptomatic treatment. These patients were followed for 2–7 years. In 19 patients given interferon-alpha, serum ALT decreased, and the mean change in peak alpha-fetoprotein values has been smaller in patients given interferon-alpha than in controls. Serum albumin levels have been higher in the group treated with interferon-alpha. Importantly, the histological activity index in the interferon-alpha patients undergoing a second biopsy after therapy was improved, and hepatitis C viral RNA has disappeared in 16% of the 45 patients treated with interferon-alpha. Hepatocellular carcinoma was detected in two interferon patients (4%), but in 17 (38%) of controls. Whether this study indicates that interferon-alpha should be used to decrease the incidence of hepatocellular carcinoma remains to be determined in larger and more effectively controlled trials (Nishiguchi et al, 1995).

REFERENCES

Alt M, Renz R, Hofschneider PH, Paumgartner G & Caselmann WH (1995) Specific inhibition of hepatitis C viral gene expression by antisense phosphorothioate oligodeoxynucleotides. *Hepatology* **22:** 707–717.

Angelico M, Gandin C, Pescarmona E et al (1995) Recombinant interferon-α and ursodeoxycholic acid *versus* interferon-α alone in the treatment of chronic hepatitis C: a randomized clinical trial with long-term follow-up. *American Journal of Gastroenterology* **90:** 263–269.

Aoki-Sei S, O'Brien MC, Ford H et al (1991) In vitro inhibition of hepatitis B virus replication by 2′,3′-dideoxyguanosine, 2′,3′-dideoxyinosine, and 3′-azido-2′,3′-dideoxythymidine in 2.2.15 (PR) cells. *Journal of Infectious Diseases* **164:** 843–851.

Bach N, Schaffner F & Lin SC (1989) High-dose recombinant interleukin-2 for chronic viral hepatitis [letter]. *Lancet* **ii:** 281.

Bain VG, Daniels HM, Chanas A et al (1989) Foscarnet therapy in chronic hepatitis B virus e antigen carriers. *Journal of Medical Virology* **29:** 152–155.

Beach JW, Jeong LS, Alves AJ et al (1992) Synthesis of enantiomerically pure (2′R,5′S)-(−)-1-[2-(hydroxymethyl)oxathiolan-5-yl]cytosine as a potent antiviral agent against hepatitis B virus (HBV) and human immunodeficiency virus (HIV). *Journal of Organic Chemistry* **57:** 2217–2219.

Beloqui O, Prieto J, Suárez M et al (1993) *N*-acetyl cysteine enhances the response to interferon-α in chronic hepatitis C: a pilot study. *Journal of Interferon Research* **13:** 279–282.

Berk L, Schalm SW, De Man RA et al (1992a) Failure of acyclovir to enhance the antiviral effect of α lymphoblastoid interferon on HBe-seroconversion in chronic hepatitis B. A multi-centre randomized controlled trial. *Journal of Hepatology* **14:** 305–309.

Berk L, Schalm SW & Heijtink RA (1992b) Zidovudine inhibits hepatitis B virus replication. *Antiviral Research* **19:** 111–118.

Bertoletti A, Chisari FV, Penna A et al (1993) Definition of a minimal optimal cytotoxic T-cell epitope within the hepatitis B virus nucleocapsid protein. *Journal of Virology* **67**: 2376–2380.

Bishop N, Civitico G, Wang YY et al (1990) Antiviral strategies in chronic hepatitis B virus infection: I. Establishment of an in vitro system using the duck hepatitis B virus model. *Journal of Medical Virology* **31**: 82–89.

Blumberg BS, Millman I, Venkateswaran PS & Thyagarajan SP (1990) Hepatitis B virus and primary hepatocellular carcinoma: treatment of HBV carriers with *Phyllanthus amarus*. (1990) *Vaccine* **8** (supplement): S86–S92.

Boman S, Ballen JL & Seggev JS (1995) Dramatic responses to intravenous immunoglobulin in vasculitis. *Journal of Internal Medicine* **238**: 375–377.

Boucher E, Jouanolle H, Andre P et al (1995) Interferon and ursodeoxycholic acid combined therapy in the treatment of chronic viral C hepatitis: Results from a controlled randomized trial in 80 patients. *Hepatology* **21**: 322–327.

Braconier JH, Paulsen O, Engman K & Widell A (1995) Combined interferon-alpha and ribavirin treatment in chronic hepatitis C: a pilot study. *Scandinavian Journal of Infectious Diseases* **27**: 325–329.

Brillanti S, Garson J, Foli M et al (1994) A pilot study of combination therapy with ribavirin plus interferon alfa for interferon-alfa-resistant chronic hepatitis C. *Gastroenterology* **107**: 812–817.

Brunetto MR, Oliveri F, Rocca G et al (1989) Natural course and response to interferon of chronic hepatitis B accompanied by antibody to hepatitis B e antigen. *Hepatology* **10**: 198–202.

Brunetto MR, Stemler M, Bonino F et al (1990) A new hepatitis B virus strain in patients with severe anti-HBe positive chronic hepatitis B. *Journal of Hepatology* **10**: 258–261.

Brunetto MR, Oliveri F, Colombatto P et al (1995) Treatment of chronic anti-HBe-positive hepatitis B with interferon-alpha. *Journal of Hepatology* **22** (supplement 1): 42–44.

Brook MG, Karayiannis P & Thomas HC (1989a) Which patients with chronic hepatitis B virus infection will respond to interferon-alpha therapy? A statistical analysis of predictive factors. *Hepatology* **10**: 761–763.

Brook MG, Petrovic L, McDonald JA et al (1989b) Histological improvement after anti-viral treatment for chronic hepatitis B virus infection. *Journal of Hepatology* **8**: 218–225.

Carman WF, Jacyna MR, Hadziyannis S et al (1989) Mutation preventing formation of hepatitis B e antigen in patients with chronic hepatitis B infection. *Lancet* **ii**: 588–591.

Caselmann WH, Eisenburg J, Hofschneider PH & Koshy R (1989) Beta- and gamma-interferon in chronic active hepatitis B. A pilot trial of short-term combination therapy. *Gastroenterology* **96**: 449–455.

Catterall AP, Moyle GJ, Hopes EA et al (1992) Dideoxyinosine for chronic hepatitis B infection. *Journal of Medical Virology* **37**: 307–309.

Chan S-W, Simmonds P, McOmish F et al (1991) Serological responses to infection with three different types of hepatitis C virus. *Lancet* **338**: 1391.

Chang C-N, Doong S-L, Zhou JH et al (1992a) Deoxycytidine deaminase-resistant stereoisomer is the active form of (±)-2′,3′-dideoxy-3′-thiacytidine in the inhibition of hepatitis B virus replication. *Journal of Biological Chemistry* **267**: 13 938–13 942.

Chang C-N, Skalski V, Hua Zhou J & Cheng (1992b) Biochemical pharmacology of (+)- and (−)-2′,3′-dideoxy-3′-thiacytidine as anti-hepatitis B virus agents. *Journal of Biological Chemistry* **267**: 22 414–22 420.

Civitico G, Wang YY, Luscombe C et al (1990a) Antiviral strategies in chronic hepatitis B virus infection: II. Inhibition of duck hepatitis B virus in vitro using conventional antiviral agents and supercoiled-DNA active compounds. *Journal of Medical Virology* **31**: 90–97.

Civitico G, Wang YY, Luscombe C et al (1990b) Antiviral strategies in chronic hepatitis B virus infection: II. Inhibition of duck hepatitis B virus in vitro using conventional antiviral agents and supercoiled-DNA active compounds. *Journal of Medical Virology* **31**: 90–97.

Clemente MG, Congia M, Lai ME et al (1994) Effect of iron overload on the response to recombinant interferon-alfa treatment in transfusion-dependent patients with thalassemia major and chronic hepatitis C. *Journal of Pediatrics* **125**: 123–128.

Cohard M, Poynard T, Mathurin P & Zarski JP (1994) Prednisone-interferon combination in the treatment of chronic hepatitis B: direct and indirect metanalysis. *Hepatology* **20**: 1390–1398.

Davis GL (1989) Interferon treatment of viral hepatitis in immunocompromised patients. *Seminars in Liver Disease* **9**: 267–272.

Davis GL, Balart LA, Schiff ER et al (1989) Treatment of chronic hepatitis C with recombinant interferon-alfa. A multicenter randomized, controlled trial. *New England Journal of Medicine* **321**: 1501–1506.

Davis HL, Schirmbeck R, Reimann J & Whalen RG (1995) DNA-mediated immunization in mice induces a potent MHC class I-restricted cytotoxic T lymphocyte response to the hepatitis B envelope protein. *Human Gene Therapy* **6:** 1447–1456.

Dean J, Bowden S & Locarnini S (1995) Reversion of duck hepatitis B virus DNA replication in vivo following cessation of treatment with the nucleoside analogue ganciclovir. *Antiviral Research* **27:** 171–178.

Di Bisceglie AM, Shindo M, Fong T-L et al (1992) A pilot study of ribavirin therapy for chronic hepatitis C. *Hepatology* **16:** 649–654.

Di Bisceglie AM, Martin P, Kassianides C et al (1989) Recombinant interferon-alfa therapy for chronic hepatitis C. A randomized, double-blind, placebo-controlled trial. *New England Journal of Medicine* **321:** 1506–1510.

Di Bisceglie AM, Rustgi VK, Kassianides C et al (1990) Therapy of chronic hepatitis B with recombinant human alpha and gamma interferon. *Hepatology* **11:** 266–270.

Di Stefano G, Busi C, Mattioli A & Fiume L (1995) Selective delivery to the liver of antiviral nucleoside analogs coupled to a high molecular mass lactosaminated poly-L-lysine and administered to mice by intramuscular route. *Biochemical Pharmacology* **49:** 1769–1775.

Dusheiko GM & Zuckerman AJ (1991) Therapy for hepatitis B. *Current Opinion in Infectious Diseases* **4:** 785–794.

Dusheiko GM, Main J, Thomas H et al (1996) Ribavirin treatment for patients with chronic hepatitis C. Results of a placebo controlled study. *Journal of Hepatology* (in press).

Farhat BA, Marinos G, Daniels HM et al (1995) Evaluation of efficacy and safety of thymus humoral factor-gamma 2 in the management of chronic hepatitis B. *Journal of Hepatology* **23:** 21–27.

Fattovich G, Brollo L, Pontisso P et al (1986) Levamisole therapy in chronic type B hepatitis. Results of a double blind randomized trial. *Gastroenterology* **91:** 692–696.

Fattovich G, Giustina G, Brollo L et al (1992) Therapy for chronic hepatitis B with lymphoblastoid interferon-α and levamisole. *Hepatology* **16:** 1115–1119.

Fattovich G, Giustina G, Alberti A et al (1994) A randomized controlled trial of thymopentin therapy in patients with chronic hepatitis B. *Journal of Hepatology* **21:** 361–366.

Fattovich G, McIntyre G, Thursz M et al (1995) Hepatitis B virus precore core variation and interferon therapy. *Hepatology* **22:** 1355–1362.

Feinstone SM, Kapikian AZ, Purcell RH et a (1975)l Transfusion associated hepatitis not due to viral hepatitis type A or B. *New England Journal of Medicine* **292:** 767–770.

Feray C, Samuel D, Thiers V et al (1992) Reinfection of liver graft by hepatitis C virus after liver transplantation. *Journal of Clinical Investigation* **89:** 1361–1365.

Fernandez H, Banks G & Smith R (1986) Ribavirin: a clinical overview. *European Journal of Epidemiology* **2:** 1–14.

Ferrell LD, Wright TL, Roberts J et al (1992) Hepatitis C viral infection in liver transplant recipients. *Hepatology* **16:** 865-876.

Fiume L, Busi C, Di Stefano G & Mattioli A (1994) Targeting of antiviral drugs to the liver using glycoprotein carriers. *Advances in Drug Delivery Reviews* **14:** 51–65.

Fiume L, Di Stefano G, Busi C et al (1995) Inhibition of woodchuck hepatitis virus replication by adenine arabinoside monophosphate coupled to lactosaminated poly-L-lysine and administered by intramuscular route. *Hepatology* **22:** 1072–1077.

Fourel I, Li J, Hantz O et al (1992) Effects of 2'-fluorinated arabinosyl-pyrimidine nucleosides on duck hepatitis B virus DNA level in serum and liver of chronically infected ducks. *Journal of Medical Virology* **37:** 122–126.

Fourel I, Cullen JM, Saputelli J et al (1994a) Evidence that hepatocyte turnover is required for rapid clearance of duck hepatitis B virus during antiviral therapy of chronically infected ducks. *Journal of Virology* **68:** 8321–8330.

Fourel I, Saputelli J, Schaffer P & Mason WS (1994b) The carbocyclic analog of 2'-deoxyguanosine induces a prolonged inhibition of duck hepatitis B virus DNA synthesis in primary hepatocyte cultures and in the liver. *Journal of Virology* **68:** 1059–1065.

Fried MW, Korenman JC, Di Bisceglie AM et al (1992) A pilot study of 2',3'-dideoxyinosine for the treatment of chronic hepatitis B. *Hepatology* **16:** 861–864.

Furman PA, Davis M, Liotta DC et al (1992) The anti-hepatitis B virus activities, cytotoxicities, and anabolic profiles of the (−) and (+) enantiomers of *cis*-5-fluoro-1-[2-(hydroxymethyl)-1,3-oxathiolan-5-yl]cytosine. *Antimicrobial Agents and Chemotherapy* **36:** 2686–2692.

Garcia de Ancos JL, Roberts DA & Dusheiko GM (1990) An economic evaluation of the costs of a interferon treatment of chronic active hepatitis due to hepatitis B or C virus. *Journal of Hepatology* **11:** s11–s18.

Gish RJ, Lau JYN, Brooks L et al (1996) Ganciclovir treatment of hepatitis B virus infection in liver transplant recipients. *Hepatology* **23:** 1–7 (abstract).

Goodarzi G, Gross SC, Tewari A & Watabe K (1990) Antisense oligodeoxyribonucleotides inhibit the expression of the gene for hepatitis B virus surface antigen. *Journal of General Virology* **71:** 3021–3025.

Guéchot J, Poupon RE, Giral P et al (1994) Relationship between procollagen III aminoterminal propeptide and hyaluronan serum levels and histological fibrosis in primary biliary cirrhosis and chronic viral hepatitis C. *Journal of Hepatology* **20:** 388–393.

Hahm KB, Han KH, Kim WH et al (1994) Efficacy of polyadenylic polyuridylic acid in the treatment of chronic active hepatitis B. *International Journal of Immunopharmacology* **16:** 217–225.

Hayashi H, Takikawa T, Nishimura N et al (1994) Improvement of serum aminotransferase levels after phlebotomy in patients with chronic active hepatitis C and excess hepatic iron. *American Journal of Gastroenterology* **89:** 986–988.

Hayashi H, Takikawa T, Nishimura N & Yano M (1995) Serum aminotransferase levels as an indicator of the effectiveness of venesection for chronic hepatitis C. *Journal of Hepatology* **22:** 268–271.

Heinrich D & Maier K-P (1995) Treatment of chronic viral hepatitis with acetylsalicylic acid. *Schweiz Med Wochenschr* **125:** 755–757.

Hendricks DA, Stowe BJ, Hoo BS et al (1995) Quantitation of HBV DNA in human serum using a branched DNA (bDNA) signal amplification assay. *American Journal of Clinical Pathology* **104:** 537–546.

Hiramatsu N, Hayashi N, Kasahara A et al (1995) Improvement of liver fibrosis in chronic hepatitis C patients treated with natural interferon-alpha. *Journal of Hepatology* **22:** 135–142.

Honkoop P, De Man RA, Heijtink RA & Schalm SW (1995) Hepatitis B reactivation after lamivudine. *Lancet* **346:** 1156–1157.

Hope RL, Weltman M, Dingley J et al (1995) Interferon-alfa for chronic active hepatitis B. Long term follow-up of 62 patients: outcomes and predictors of response *Medical Journal of Australia* **162:** 8–11.

Iizuka A, Watanabe T, Kubo T et al (1994) M13 bacteriophage DNA inhibits duck hepatitis B virus during acute infection. *Hepatology* **19:** 1079–1087.

Ilan Y, Nagler A, Adler R et al (1993) Adoptive transfer of immunity to hepatitis B virus after T cell-depleted allogeneic bone marrow transplantation. *Hepatology* **18:** 246–252.

Ilan Y, Nagler A, Shouval D et al (1994) Development of antibodies to hepatitis B virus surface antigen in bone marrow transplant recipient following treatment with peripheral blood lymphocytes from immunized donors. *Clinical and Experimental Immunology* **97:** 299–302.

Kaneko S, Miller RH, Di Bisceglie AM et al (1990) Detection of hepatitis B virus DNA in serum by polymerase chain reaction. *Gastroenterology* **99:** 799–804.

Kassianides C, Hoofnagle JH, Miller RH et al (1989) Inhibition of duck hepatitis B virus replication by 2′,3′-dideoxycytidine. A potent inhibitor of reverse transcriptase. *Gastroenterology* **97:** 1275–1280.

Kato N, Hijikata M, Nakagawa M et al (1991) Molecular structure of the Japanese hepatitis C viral genome. *FEBS Letters* **280:** 325–328.

Korba BE & Gerin JL (1992) Use of a standardized cell culture assay to assess activities of nucleoside analogs against hepatitis B virus replication. *Antiviral Research* **19:** 55–70.

Kos T, Molijn A, Blauw B & Schellekens H (1991) Baculovirus-directed high level expression of the hepatitis delta antigen in *Spodoptera frugiperda* cells. *Journal of General Virology* **72:** 833–842.

Krogsgaard K (1994) Does corticosteroid pretreatment enhance the effect of interferon-alfa treatment in chronic hepatitis B. *Journal of Hepatology* **20:** 159–162.

Kruger M, Tillmann C, Trautwein K et al (1995) Famciclovir treatment of hepatitis B virus recurrence after orthotopic liver transplantation—a pilot study. *Hepatology* **22:** 449 (abstract).

Lake JR & Wright TL (1991) Liver transplantation for patients with hepatitis B: what have we learned from our results. *Hepatology* **13:** 796–799.

Lau JYN, Lai CL, Wu PC et al (1991) A randomised controlled trial of recombinant interferon-gamma in Chinese patients with chronic hepatitis B virus infection. *Journal of Medical Virology* **34:** 184–187.

Lee B, Luo WX, Suzuki S et al (1989) In vitro and in vivo comparison of the abilities of purine and pyrimidine 2′,3′-dideoxynucleosides to inhibit duck hepadnavirus. *Antimicrobial Agents and Chemotherapy* **33:** 336–339.

Levin S, Leibowitz E, Torten J & Hahn T (1989) Interferon treatment in acute progressive and fulminant hepatitis. *Israel Journal of Medical Science* **25**: 364–372.

Liaw Y-F, Sheen I-S, Chen T-J et al (1991) Incidence, determinants and significance of delayed clearance of serum HBsAg in chronic hepatitis B virus infection: a prospective study. *Hepatology* **13**: 627–631.

Liaw Y-F, Lin S-M, Chen T-J et al (1994) Beneficial effect of prednisolone withdrawal followed by human lymphoblastoid interferon on the treatment of chronic type B hepatitis in Asians: A randomized controlled trial. *Journal of Hepatology* **20**: 175–180.

Lin C-Y (1995) Treatment of hepatitis B virus-associated membranous nephropathy with recombinant interferon-alpha. *Kidney International* **47**: 225–230.

Lisker-Melman M, Webb D, Di-Bisceglie AM et al (1989) Glomerulonephritis caused by chronic hepatitis B virus infection: treatment with recombinant human interferon-alpha. *Annals of Internal Medicine* **111**: 479–483.

Lofgren B, Nordenfelt E & Oberg B (1989) Inhibition of RNA- and DNA-dependent duck hepatitis B virus DNA polymerase activity by nucleoside and pyrophosphate analogs. (1989) *Antiviral Research* **12**: 301–310.

Lok AS, Lai CL, Wu PC et al (1989) Treatment of chronic hepatitis B with interferon: experience in Asian patients. *Seminars in Liver Disease* **9**: 249–253.

Mabit H, Dubanchet S, Capel F et al (1994) *In vitro* infection of human hepatoma cells (HepG2) with hepatitis B virus (HBV): spontaneous selection of a stable HBV surface antigen-producing HepG2 cell line containing integrated HBV DNA sequences. *Journal of General Virology* **75**: 2681–2689.

McKenzie R, Fried NW, Sallie R et al (1995) Hepatic failure and lactic acidosis due to fialuridine (FIAU), an investigational nucleoside analogue for chronic hepatitis B. *New England Journal of Medicine* **333**: 1099–1105.

McMillan JS, Shaw T, Angus PW & Locarnini SA (1995) Effect of immunosuppressive and antiviral agents on hepatitis B virus replication *in vitro*. *Hepatology* **22**: 36–43.

McOmish F, Chan S-W, Dow BC et al (1993) Detection of three types of hepatitis C virus in blood donors: Investigation of type-specific differences in serologic reactivity and rate of alanine aminotransferase abnormalities. *Transfusion* **33**: 7–13.

Marcellin P, Ouzan D, Degos F et al (1989a) Randomized controlled trial of adenine arabinoside 5'-monophosphate in chronic active hepatitis B: comparison of the efficacy in heterosexual and homosexual patients [see comments]. *Hepatology* **10**: 328–331.

Marcellin P, Pialoux G, Girard PM et al (1989b) Absence of effect of zidovudine on replication of hepatitis B virus in patients with chronic HIV and HBV infection [letter]. *New England Journal of Medicine* **321**: 1758

Marcellin P, Loriot MA, Boyer N (1990a) Recombinant human interferon-gamma in patients with chronic active hepatitis B: pharmacokinetics, tolerance and biological effects. *Hepatology* **12**: 155–158.

Marcellin P, Martinot-Peignoux M, Loriot MA et al (1990b) Persistence of hepatitis B virus DNA demonstrated by polymerase chain reaction in serum and liver after loss of HBsAg induced by antiviral therapy. *Annals of Internal Medicine* **112**: 227–228.

Marcellin P, Samuel D, Areias J (1994) Pretransplantation interferon treatment and recurrence of hepatitis B virus infection after liver transplantation for hepatitis B-related end-stage liver disease. *Hepatology* **19**: 6–12.

Marcellin P, Pouteau M, Loriot MA et al (1995) Adenine arabinoside 5'-monophosphate in patients with chronic hepatitis B: comparison of the efficacy in patients with high and low viral replication. *Gut* **36**: 422–426.

Martin P, Muñoz SJ, Di Bisceglie AM et al (1991) Recurrence of hepatitis C virus infection after orthotopic liver transplantation. *Hepatology* **13**: 719–721.

Martín J, Quiroga JA, Bosch O & Carreño (1994) Changes in cytokine production during therapy with granulocyte-macrophage colony-stimulating factor in patients with chronic hepatitis B. *Hepatology* **20**: 1156–1161.

Mason WS, Cullen J, Saputelli J (1994) Characterization of the antiviral effects of 2' carbodeoxyguanosine in ducks chronically infected with duck hepatitis B virus. *Hepatology* **19**: 398–411.

Matthes E, von Janta-Lipinski M, Will H et al (1992) Inhibition of hepatitis B virus production by modified 2',3'-dideoxy-thymidine and 2',3'-dideoxy-5-methylcytidine derivatives. *In vitro* and *in vivo* studies. *Biochemical Pharmacology* **43**: 1571–1577.

Milich DR, Jones JE, Hughes JL et al (1990) Is a function of the secreted hepatitis B e antigen to induce immunologic tolerance *in utero*. *Proceedings of the National Academy of Science of the USA* **87**: 6599–6603.

Milich DR, Wolf SF, Hughes JL & Jones JE (1995) Interleukin 12 suppresses autoantibody production by reversing helper T-cell phenotype in hepatitis B e antigen transgenic mice. *Proceedings of the National Academy of Science of the USA* **92**: 6847–6851.

Minuk GY & LaFreniere R (1988) Interleukin-1 and interleukin-2 in chronic type B hepatitis. *Gastroenterology* **94**: 1094–1096.

Minuk GY, German GB, Bernstein C et al (1992) A pilot study of steroid withdrawal followed by oral acyclovir in the treatment of chronic type B hepatitis. *Clinical Investigative Medicine* **15**: 506–512.

Mizutani T, Kato N, Hirota M et al (1995) Inhibition of hepatitis C virus replication by antisense oligonucleotide in culture cells. *Biochemical and Biophysical Research Communications* **212**: 906–911.

Mutchnick MG, Appelman HD, Chung HT et al (1991) Thymosin treatment of chronic hepatitis B: a placebo-controlled pilot trial. *Hepatology* **14**: 409–415.

Mutchnick MG, Ehrinpreis MN, Kinzie JL & Peleman RR (1994) Prospectives on the treatment of chronic hepatitis B and chronic hepatitis C with thymic peptides and antiviral agents. *Antiviral Research* **24**: 245–257.

Naoumov NV, Thomas MG, Mason AL et al (1995) Genomic variations in the hepatitis B core gene: a possible factor influencing response to interferon-alfa treatment. *Gastroenterology* **108**: 505–514.

Nishiguchi S, Kuroki T, Nakatani S et al (1995) Randomised trial of effects of interferon-α on incidence of hepatocellular carcinoma in chronic active hepatitis C with cirrhosis. *Lancet* **346**: 1051–1055.

Ojwang JO, Bhattacharya BK, Marshall HB et al (1995) Inhibition of episomal hepatitis B virus DNA in vitro by 2,4-diamino-7-(2-deoxy-2-fluoro-β-D-abinofuranosyl)pyrrolo[2,3-d]pyrimidine. *Antimicrobial Agents and Chemotherapy* **39**: 2570–2573.

Olynyk JK, Reddy KR, Di Bisceglie AM et al (1995) Hepatic iron concentration as a predictor of response to interferon alfa therapy in chronic hepatitis C. *Gastroenterology* **108**: 1104–1109.

Onji M, Kondoh K & Horiike N et al (1987) Effect of recombinant interleukin 2 on hepatitis e antigen positive chronic hepatitis. *Gut* **28**: 1648–1652.

Oon CJ (1995) Natural lymphoblastoid α-interferon in the prevention of hepatocellular carcinoma in high-risk hepatitis B surface antigen (HBsAg) positive carriers: a 5-year follow-up. *Proceedings of the Second International Symposium on Lymphoblastoid Alpha-Interferon*. Barcelona, Spain, October 1994.

Par A, Paal M & Hollis I et al (1989) Immunomodulatory effect of isoprinosine in chronic active hepatitis B virus positive hepatitis: a comparitive study with levamisole. *International Journal of Immunotherapy* **5**: 43–50.

Pardo M, Castillo I, Navas S & Carreño V (1995) Treatment of chronic hepatitis C with cirrhosis with recombinant human granulocyte colony-stimulating factor plus recombinant interferon-alpha. *Journal of Medical Virology* **45**: 439–444.

Perrillo RP, Schiff ER, Davis GL et al (1990) A randomized, controlled trial of interferon-alfa-2b alone and after prednisone withdrawal for the treatment of chronic hepatitis B. The Hepatitis Interventional Therapy Group [see comments]. Comment in: *New England Journal of Medicine* 1990 Aug 2; **323(5)**: 337–9. *New England Journal of Medicine* **323**: 295–301.

Perrillo R, Tamburro C, Regenstein F et al (1995) Low-dose, titratable interferon alfa in decompensated liver disease caused by chronic infection with hepatitis B virus. *Gastroenterology* **109**: 908–916.

Pol S (1995) Immunotherapy of chronic hepatitis B by anti HBV vaccine. *Biomedical Pharmacotherapy* **49**: 105–109.

Pol S, Driss F, Michel M-L et al (1994) Specific vaccine therapy in chronic hepatitis B infection. *Lancet* **344**: 342

Poterucha JJ, Rakela J, Lumeng L et al (1992) Diagnosis of chronic hepatitis C after liver transplantation by the detection of viral sequences with polymerase chain reaction. *Hepatology* **15**: 42–45.

Quiroga JA, Mora I, Porres JC & Carreño V (1988) Elevation of 2′,5′-oligoadenylate synthetase activity and HLA-I associated beta 2-microglobulin in response to recombinant interferon-gamma administration in chronic HBeAg-positive hepatitis. *Journal of Interferon Research* **8**: 755–763.

Rakela J, Wood JR, Czaja AJ et al Parent K (1990) Long-term versus short-term treatment with recombinant interferon-alfa-2a in patients with chronic hepatitis B: a prospective, randomized treatment trial. *Mayo Clinic Proceedings* **65:** 1330–1335.

Read AE, Donegan E, Lake J et al (1991) Hepatitis C in liver transplant recipients. *Transplant Proceedings* **23:** 1504–1505.

Reichard O, Andersson J, Schvarcz R & Weiland O (1991) Ribavirin treatment for chronic hepatitis C. *Lancet* **337:** 1058–1061.

Reichard O, Glaumann H & Weiland O (1994) Long-term histological outcome in patients with chronic hepatitis C treated repeatedly with interferon-alpha-2b without sustained response. *Scandinavian Journal of Infectious Diseases* **26:** 383–389.

Reichen J, Bianchi L, Frei PC et al (1994) Efficacy of steroid withdrawal and low-dose interferon treatment in chronic active hepatitis B. Results of a randomized multicenter trial. *Journal of Hepatology* **20:** 168–174.

Rensen PCN, van Dijk MCM, Havenaar EC et al (1995) Selective liver targeting of antivirals by recombinant chylomicrons—a new therapeutic approach to hepatitis B. *Nature Medicine* **1:** 221–225.

Ruiz-Moreno M, Jimenez J, Porres JC et al (1990) A controlled trial of recombinant interferon-alpha in Caucasian children with chronic hepatitis B. *Digestion* **45:** 26–33.

Schvarcz R, Hansson BG, Lernestedt J-O & Weiland O (1994) Treatment of chronic replicative hepatitis B virus infection with short-term continuous infusion of foscarnet. *Infection* **22:** 330–332.

Schvarcz R, Yun ZB, Sönnerborg A & Weiland O (1995) Combined treatment with interferon-alpha-2b and ribavirin for chronic hepatitis C in patients with a previous non-response or non-sustained response to interferon alone. *Journal of Medical Virology* **46:** 43–47.

Shaw T, Amor P, Civitico G et al (1994) In vitro antiviral activity of penciclovir, a novel purine nucleoside, against duck hepatitis B virus. *Antimicrobial Agents and Chemotherapy* **38:** 719–723.

Stevenson W, Gaffey M, Ishitani M et al (1995) Clinical course of four patients receiving the experimental antiviral agent fialuridine for the treatment of chronic hepatitis B infection. *Transplant Proceedings* **27:** 1219–1221.

Suou T, Hosho K, Kishimoto Y et al (1995) Long-term decrease in serum N-terminal propeptide of type III procollagen in patients with chronic hepatitis C treated with interferon alfa. *Hepatology* **22:** 426–431.

Takano S, Ito Y, Yokosuka O et al (1994) A multicenter randomized controlled dose study of ursodeoxycholic acid for chronic hepatitis C. *Hepatology* **20:** 558–564.

Teran JC, Mullen KD, Hoofnagle JH & McCullough AJ (1994) Decrease in serum levels of markers of hepatic connective tissue turnover during and after treatment of chronic hepatitis B with interferon-α. *Hepatology* **19:** 849–856.

Tsiquaye KN, Slomka MJ & Maung M (1994) Oral famciclovir against duck hepatitis B virus replication in hepatic and nonhepatic tissues of ducklings infected in ovo. *Journal of Medical Virology* **42:** 306–310.

Tur-Kaspa R, Teicher L, Laub O et al (1990) Interferon-alpha suppresses hepatitis B virus enhancer activity and reduces viral gene transcription. *Journal of Virology* **64:** 1821–1824.

Unander DW, Webster GL & Blumberg BS (1995) Usage and bioassays in *Phyllanthus* (Euphorbiaceae). IV. Clustering of antiviral uses and other effects. *Journal of Ethnopharmacology* **45:** 1–18.

Utili R, Sagnelli E, Gaeta GB et al (1994) Treatment of chronic hepatitis B in children with prednisone followed by interferon-alfa: a controlled randomized study. *Journal of Hepatology* **20:** 163–167.

Varagona G, Brown D, Kibbler H et al (1992) Response, relapse and retreatment rates and viraemia in chronic hepatitis C treated with interferon-α 2b. A phase III study. *European Journal of Gastroenterology and Hepatology* **4:** 707–712.

von Weizsäcker F, Blum HE & Wands JR (1992) Cleavage of hepatitis B virus RNA by three ribozymes transcribed from a single DNA template. *Biochemical and Biophysical Research Communications* **189:** 743–748.

Wang Y-J, Lee S-D, Hsieh M-C et al (1994) A double-blind randomized controlled trial of colchicine in patients with hepatitis B virus-related postnecrotic cirrhosis. *Journal of Hepatology* **21:** 872–877.

Wang MX, Cheng HW, Li YJ et al (1995a) Herbs of the genus *Phyllanthus* in the treatment of chronic hepatitis B: observations with three preparations from different geographic sites. *Journal of Laboratory and Clinical Medicine* **126:** 350–352.

Wang Y, Luscombe C, Bowden S et al (1995b) Inhibition of duck hepatitis B virus DNA replication by antiviral chemotherapy with ganciclovir–nalidixic acid. *Antimicrobial Agents and Chemotherapy* **39:** 556–558.

Wen Y-M, Xiong S-D & Zhang W (1994) Solid matrix–antibody–antigen complex can clear viraemia and antigenaemia in persistent duck hepatitis B virus infection. *Journal of General Virology* **75:** 335–339.

Whalen RG & Davis HL (1995) DNA-mediated immunization and the energetic immune response to hepatitis B surface antigen. *Clinical Immunology and Immunopathology* **75:** 1–12.

Wong JB, Koff RS, Tinè F & Pauker SG (1995) Cost-effectiveness of interferon-α-2b treatment for hepatitis B e antigen-positive chronic hepatitis B. *Annals of Internal Medicine* **122:** 664–675.

Wright TL, Donegan E, Hsu HH et al (1992) Recurrent and acquired hepatitis C viral infection in liver transplant recipients. *Gastroenterology* **103:** 317–322.

Yamaguchi S, Onji M, Kondoh H et al (1988) Immunologic effects on peripheral lymphoid cells from patients with chronic hepatitis type B during administration of recombinant interleukin 2.*Clinical and Experimental Immunology* **74:** 1–6.

Yokota T, Konno K, Chonan E et al (1990) Comparative activities of several nucleoside analogs against duck hepatitis B virus in vitro. *Antimicrobial Agents and Chemotherapy* **34:** 1326–1330.

Zignego AL, Samuel D, Gigou M et al (1993) Patterns of hepatitis delta reinfection after liver transplantation and their evolution during a long term follow-up. *Progress in Clinical and Biological Research* **382:** 409–417.

9

Hepatitis B and C viruses and primary liver cancer

CHRISTIAN BRECHOT

A large number of epidemiological and molecular studies have clearly indicated the major importance of environmental factors in the development of primary liver cancers in humans. A striking feature of hepatocellular carcinoma (HCC) is a marked diversity of prevalence among different geographical areas; thus, altogether, primary liver cancer is the eighth most frequent tumour world-wide, the highest incidence being shown in sub-Saharan Africa and South East Asia (Kew and Popper, 1984). Chronic infections by hepatitis B (HBV) and C (HCV) are major risk factors (Figure 1). Although this review will mostly analyse the impact of HBV and HCV chronic infections it is, however, important to emphasize that some chemical carcinogens are also involved, as well as poorly defined hormonal factors which would account for a higher incidence of the tumour in man. Finally, the role of genetic factors has not yet been properly addressed owing to several confounding variables such as intrafamilial transmission of HBV.

The mechanisms involved in virally related liver carcinogenesis still remain

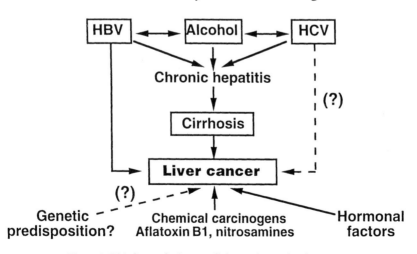

Figure 1. Risk factors for hepatocellular carcinoma development.

Baillière's Clinical Gastroenterology—
Vol. 10, No. 2, July 1996
ISBN 0–7020–2094–X
0950–3528/96/020335 + 39 $12.00/00

Copyright © 1996, by Baillière Tindall
All rights of reproduction in any form reserved

a matter of debate. This review will therefore discuss the molecular basis for HBV- and HCV-related liver carcinogenesis. It will also address how these viral infections can co-operate with other environmental factors such as alcohol and chemical carcinogens. We will focus on hepatocellular carcinoma (HCC), the major histological form of primary liver cancer and the one which has been shown to be associated with HBV and HCV infections.

THE 'INDIRECT' EFFECTS OF CHRONIC HBV AND HCV INFECTIONS: THE ROLE OF CIRRHOTIC LESIONS

Cirrhosis, which is present in about 90% of patients with HCC tumours in most areas, is recognized as an important risk factor. Early clinical observations in Africa showed the evolution of acute hepatitis (AH) to chronic active hepatitis (CAH), cirrhosis and, eventually, liver cancer (Kew and Popper, 1984; Kew, 1989). The importance of this association has since been confirmed but its prevalence is considered to be lower in Africa (about 50% of cases) than in Asia, Europe and America (80–100%). Infections by HBV and HCV are characterized by the risk of chronic infection: about 5% and 40–80% for HBV in adults and newborns, respectively, and 60–80% for HCV. Chronic infection will be associated with pleiotropic liver lesions of varying severity but will lead to cirrhosis in about 20–30% of cases. Several recent prospective studies have shown a 3–5% incidence rate per year of HCC development (Figure 2); thus, 30–50% of cirrhotic patients will show HCC after a 10-year follow-up! (Colombo, et al, 1991; Colombo and Romeo, 1994). It has also been suggested that HCC incidence might be higher in HCV-infected as compared with HBV-infected cirrhotic patients, but this is still debated. This information stresses the importance of under-standing the mechanisms accounting for the role of cirrhosis; still, it is striking that the molecular basis of the promoting effect of cirrhosis is far from clear, although it is generally related to 'liver cell regeneration' (Farshid and Tabor, 1992; Hsia et al, 1992; Tabor et al, 1992). During cirrhosis, irreversible nodular changes appear in which hepatocytes lose their normal plate arrangement, are surrounded by extensive fibrosis, and show evidence of increased DNA synthesis (Tarao et al, 1992). The pattern of growth-regulating molecules in cirrhosis is thus likely to be very different from those known to be involved after partial hepatectomy. It also not known whether those cells which exhibit increased DNA synthesis are derived from normal hepatocytes, as in regeneration occurring after partial hepatectomy, or would originate from putative 'stem cells', including 'oval cells' described in animal models of chemical carcinogenesis (Sell, 1993). It is also important to realize that chronic viral hepatitis per se, before the appearance of histological features of 'cirrhosis' probably plays a major role: chronic viral infections are indeed associated with a distinct pattern of inflammation, liver cell necrosis and fibrotic tissue accumulation. This implies abnormal synthesis of several cytokines, some of them with a marked impact on liver cell proliferation. With this view, several studies have clearly pointed out the increased risk of HCC among patients with

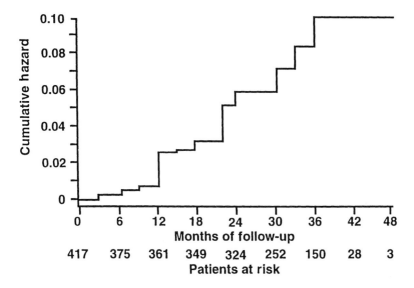

Figure 2. HCC and cirrhosis. The figure, which is based on one European report, shows the high rate of HCC in patients with liver cirrhosis. Reproduced from Colombo et al (1991, *New England Journal of Medicine* **325**: 675–680) with permission.

established cirrhosis and ongoing active chronic hepatitis. Finally, besides liver cell regeneration, hepatic failure associated with chronic hepatitis and cirrhosis will modify the metabolism of some potential chemical carcinogens and thus might also promote liver carcinogenesis.

Unfortunately, we lack accurate animal models of liver cirrhosis, although baboons chronically intoxicated with alcohol can show some characteristic features of liver cirrhosis. The liver lesions observed in rats after carbon tetrachloride (CCl_4) treatment bear little resemblance to cirrhosis. Animal models of hepadnavirus infection and HBV transgenic mice have, however, provided much important information on these issues. Woodchucks and ground squirrels chronically infected by the woodchuck hepatitis virus (WHBV) and the ground squirrel hepatitis virus (GHBV), respectively, develop HCCs against a background of CAH without cirrhosis; this observation emphasizes the absence of a strict 'requirement' for cirrhosis in liver carcinogenesis (see the review of Buendia, 1994). The availability of transgenic mice containing different HBV DNA inserts has also provided major information on these issues (reviewed recently by Chisari, 1995); these animals have indeed been very useful for demonstrating the importance of liver cell regeneration secondary to necrosis hepatocytes in the absence of a direct 'mutagenic' agent. In particular, targeting in the liver with an albumin promoter accumulation of the large PreS1/S2/S HBV envelope protein encoded by the sequences of HBV (Figure 3) has a direct toxic effect and leads to cell necrosis independently of an immune response to the viral protein and inflammation; liver cancer develops after an average of 18 months, probably as a consequence of the continuous cell

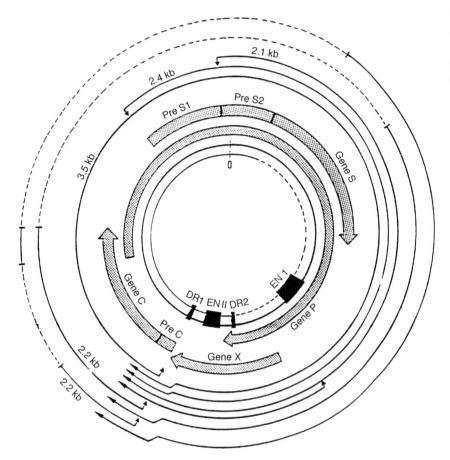

Figure 3. Structure of HBV DNA. The figure shows the four major open reading frames and the various HBV RNAs.

regeneration (Chisari et al, 1989; Toshkov et al, 1994). This is one case in which liver cancer cells emerge in the apparent absence of genetic priming events such as those involved in chemical carcinogenesis (Huang and Chisari, 1995). In addition, these mice show increased sensitivity to chemical carcinogens, a situation reminiscent of human exposure to both HBV and chemical carcinogens (Bannasch et al, 1989; Sell et al, 1991) and extensive oxidative DNA damage (Hagen et al, 1994).

'DIRECT' EFFECTS OF HBV ON THE LIVER CELL PHENOTYPE: IMPLICATIONS IN LIVER CARCINOGENESIS

Although there is general agreement on the importance of cirrhosis in the carcinogenic process, the existence of a direct effect of HBV in liver cell transformation is still controversial. The demonstration that HBV DNA integrated into the DNA of tumour cells from patients with HCC led to attempts to identify the cellular sequences adjacent to the sites of HBV DNA integration (Bréchot et al, 1980; Chakraborty et al, 1980; Edman et al, 1980; Marion et al, 1980; Koshy et al, 1983; Monjardino et al, 1983; Koshy et al, 1991; Koshy and Wells, 1991); see also reviews by Buendia, et al (1994) and Paterlini and Bréchot (1994). By analogy with tumours induced by retroviruses, it was expected that HBV DNA would be integrated in the vicinity of oncogenes, which had recently been identified. In fact, this was not the case—in sharp contrast to results subsequently obtained in woodchuck HCC. While this is now often taken as evidence against a direct role for HBV and for the sole responsibility of cirrhosis in liver cancer, there are in fact several lines of evidence that HBV is directly involved in HCC. Indeed, integration of HBV DNA can lead to chromosomal re-arrangements at the site of integration (Matsubara and Tokino, 1990), and evidence of insertional mutagenesis has been obtained in some humans with HCC and about 50% of woodchucks with HCC. Integration of the viral DNA also frequently leads to the synthesis of the X and truncated envelope viral proteins which have been implicated in liver carcinogenesis. We will now review current evidence supporting these hypotheses (Figure 4).

HBV DNA sequences in the liver of hepatitis B surface antigen-positive HBV carriers

HBV DNA was initially characterized by means of the Southern blot procedure. Viral DNA sequences were then cloned to define their structure more accurately, and viral RNAs were analysed in detail. The distinction between free and integrated HBV DNA in the Southern blot procedure is based on the use of different restriction enzymes which either do not cut most HBV genomes, or cut at one or two sites. Using this strategy, it has been shown that HBV DNA sequences are integrated into cellular DNA in most (about 90%) but not all liver tumour samples from hepatitis B surface antigen (HBsAG)-positive patients (Bréchot, 1987). The Southern blotting usually suggested monoclonal or oligoclonal proliferation of the cells containing HBV DNA (Miller and Robinson, 1986; Blum et al, 1987; Bréchot, 1987). The restriction DNA profile differs from one tumour to the next and generally reveals several different integration sites; however, clonally expanded cells containing a single integration site are found in some cases (Bréchot, 1987). It is noteworthy that, even in HBsAg-positive PLCs, HBV DNA is sometimes not detectable in all tumour cells, suggesting that integration in some HBsAg-positive patients is not always necessary to maintain a transformed phenotype (Bréchot and Paterlini, unpublished observations).

Integration of HBV DNA is not restricted to tumour cells: clonally expanded cells containing integrated HBV DNA molecules can be identified in the non-tumourous, cirrhotic, livers of patients with HCC (Bréchot et al, 1981; Takada et al, 1990). However, the restriction profile

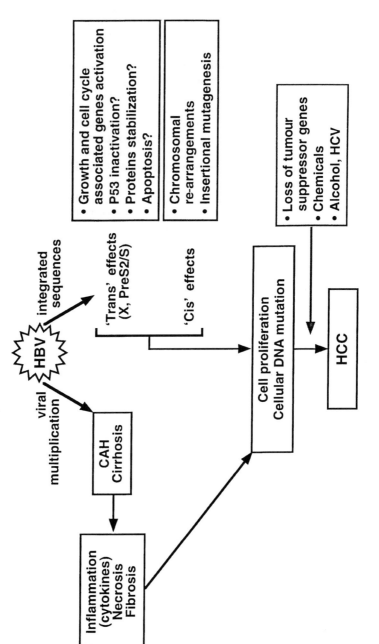

Figure 4. Molecular mechanisms involved in HBV-related liver carcinogenesis: summary of the different pathways involved.

differs from that of tumour, suggesting the co-existence of different clones in the liver prior to tumour development; alternatively, secondary chromosomal re-arrangements might have occurred during the tumour growth (Robinson, 1990). Integration has also been demonstrated in chronic HBV carriers (both adults and children) with no evidence of HCC (Bréchot et al, 1981; Shafritz et al, 1981; Kam et al, 1982; Hadziyannis et al, 1983; Yaginuma et al, 1987; Yasui et al, 1992). Although the restriction profiles in these cases can be consistent with clonal expansion of infected cells, another pattern is more frequent. This suggests either little or no proliferation of cells containing HBV sequences (Bréchot, 1987). Some studies have even suggested that such a restriction profile consistent with HBV DNA integration can be observed at the acute stage of HBV infection and in subjects with a severe form of acute hepatitis (Lugassy et al, 1987). Thus, integration precedes the development of the tumour. Comparative analysis of the various restriction profiles at different times in the course of HBV infection suggests a progressive clonal expansion of some infected cells which is detectable only in patients who have been infected for a long time. Integration of HBV DNA is not necessary for its replication, but occurs when cellular DNA replicates during liver cell proliferation secondary to necrosis of adjacent hepatocytes (Hino et al, 1991).

Free viral DNA is also frequently detected by Southern blotting (Bréchot et al, 1981; Scotto et al, 1985; Matsubara and Tokino, 1990; Robinson, 1990; Matsubara, 1991). The presence of HBV DNA replicative intermediates is generally associated with an HBV viraemia, although in some patients (particularly those with HCC) replicative forms can be detected in the liver while HBV DNA is undetectable (by dot blot) in the serum; this suggests defective viral encapsidation and/or secretion of viral particles (Raimondo et al, 1988). Free monomeric HBV DNA can also be detected, mostly at the end of viral multiplication, in acute or chronic infection. Finally, free oligomeric HBV DNA forms with complex structures have been found in a few acutely infected patients; their significance is not known, but it is feasible that they could be intermediates in the integration process (Bréchot et al, 1984; Lugassy et al, 1987). Viral oligomers have been detected in woodchucks infected by WHV (Rogler and Summers, 1982).

It is, however, important to note the technical limitations of the Southern blot assay for the analysis of HBV DNA status; in particular, it is often difficult to detect integrated sequences in hepatocytes which have undergone little or no clonal expansion when free viral DNA is also present (Bowyer et al, 1987; Bréchot, 1987). Furthermore, the Southern technique provides no information as to the identity of the infected cells.

A combination of immunohistochemical and in situ hybridization procedures has been used to settle this latter point. HBV DNA replication, as shown by the detection of HBV DNA replicative forms (in the cytoplasm) and HBcAg (mostly in the nucleus), as well as HBsAg synthesis, are generally found in different hepatocytes (Fournier et al, 1982; Alberti et al, 1984; Burrell et al, 1984; Mondelli et al, 1984). At the time of tumour development, the degree of viral DNA replication has usually decreased and HBsAg can be detected in about 20% of cases in tumour cells (Wang et al, 1991a); HBcAg is very rarely detectable (Raimondo et al, 1988; Wang et al, 1991a). In contrast, in the adjacent non-tumour cirrhotic liver, both HBsAg and HBcAg are detectable. These observations have led to suggestions that different cell populations are infected by HBV: the differentiating status of some hepatocytes might be compatible with HBV DNA replication and HBcAg expression and would thus be targets for the immune response; in contrast, other liver cells might not support a complete replicative cycle, only express HBsAg, and they might be progressively selected during chronic HBV carriage (London and Blumberg, 1982). When HCC occurs, the tumour cells are no longer permissive for the viral DNA replication and do not express HBcAg; however, as discussed latter, recent evidence suggests that they frequently express the viral X protein.

The availability of the HBV DNA probes, together with improvements in serological tests for hepatitis e antigen (HBeAg), has allowed a precise appraisal of the course of HBV infection to be made. During chronic HBV infection, one can schematically distinguish two phases: the viral multiplication phase, as shown by the detection of serum HBeAg and HBV DNA, is highly variable from one patient to the next, and is followed by an HBV carriage phase, as shown by HBsAg positivity and the absence of markers of HBV multiplication. Re-activation of viral multiplication may, however, occur, together with an exacerbation of liver cell necrosis. As mentioned earlier, HBV multiplication has generally declined markedly when HCC develops, at least in Western countries, Africa and Japan; in Taiwan, HBV multiplication persists when HCC occurs (Chen et al 1986; Loncarevic et al, 1990a). In Western countries and Africa, some investigators have shown the persistence of replicative intermediates in the tumour liver cells of patients with HCC and suggested that they might not be normally encapsidated (Raimondo et al, 1988); however, it is not known whether this leads to further integration of viral DNA into cellular DNA and thereby modifies the course of tumour development.

HBV DNA can also be detected in types of cell other than hepatocytes; classical Southern blot analysis, PCR and in situ hybridization have revealed it in mononuclear blood cells (Romet-Lemonne et al, 1983; Elfassi et al, 1984; Pontisso et al, 1984; Hadchouel et al, 1985; Pasquinelli et al, 1986), biliary and smooth muscle cells (Blum et al, 1983) and in the pancreas, kidney (Shimoda et al, 1981; Dejean et al, 1984a,b; Yoffe et al, 1986; Omata, 1990; Yoffe et al, 1990; Galun et al, 1992) and sperm cells (Hadchouel et al, 1985; Naumova and Kisselev, 1990). The most frequently identified viral DNA form is a 3.2 kb DNA molecule whose migration in agarose gels is consistent with a linear structure; viral oligomers have also been shown in mononuclear blood cells, but the integration of HBV DNA suggested by some Southern blot analyses has not been clearly established. Infection of mononuclear blood cells is an early event in the course of HBV infection: indeed, a combination of classical Southern blot analysis and PCR has been used to detect viral DNA (together with HBV transcripts) in both acutely infected subjects (Pasquinelli et al, 1986, 1988) and chronically infected subjects (Baginski et al, 1991). In woodchucks, mono-nuclear bone marrow cells are the first to show evidence of WHV DNA in an experimental acute infection (Korba et al, 1987, 1988a,b 1989a,b). Taken together, these results show that the tropism of the virus is broader than previously thought, but that replication of HBV DNA occurs mostly in liver cells. It is also important to note that, in 1996, the implications of the presence of HBV DNA in these various types of cell are still unknown.

Structure of integrated HBV and flanking cellular DNA sequences

Integrated HBV DNA sequences have been characterized in cell lines derived from hepatocellular carcinomas, and directly in tumour tissues.

Structure of integrated viral DNA

There is no single structure, but some common features can be seen in independent cases. At least one region of the viral genome is preferentially involved in integration: the region of the cohesive end part of HBV DNA and the direct repeats DR1 and DR2, at which synthesis of the minus and plus DNA strands, respectively, are initiated (Koshy et al, 1983; Dejean et al, 1984a,b; Fowler et al, 1986; Nagaya et al, 1987; Shih et al, 1987; Zhou et al, 1987; Buendia, 1992; Quade et al, 1992). In a survey of 17 clones (Nagaya et al, 1987), half of the integrations occurred in the cohesive end overlap or in sequences close to or included in DR1 and DR2. When duplicated HBV DNA sequences are identified (in a 'head-to-tail' or 'tail-to-tail' arrangement) the virus–virus junctions are also frequently located in this cohesive end region of the genome. In PLC/PRF5 cells integration was reported to occur frequently in the single-stranded part of the HBV DNA (Koshy et al, 1983), but this result was subsequently challenged by the analysis of other integrants from the same cell line.

Uninterrupted linear HBV DNAs, with insertions in the X and C open reading frames (ORFs) and small deletions (10–100 bp) at the virus/host junction, have been shown in some tumours, but this is a rather rare event; in the PLC/PRF5 cell line, for example, none of the seven integrants yielded such structures. More frequently, complex re-arrangements of the viral sequences occur in tumours, with deletions, insertions or duplications (Mizusawa et al, 1985, Yaginuma et al, 1987). Short HBV sequences or, in contrast, greater-than-unit-length genomes can be shown. It is important to note that such re-arrangements are not specific to tumour samples but can also be detected in liver samples from patients with chronic active hepatitis and apparently free of HCC (Tanaka et al, 1988).

The S ORF is often conserved, and its integrity has been confirmed in a few cases by the expression of HBsAG upon transfection of the clones containing the integrated HBV DNA (Dejean et al, 1984b, Freytag von Loringhoven et al, 1985). In contrast, the core gene is frequently deleted (Koike et al, 1983; Koch et al, 1984a,b; Shaul et al, 1984; Choo et al, 1986; Zhou et al, 1987; Chang et al, 1991; Takada et al, 1992a,b), while the X ORF is frequently truncated by insertion in the cohesive end region of the viral genome. A frequent observation is therefore insertion in the cohesive end on one side while the other junction is located between the C and the PreS genes, and integration of an HBV DNA molecule extending from PreS to X genes has been observed in several cases. Another relatively common feature of independent HCCs is the apparent conservation, even in complex HBV DNA structures, of PreS2/S ORFs truncated at the 3' part of the S gene, possibly leading to truncated PreS2/S proteins with a transactivating effect (Nagaya et al, 1987; Meyer et al, 1992a,b). The sequences located 5' to the PreS and S genes might therefore also be prone to recombination with the host genome, possibly in correlation with transcriptional activity. It is interesting that none of the integrated HBV genomes so far reported have structures which would allow them to be transcribed into pre-genomic RNA, the template for HBV DNA replication. Finally, intriguing results have been reported for the PLC/PRF5 cell line; for example, a 182 bp sequence detected at one of the virus/host junctions is only 40% homologous to HBV, is apparently not a cellular sequence, and might be implicated in several independent integrations (Berger and Shaul, 1987). Furthermore, one analysis suggested integration of four different adw HBV DNA molecules in this one cell line. While these are potentially very interesting observations, their implications are unclear as similar results have not been reported in vivo. Along the same lines, evidence has been presented for in vivo recombination between free and integrated viral DNA together with multiple integration events (Georgi-Geisberger et al, 1992).

Structure of the viral/cellular DNA junctions

Again, there is no single pattern. Most results are consistent with an illegitimate recombination event between the viral and cellular DNA, frequently associated with a short deletion of cellular DNA at the site of integration (Berger and Shaul, 1987; Nakamura et al, 1988; Takada et al, 1990; Takada and Koike, 1990). In some integrants there is partial sequence homology between the deleted cellular DNA and the viral genome close to the integration site, and it might be involved in this process (Koch et al, 1984a,b; Mizusawa et al, 1985; Rogler et al, 1985; Yaginuma et al, 1985; Hino et al, 1986; Tokino et al, 1987). In contrast, integration of an uninterrupted linear HBV DNA led to duplication of a 12 bp cellular DNA segment at the integration site, a feature reminiscent of retrovirus integration (Yaginuma et al, 1985), but this observation has remained anecdotal. There is so far no evidence of a single cell sequence being a target for HBV DNA integration. In several integrants, however, integration frequently occurs in repeat sequences (Alu or satellite III DNA sequences) (Shaul et al, 1986; Berger and Shaul, 1987; Matsumoto et al, 1988) possibly implicated in non-homologous recombination. In this regard, a detailed analysis of the PLC/PRF5 cell line has shown that eight of the nine integrated HBV DNAs are present in the H3 component of the human genome; it represents about 4% of total cellular DNA, has a base composition (51% GC) close to that of HBV DNA (49% GC), and includes Alu repeats (Zerial et al, 1986). This observation suggests preferential targeting of HBV DNA integration as is the case of some retroviruses, but has not yet been extended to HBV DNA sequences from other HCCs. Duplication and inversion of integrated HBV DNA can also involve adjacent cells' DNA in some tumours (Nagaya et al, 1987; Matsubara and Tokino, 1990). An amplification and translocation of the HBV DNA sequence, together with the adjacent host cell DNA, from one cellular domain to another, has also been shown in PLC/PRF5 cells (Bowcock et al, 1985; Ziemer et al, 1985).

Mechanisms possibly involved in HBV DNA integration

Taken together, the results presented above are consistent with several different modes of viral integration; in some tumours, where the cohesive end and the core sequences are located on the two extremities of the integrant, one of the virus/host junctions is generated by insertion of the 5′ end of the linear minus-strand replicative intermediate, while the other junction shows either no specific location in the viral genome or is preferentially inserted into the PreS ORFs; whether the location of this second junction in the HBV DNA is a secondary recombination event (deletion?) or rather reflects integration of subgenomic replicative intermediates is not known (Yaginuma et al, 1985; Dejean et al, 1986; Nagaya et al, 1987; Yaginuma et al, 1987). Alternatively, the substrate for the integration may be an open relaxed circular or linear form of HBV DNA (Shih et al, 1987; Hino et al, 1989), the insertion being generated by strand invasion and displacement. In other cases, re-arrangements creating complex oligomeric HBV DNA structures may have occurred before integration, and free oligomers have been detected in the liver of woodchucks with HCC, humans with acute hepatitis, and in mononuclear blood cells (see previous section). Whatever the substate for integration, non-homologous recombination probably involves topoisomerase I, which has cleavage sites near DR1 in HBV and WHV (Wang and Rogler, 1991; Wang et al, 1991a,b,c).

The frequent insertion of HBV DNA in the cohesive overlap might have important consequences for molecular events occurring after integration. Indeed, it has been proposed that, once integrated, the cohesive end of the viral genome might be 'reactivated' by proteins such as the terminal DNA-binding protein (Nagaya et al, 1987). This might generate further re-arrangements of the integrated HBV sequences as well as recombination between HBV genomes inserted on different chromosomes, resulting in chromosomal translocation (Hino et al, 1991). In line with this hypothesis, an in vitro assay showed indirect evidence of increased recombination events due to HBV DNA in the presence of liver cell protein extracts from patients with HCC (Hino et al, 1984, 1986, 1989, 1991, 1992).

If these molecular events are relevant in vivo, 're-activation' of HBV recombination should be prevented by the immediate encapsidation of the viral polymerase. In this regard it has been hypothesized that abnormal encapsidation of the replicative HBV DNA may occur in tumours (Raimondo et al, 1988; Loncarevic et al, 1990a,b).

Consequences of HBV DNA integration (Figures 4 and 5)

Chromosomal DNA instability. HBV DNA integration sites have been mapped to different chromosomes, although an increased rate of insertions on chromosomes 11 and 17 has been observed (Rogler et al, 1985; Hino et al, 1986; Nagaya et al, 1987; Slagle et al, 1991; Tokino and Matsubara, 1991; Meyer et al, 1992b). Integration can lead to small deletions (a few base pairs) in the cellular DNA, but several large chromosomal deletions (chromosome 11p14, 4q32, 11q13 in particular) (Wang and Rogler; 1988; Urano et al, 1991) have been shown. Translocations have been also described at the site of HBV DNA integration (chromosomes 17/X; 5/9; 17/18 (17q21–22/18q11.1–q11.2)) (Hino et al, 1986; Tokino et al, 1987; Pasquinelli et al, 1988; Murakami et al, 1991; Nishida et al, 1993; Fujimoto et al, 1994; Yeh et al, 1994). In one tumour, integrated HBV sequences were found to be co-amplified with the *hst-1* oncogene (Hatada et al, 1988). These results, combined with those concerning the modes of HBV DNA integration, have led to suggestions that HBV DNA integration might increase the likehood of chromosomal re-arrangements (Hino et al, 1991; Tatzelt et al, 1993), possibly with a contribution by tumour suppressor genes or oncogenes. However, there has been no direct evidence so far of such a gene at a deletion site or at a translocation breakpoint. On the same lines, integrated HBV DNA sequences have been shown to co-amplify with the transforming gene *hst-1* in a human HCC (Hatada et al, 1988).

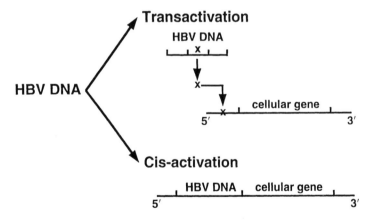

Figure 5. HBV and HCC: the cis and trans effects of HBV.

Synthesis of the X and truncated PreS2/S proteins.

HBV X (Figures 6 and 7)

Despite the frequent re-arrangements of integrated HBV DNA sequences, an intact X protein or a truncated form retaining its biological effects can be synthesized from a large number of integrants. X is an essential gene for the establishment of in vivo WHV infection in the woodchuck. X is expressed at a low level throughout all stages of the viral infection, as evidenced by the detection of anti-X antibodies (Haruna et al, 1991); it is generally believed that the titres of anti-X will parallel the level of viral multiplication. In vitro X is a major regulator of HBV promoters such as PreS1 and capsid; still, it is indispensable for viral genome replication in vivo, and this discrepancy with the in vitro observations is not understood (Zoulim et al, 1994). In addition, X has been shown to modulate the expression of several other viral sequences such as HIV1 LTR, SV40 etc. (Kekulé, 1994; Koike, 1995).

There are several lines of evidence which point to an important role for X in liver carcinogenesis (Kekulé, 1994). Expression of X RNA has been

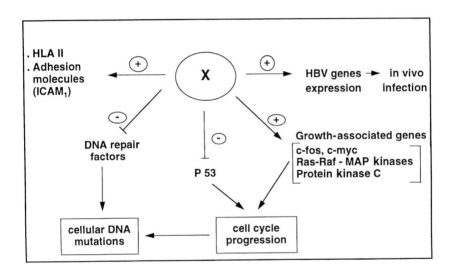

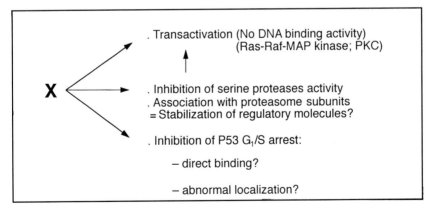

Figures 6 and 7. HBV X and liver carcinogenesis: summary of the various molecular effects of HBV X protein.

shown to be maintained in tumourous hepatocytes, even though S and C viral transcripts were not detectable any more. Some reports have also demonstrated the presence of the protein in the tumourous hepatocytes, but these studies have been hampered by the low performance of most available anti-X antibodies. There are also in vivo studies in transgenic mice which showed development of HCCs in animals expressing the X protein at a high level under the control of the X promoter (Kim et al, 1991; Koike et al, 1994b). It is now clear, however, that such HCCs will develop only in mice with an intrinsic genetic susceptibility to tumour development (Lee et al, 1990). Finally some reports, also based on transgenic mice, suggest a cooperative effect between HB X and chemical carcinogens in the occurrence of HCC. In vitro studies are also consistent with a role for X in some steps of cellular transformation. Expression of X can induce foci in some experimental conditions in NIH 3T3 cells. The most convincing evidence, however, comes from studies in different types of cell which demonstrated progression of the cell through G1/S and G2/M transitions upon X expression (Koike et al, 1994a; Koike, 1995); these reports have also emphasized the importance of the ras-raf-MAP kinase transduction pathway induced by X in this phenotypic effect (Benn and Schneider, 1994, 1995).

There are several potential mechanisms which have been proposed to account for the induction by X of cell cycle progression and, in cooperation with other factors, transformation. Their respective impact is still debated since many results have been obtained in in vitro models whose actual relevance is controversial; it is also important to emphasize that a major problem for such studies is the difficulty in obtaining an efficient expression of the X protein. Yet, the available data can be summarized as follows: there is evidence for transcriptional activation of several cellular genes upon X expression, such as growth-related c-*fos* and c-*myc* oncogenes, but also genes encoding adhesion (ICAM-1) ald HLAII molecules (Rossner, 1992). This transcriptional activation is mediated by different transcription factors such as NF-KB, AP-1, CREB, but does not involve direct binding of X to DNA sequences; instead, X might activate transcription by two distinct pathways: direct binding to elements of the transcriptional machinery, such as TATA binding protein and RNA polymerase II subunits, and activation of transduction signals such as the ras-raf-MAP kinase and protein kinase C (Kekulé et al, 1993) cascades. In this view an important point to clarify is the precise subcellular localization of X; while some recent studies have suggested a dual localization—nuclear and cytoplasmic, with distinct biological effects (Doria et al, 1995)—this is still debated, and most evidence points to a major cytoplasmic signal.

There are, however, other interesting biochemical properties of X to consider: X has been shown to inhibit the activity of some serine protease inhibitors (Takada et al, 1994) and components of the proteasome complex (Fischer et al, 1994). One can therefore hypothesize that X might modulate the degradation, and thus the turn-over, of some cellular proteins involved in transcription and/or cell cycle progression regulation. X might also directly impair regulation of the G1/S transition by interacting with P53 (Feitelson et al, 1993; Truant et al, 1995; Ueda et al, 1995); P53 is indeed acting as a major negative regulator of the entry into S phase as long as DNA repair, induced by ionizing radiations for example, has not been completed (Levine, 1993). It is a transcriptional activator and induces expression of one of the cyclin-dependent kinase (CDK) inhibitors (CKI)—P21—which will, in turn, inhibit kinase activity of several cyclin-CDK complexes and block cell-cycle progression. Finally, P53 is also involved in cell apoptosis by unknown mechanisms. Some reports have suggested direct binding to, and inhibition of, activity of P53 by X. It is important to note that, although of potential major impact, the direct binding of X to P53 has not yet been confirmed (Henkler et al, 1995); it has also been hypothesized that X might modify the cellular localization of P53 by inhibiting its entry into the nucleus at G1-S, thereby preventing negative regulation of this transition. X might further interact with DNA repair by binding to a cellular DNA repair protein (Lee et al, 1995). Finally, there is some recent evidence which would directly implicate X in apoptosis. Thus, altogether, there are now several directions to be thoroughly investigated. A major issue is to demonstrate that these various molecular effects are relevant in vivo. However, the available evidence is consistent with an important role for the X protein in liver carcinogenesis. With this view it is important to note that X is expressed from free replicating viral DNA as well as integrated HBV sequences, and thus X expression can be detected in the early stages of HBV infection; it not clear, however, whether the biological effects of free X and X generated from an HBV integrant are actually identical.

PreS2/S

Truncated forms of the PreS2/S envelope protein, generated from deleted integrated viral genomes might be also involved in liver cell transformation (Hildt et al, 1993; Lauer et al, 1994). It has been reported, from sequence data available in the literature, that up to 25% of HCCs would contain viral genomes whose structure might encode such deleted proteins (Schlüter et al, 1994); there is in vitro evidence for a transactivating effect of PreS2/S proteins lacking their C-terminal domain on cellular genes such as c-*myc* and c-*fos*. This transactivating effect must be indirect since truncated PreS2/S proteins are exclusively cytoplasmic, anchored into the membrane of the endoplasmic reticulum by the transmembrane domains of the S sequence; in fact, the mechanisms involved are not known, although it has been suggested that the generation of free radical oxides might be involved. More direct evidence for the role of PreS2/S comes from the demonstration of its co-operative effect with c-Ha ras in cell transformation (Lüber et al, personal communication).

Insertional mutagenesis (cis-activation). Two different situations must be distinguished: in HCCs in woodchucks infected by WHV, insertion of the WHV DNA into the c-*myc* or N-*myc* oncogenes is frequent (identified in half the tumours so far analysed) (Fourel et al, 1990a,b; Buendia, 1992, 1994; Buendia et al, 1994; Etiemble et al, 1994) (Figure 8). There is

- ⎡100% of HCC in neonatally WHV infected animals
  ⎣Rapid development (< 2 years)

- 50% of tumours= ⎡- viral insertion in myc family gene ⎡- c-*myc*
                  ⎣- ↗↗ myc expression   ⎢- N-*myc*
                                                         ⎣- N-*myc* 2

- Transgenic mice with WHV—c-*myc*:
    - 100% develop HCC in 20 months
    - Expression of c-*myc* ⎡- 3-10 days after birth
                           ⎣- Pre-neoplasic and neoplasic nodules

TRANSGENE   c-*myc*
      WHV

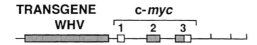

Figure 8. Woodchucks and HCC: summary of the evidence for frequent cis-activation of N-*myc* and c-*myc* genes upon WHV DNA integration. From information given in Hsu et al (1988), Fourel et al (1990b) and Etiemble et al (1994).

convincing evidence, in vitro in cell culture and in vivo in transgenic mice, for the direct transforming property of constructs containing these integrants; these observations have also underlined that, in these wood-chuck tumours, the sites of integration of WHV DNA into c-*myc* are identical to those utilized by some oncogenic retroviruses in experimentally induced animal tumours.

In contrast, in human tumours, a direct cis-acting promoter insertion mechanism has been definitely shown in only two cases, and both tumours developed on a histologically non-cirrhotic liver with evidence of clonal proliferation of cells containing a single HBV integration site.

In the first case, HBV DNA integration occurred in an exon of the retinoic acid receptor B gene (RAR B); 29 amino acids of the viral PreS1 gene were fused to the DNA-binding and hormone-binding domains of the RAR, which is a member of the steroid–thyroid receptor gene family (Dejean et al, 1986; Dejean and De Thé, 1990). The major role of retinoic acid and retinoids in cell differentiation and proliferation is well established, and it is plausible that viral insertion, by generating a chimeric HBV/RAR B protein, was involved in the liver cell transformation. The transformation of erythrocytic progenitor cells by retrovirus carrying the hybrid HBV RAR B construct is indeed consistent with this hypothesis (Garcia et al, 1993). In addition, the identification of RAR B led to the detection of a family of genes encoding, in particular, the RAR A receptor. The chromosomal translocation t (Kekulé et al, 1990, Takada and Koike, 1990) in the pro-myelocytic form of acute leukaemia has now been shown to fuse RAR A to a new cellular gene (PML) (De Thé et al, 1990, 1991).

In the second case, the human cyclin A-encoding gene was identified by our group in an early liver cancer developing on a histologically normal liver (Wang et al, 1990, 1992a). We have now cloned and sequenced the entire normal cyclin A gene and shown that integration of HBV DNA occurs in the second intron (Figure 9). We have also recently demonstrated that the insertion of HBV DNA markedly modifies the cyclin A expression pattern. Northern blot analysis of the original tumour (referred to as 'HEN') showed an intense accumulation of cyclin A and HBV transcript (Wang et al, 1992a). A cDNA library was generated from the original tumour tissue, and this allowed us to determine the structure of the two (1.7 and 2.7 kb) RNAs identified in this tissue with both HBV and cyclin A probes. They are both synthesized from the HBV PreS2/S promoter and, after splicing in the middle of the S gene, joined the exon 3–8 of the cyclin A gene (Wang et al, 1992a). The Pres2/S promoter is known to drive the expression of the middle and large proteins of the viral surface antigen. It functions constitutively, and the expression of HBsAg is often maintained in liver cancers despite de-differentiation of the transformed hepatocyte. Northern blots

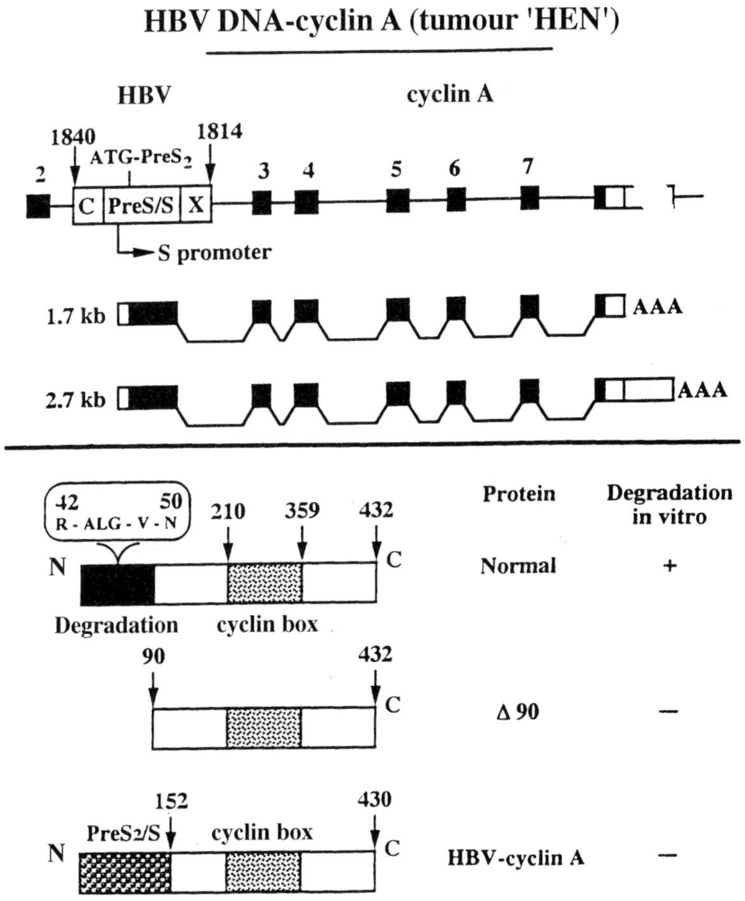

HBV DNA-cyclin A (tumour 'HEN')

Figure 9. HBV DNA insertion into the cyclin A gene. The figure shows the structure of the re-arranged cyclin A gene upon insertion of HBV DNA and the two hybrid HBV/cyclin A RNAs generated by the integration (upper part). The lower part shows the structure of the hybrid protein generated from these RNAs, as compared to normal cyclin A.

showed no evidence of transcription of the unoccupied cyclin A allele in the tumour, but there was no sign of a gross re-arrangement at the cyclin A locus; this might therefore solely reflect a low rate of cyclin A RNA transcription in a tumour with a low proliferation index (Wang et al, 1992a).

Cyclin A plays a major role in both G2/M and G1/S check-points of the cell cycle (Desdouets et al, 1995). Cyclin A is indeed implicated in the initiation and accomplishment of the S transition phase; recent data from our laboratory, based on inactivation of cyclin A gene by homologous recombination, have demonstrated that cyclin A is an essential gene for cell-cycle progression (Murphy et al, submitted). Analysis of the protein potentially encoded in the tumour by the hybrid RNAs yielded several points of interest: they code for a 430-amino acid chimeric protein, in which the N-terminal 152 amino acids of cyclin A are replaced by 150 amino acids from the PreS2 and S viral proteins, while the C-terminal two-thirds of cyclin A, including the cyclin box, remain intact. The cyclin A degradation sequences located in the N-terminal part of the protein are therefore deleted. Using an in vitro degradation assay with frog oocytes, we verified that HBV/cyclin A is not degradable (Wang et al, 1992a). It is, however, striking that despite the large amount of HBV/cyclin RNAs in tumour tissue, we failed to detect hybrid protein in these samples by means of Western blotting. This might be due to modifications in the structure of the protein to low-level expression in tumour cells (possibly necessary to avoid a cytotoxic effect of cyclin A) (Wang et al, 1992a).

Several hypotheses can be proposed to account for the potential role of the HBV/cyclin in cell transformation: the absence of degradation of a molecule retaining the ability to complex to and activate cdk kinases might lead to unregulated and premature DNA synthesis and thus to cell proliferation. It is also quite plausible that the location of the HBV/cyclin A protein is changed, given the membrane location of PreS2/S molecules in HBV-infected cells. Finally, it is noteworthy that the PreS2/S viral sequences present in HBV/cyclin A are deleted in their C-terminal part and thus have a similar structure to the deleted PreS2/S proteins we have described in the previous section. We have now obtained in vitro results which demonstrate the transforming property of the HBV-cyclin A protein (Patil et al, in preparation). These data confirm that at least in some tumours, the analysis of HBV insertion sites can lead to the identification of the cellular genes essential for cell-cycle progression and/or differentiation.

The results obtained with this tumour contrast with those obtained with liver cancers, in which no HBV DNA is integrated in the cyclin A gene: only 6/43 showed a significant increase in the amount of cyclin A transcripts, and none yielded evidence of a re-arrangement of the cyclin A gene (De Mitri et al, 1995). This phenomenon must therefore be viewed as a rare event, at least in liver cancer. On the other hand, our group has shown that the expression of cyclin A RNA or protein is an interesting marker of tumour cell proliferation in vivo (Paterlini et al, 1993, 1994).

Two further cases of cis activation of a cellular gene have recently been shown; in the PLC/PRF/5 cell line, HBV DNA inserted into the gene encoding human mevalonate kinase; the results are reminiscent of those obtained with the cyclin A gene since hybrid transcripts are synthesized from the PreS2/S promoter and fused to the cellular sequence. Mevalonate kinase had previously been identified only in the rat; by phosphorylating cholesterol, it regulates the synthesis of isoprenoid compounds which are involved in cell proliferation (Graef et al, 1995). In addition, it has recently been shown in a human HCC that HBV DNA has inserted into a gene homologous to the epidermal growth factor receptor encoding gene (Zhang et al, 1992).

It is interesting to note that, in the four cases so far reported, the study of integrated HBV DNA has led to the identification a new gene encoding a protein with a major role in cell proliferation or differentiation. In addition, in three of these samples, sufficient material was available to demonstrate that the viral insertion modified the expression of the gene, with synthesis of hybrid transcripts potentially encoding fusion proteins. While this result strongly argues for a role of HBV DNA insertion in liver cell trans-formation, these findings have remained isolated. Why insertional muta-genesis is frequent in woodchuck HCCs and rare in human tumours is not clear. It is, however, important to bear in mind that human HCC is a hetero-geneous group of tumours; in particular, the small subgroup of patients with tumours arising on non-cirrhotic livers may differ, with regard to the sites of HBV DNA integration, from those with tumour developing on a cirrhotic liver. As a result, the number of tumours so far analysed in detail may still be too limited. Finally, insertion of the viral DNA can occur at distance from the activated gene (Fourel et al, 1994).

Escape of cells containing the integrated HBV DNA from the immune response. Besides the direct effects of HBV on the hepatocyte, integration frequently interrupts the HBcAg gene; in addition, viral DNA replication usually markedly decreases at the time of tumour development, leading to a fall in HBcAg synthesis (Pontisso et al, 1984; Raimondo et al, 1988, Loncarevic et al, 1990a). In view of the role of HBc and HBe epitopes in the immune response to infected cells, it is plausible that cells containing integrated HBV DNA might 'escape' immune destruction, thus conferring a selective growth advantage in the chronic course of infection. In fact, in vivo studies in mice inoculated with cell lines expressing different regions of the HBV genome have provided good support to this hypothesis (Chang et al, 1995).

HEPATOCELLULAR CARCINOMA IN HEPATITIS B SURFACE ANTIGEN-NEGATIVE PATIENTS

There are striking geographical variations in the association between HCC and chronic infection by HBV. In Western countries (i.e. Northern Europe, USA) and in Japan only 15–20% of tumours occur in HBsAg-positive patients, and other environmental factors such as alcohol and infection by hepatitis C virus (HCV) are clearly major risk factors. A number of epidemiological studies have shown a high prevalence of anti-HBs and anti-HBc antibodies in HBsAg-negative subjects (about 40–50% in France), indicating exposure to the virus (Kew and Popper, 1984; Bréchot, 1987; Loncarevic et al, 1990a). These antibodies generally reflect resolved HBV infection; in HBsAg-negative subjects with HCC, however, HBV DNA sequences can be detected in the tumours, demonstrating the persistence of the viral infection and suggesting its implication in liver carcinogenesis (Bréchot, 1987). It is important to realize that the improvement in the sensitivity of tests for HBsAg, together with the introduction of sensitive tests for HBV DNA, has modified the criteria for the diagnosis of HBV infection; there is indeed a spectum of chronic HBV infections with a low replication rate which might also be a risk factor for liver cancer (Bréchot et al, 1985; Liang et al, 1991).

In the following section we will review the main issues raised by these observations.

The prevalence of HBV DNA in liver tumours of HBsAg-negative patients (Tables 1 and 2)

The actual prevalence of these HBV DNA-positive HCCs in HBsAg-negative subjects has been a matter of debate owing to the low copy number per cell of viral DNA sequences (estimated at 0.1 to 0.01). Studies performed in different geographical areas have given very different results,

Table 1. Detection of HBV DNA in HBsAg-negative patients with HCC.

Country	Serum	Tumour	Reference
France	11/22	19/34	Paterlini et al (1990, 1993, 1994)
Italy	ND	7/11	Paterlini et al (1990)
Spain	12/54	ND	Ruiz et al (1992)
Germany	ND	8/12	Unsal et al (1994)
Japan	8/22	ND	Ohkoshi et al (1991)
South Africa	ND	11/18	Paterlini et al (1991)
Senegal	18/31	ND	Coursaget et al (1991)
Mozambique	ND	4/11	Dazza et al (1991)
USA	25/105	14/38	Liang et al (1992)
India	3/22[a]	11/22	Ramesh et al (1994)

[a] Serum HBV DNA tested by dot blot.

Table 2. Detection of HBV RNAs in HBsAg-negative and HBsAg-positive HCC.

		HBV RNA[a]		
		S	X	C
HBsAg-negative patients (9)	9T[b]	0	7	0
	8NT[c]	0	7	0
HBsAg-positive patients (6)	6T	5	6	5
	6NT	6	6	6

[a] S, X and C HBV RNA accumulation.
[b] T = tumourous tissue.
[c] NT = non-tumourous tissue.

probably because of different technical conditions (specificity and sensitivity) as well as distinct epidemiological situations. Thanks to the sensitivity of the polymerase chain reaction (PCR), the previous observations have been confirmed. In addition, PCR has been used to demonstrate transmission of HBV particles present in the serum of these HBsAg-negative patients to chimpanzees, and to determine the nucleotide sequence of the HBV genomes. For example, in a study performed in patients from areas of high (South Africa) and low (France, Italy) HBV prevalence, HBV DNA was detected in 37/63 HBsAg-negative patients, including 15 of 24 serologically recovered and 13 of 32 patients with no detectable HBV serological markers (Paterlini et al, 1990, 1991, 1993; Unsal et al, 1994). Similar results were also obtained recently in Spain, Africa and in the United States (Table 3). It is striking that there was no real correlation between the serological HBV profiles and the presence or absence of HBV DNA in serum or tumour specimens. Taken together, these studies show that HBV infection persists in a large number of subjects with HBsAg-negative HCCs.

Table 3. Association of HCC to HCV: prevalence of anti-HCV.

	Country	Patients	General population
High prevalence areas	Japan	70–80%	1.5%
	Italy	58–76%	0.8–1%
	Spain	50–75%	0.8–1%
'Intermediate' areas	France	20–50%	1.4–1%
	Greece	13–39%	1.4%
	Romania	45%	?
	Switzerland	36%	?
	Austria	36%	?
	Rwanda	38%	17%
Low prevalence areas	Senegal	10.9%	5%
	Mozambique	7.6%	7.3%
	South Africa	30% (?)	1% (?)

Structure of HBV DNA in tumours

With regard to the state of HBV DNA, its low copy number per cell has hampered the interpretation of the results of Southern blotting. However, using our PCR test and distinct primers distributed on the S, Pre/S, C and X HBV genes, we were able to provide further information. For several patients, a positive result was obtained with only some of the HBV primers, a finding consistent with the presence of defective HBV DNA. In other cases, the tumour DNA scored positive with all the HBV primers, a fact consistent with the presence of free or integrated HBV DNA and no gross re-arrangements. Interestingly, defective HBV genomes have been identified more frequently in tumours than in non-tumour tissues. In addition, they have also been shown more frequently in completely seronegative individuals than in anti-HBs- and anti-HBc-positive subjects; this observation probably reflects a technical point since the presence of defective HBV DNA can be obscured by concomitant complete viral genomes.

The PCR profiles obtained with DNA from tumour, non-tumour and serum samples from the same European patients showed marked differences. In the serum and non-tumour samples, amplification was achieved with all the primers tested; in contrast, tumour DNA repeatedly gave negative results with at least one primer. These findings demonstrate that the HBV DNA sequences in the tumour do not derive from contaminating non-tumour cells or serum-derived particles. They are also consistent with the clonal expansion of cells containing defective and integrated HBV DNA (Paterlini et al, 1993).

Among the factors which might account for the negativity of serological HBsAg tests are a low level of infectious HBV particles at the time of contamination, an abnormal host immune response to the virus, and genetic variations of the HBV genomes (review in Bréchot, 1993; Carman et al, 1993; Preisler-Adams et al, 1993).

Transcription of the HBV DNA sequences

Northern blot analysis has not proven sensitive enough for the detection of HBV RNAs in these tumours. In contrast, cDNA synthesis followed by PCR with primers on the S gene (RT–PCR) revealed HBV RNA sequences in most of HBV DNA-positive tumours from HBsAg-negative patients. However, owing to the compact organization of the HBV genome it was not possible to determine precisely which viral transcripts were synthesized. In a recent study (Paterlini et al, 1994), we investigated the HBV RNAs with primers located on the S-, C- and X-encoding sequences. X, but not C and S, transcripts were identified in tumour tissues from seven of the nine HbsAg (−) HBV DNA (+) patients studied (Table 2) (Paterlini et al, 1994). More recently we could further confirm these observations by detecting the X protein in these tumourous liver cells (Paterlini et al, unpublished observations). This may provide a clue to the pathogenesis of these tumours in view of the potential transforming properties of the X protein envisaged in HBsAg-positive liver cancers. This view is consistent with several pieces of evidence which show persistence of HBV DNA long after recovery from acute viral hepatitis (Michalak, 1994) and in patients with chronic hepatitis (Bréchot et al, 1985; Mason et al, 1992; Chazouillères et al, 1994).

Potential role of HBV in the pathogenesis of HBsAg-negative HCC

Taken together, the results demonstrate a high rate of persistent HBV infection in patients with HCC negative for serum-HBsAg, many of whom also lack detectable antibodies to the virus. They also show clonal expansion of the tumour cells containing the integrated viral DNA and the preferential transcription in these cells of HBV RNA sequences encoding the viral X protein. While these findings strongly argue for a role for HBV in the development of these tumours, one highly paradoxical result still remains to be explained: why is the copy number of HBV DNA per cell so low if clonal expansion of infected cells occurs? One hypothesis is that HBV might act as an 'initiating' agent, and that maintenance of the transformation process does not require the persistence of HBV DNA; in addition, there may be chromosomal re-arrangements which eliminate the viral DNA from the tumour clones. This explanation has also been put forward to account for human and bovine papillomavirus—and some retrovirus-related tumours (Galloway and McDougall, 1983; Smith and Campo, 1988; Morgan et al, 1990).

The involvement of HBV in HBsAg-negative liver cancers is also reinforced by two lines of evidence. In the woodchuck model of HCC, 17% of animals infected by the WHV developed primary liver cancers despite negativation of the assay for WHV surface antigen in the serum and the appearance of antibodies to the surface and capsid viral antigenes; in addition, WHV DNA was detected in the tumour tissues of these animals with a much lower copy per cell number than in WHsAg-positive woodchucks (about 1 and 1000 molecules per cell, respectively) (Korba et al, 1989a,b; Gerin et al, 1991) an observation quite similar to that we have discussed in previous sections in human HCCs. Ground squirrel might also turn out to be an interesting model for this issue since GSHV DNA sequences have been identified in HCCs developing in completely seronegative animals (Transy et al, 1992). Another line of evidence for a direct role of HBV in liver cancer stems from the detection of HBV DNA in a significant number (7/12) of HCCs in HBsAg-negative patients, developing on non-cirrhotic, histologically-close-to-normal livers; thus, cirrhosis cannot solely account for the induction of the cancer in these cases (Paterlini et al, 1991).

HBV IN HBsAG-POSITIVE AND -NEGATIVE PRIMARY LIVER CANCERS: HYPOTHETICAL MECHANISMS

In the previous sections we have presented evidence for the involvement of HBV in both HBsAg-positive and -negative liver cancers. Obviously, other factors (such as HCV, alcohol, chemical carcinogens and hormonal factors) should also be included in the multifactorial process involved in liver carcinogenesis. A major difference between HBsAg-positive and HBsAg-negative HBV DNA-positive PLCs is related to the number of viral DNA sequences per cell and the rate of HBV DNA replication (Figure 10). In HBsAg-positive chronic carriers, HBV multiplication is sustained for enough time to induce liver cell necrosis and thus secondary proliferation of adjacent liver cells (i.e. regeneration). In these subjects, HBV may therefore act at two complementary steps of liver cell transformation: it might exert a direct role by a combination of transactivation and integration; in addition, it can induce promotion and clonal expansion of the initiated 'cells' by inducing liver cell necrosis and regeneration (Figures 4 and 10)).

In contrast, in HBsAg-negative HBV DNA-positive patients, the number of HBV DNA copies per cell is low, and viral DNA replication is barely detectable. In most of these cases, therefore, it is unlikely that HBV is

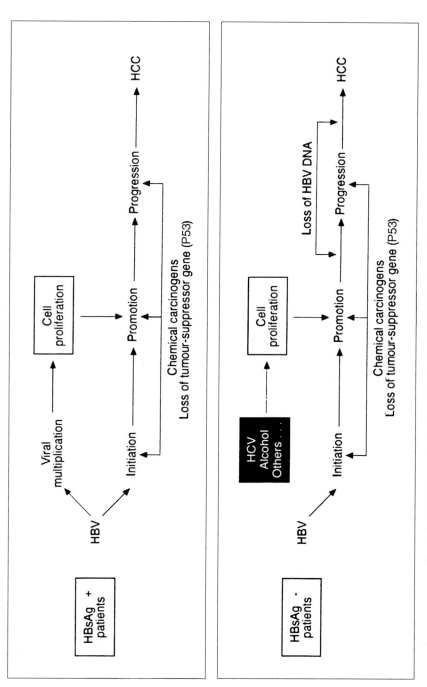

Figure 10. Model to explain the hypothetical role of HBV in HBs Ag-positive and negative HCCs.

solely involved in liver cell necrosis, chronic active hepatitis and cirrhosis. Instead, other factors such as HCV, alcohol or other still unrecognized agents might be responsible for cirrhosis and thus promotion of the neoplastic transformation. On the other hand, we have presented evidence for the persistence of integrated viral DNA which may exert a direct effect via integration and/or transactivation. HBV might, therefore, be able to initiate liver cell transformation in a limited number of clonally extended cells; the subsequent development of an HCC would be dependent on the effect of co-factors able to promote liver cell regeneration via development of cirrhosis.

HEPATITIS C VIRUS AND HCC

Hepatitis C virus (HCV) is the main aetiological factor of post-transfusional and sporadic non-A/non-B hepatitis. This viral infection is characterized by an extremely high rate (60–80%) of chronic carrier state development, associated with a low grade, yet persisting, viral multi-plication (Kato, 1993; Gretch, 1994; Magrin, 1994; Duvoux, 1995; Nousbaum, 1995). Among HCV chronically infected patients the severity of the liver lesion markedly varies, ranging from very mild chronic hepatitis to cirrhosis and hepatocellular carcinoma. Several studies have, however, noted the high rate of cirrhosis (about 20%) and HCC after long-term evolution (10–30 years) (Kiyosawa, 1990; Tremolada, 1992; Koretz, 1993; Tong, 1995). However, detailed analysis of the natural course of HCV infection is not available (Seef, 1992). It is also still debated whether or not acute HCV infection, by itself, can induce fulminant hepatitis (FH): HCV related FH have been indeed reported in Japan (Yanagi, 1990) and Taiwan (Chu, 1994) while, among cases identified in France and United States, HCV was always associated to HBV infections (Wright, 1991; Féray, 1993; Liang, 1993).

The pathogenetic mechanisms of HCV infection are poorly known; in particular, the respective importance of the viral and host factors is still unclear.

HEPATITIS C VIRUS GENOME AND VIRAL PARTICLES (Figure 11)

HCV is now recognized as a member of the Flaviviridae, together with the Pestiviruses and Flaviviruses (Matsuura and Miyamura, 1993; Santolini et al, 1994). Its genome is a positive, single-stranded RNA molecule with a length averaging 9.4 kb. It includes two untranslated regions at the 5' and 3' ends, and a large open reading frame encoding a 3010–3030 amino acid polyprotein (Figure 11). This polyprotein is post-translationally processed into structural and non-structural proteins, the cleavage being dependent on host- and virus-encoded enzymes (Grakoui and Wychowski, 1993; Lin et al, 1994; Bartenschlager et al, 1995; Hahm et al, 1995; Tanji et al, 1995).

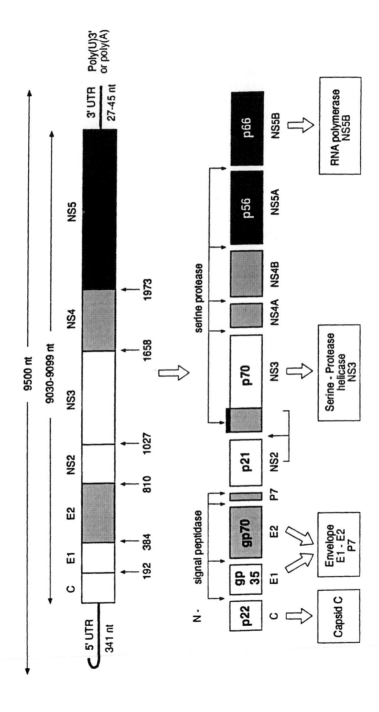

Figure 11. Structure of the HCV genome. The figure illustrates the structure of HCV RNA and the cleavage of the viral polyprotein in structural and non-structural proteins.

The structural proteins, encoded in the N terminal region, include the core protein followed by two envelope glycosylated proteins: E1 and E2; a p7 protein, also encoded by the E2 region and processed from an E2-p7 precursor, has recently been described, but its role is unknown. The non-structural domain encodes six proteins: NS2, 3, 4A, 4B, 5A and 5B. NS3 shows, in fact, three enzymatic activities: serine-proteinase, helicase and ATP-dependent nucleotide triphosphatase. A second protease is encoded by NS2 and the N-terminal sequence of NS3 (Hirowatari et al, 1995). NS4 A forms a heterodimeric complex with NS3, acting as a necessary cofactor for the NS3 proteinase activity (Failla et al, 1994). Finally, NS5 B contains the GDD motif conserved among RNA-dependent RNA polymerases and probably acts as the HCV RNA polymerase. The functions of NS2 and NS4B are as yet unknown. It is important to note that, until recently, the potential function of these viral proteins was only tentatively deduced from sequence analysis. Recently, purification of recombinant NS3 and NS5 has allowed us to demonstrate the serine proteinase and helicase activities of NS3 as well as the polymerase activity of NS5. This will open up new possibilities for the design of drugs capable of inhibiting HCV polyprotein processing and HCV RNA replication.

Current knowledge of the role of HCV in liver carcinogenesis (summary)

Epidemiological data (Colombo and Romeo, 1994)

A large number of studies have shown that HCV is, in most geographical areas, an important risk factor for HCC (Table 3). Still, there are several geographical areas where the figures are quite preliminary. In Japan and Southern Europe, figures for anti-HCV prevalence of 80 and 60% have been shown, respectively; in Northern Europe, recent data suggest that approximately 30% of HCCs are associated with chronic HCV infection. In subSaharan Africa and South-East Asia, where HBV-associated HCCs are prevalent, the impact of HCV is much lower (about 10%). Prospective studies have also further reinforced the role of HCV in different geographical areas.

Molecular studies

HCV RNA sequences can be detected in the tumourous tissues of patients with liver cancer. Sequencing of the hypervariable part of the E2 envelope region has confirmed that HCV RNA sequences indeed persist in the tumour cells and do not merely reflect contamination by non-tumour cells or serum particles; instead, mutations identified in the HCV RNA sequences from tumour as compared to non-tumour cells reflect infection by an identical HCV isolate, followed by replication at a different rate of the HCV genome when tumour develops (Paterlini and Bréchot, 1994; Sullivan and Gerber, 1994; Kurosaki et al, 1995). In contrast to HBV, the HCV genome does not integrate into cellular DNA, and replication is thus necessary for its persistence. Studies based on PCR for the detection of negative HCV strand, as well as for the identification of different HCV proteins into tumour cells, have been consistent with replication of the HCV genome; such studies are, however, complicated by technical pitfalls when searching for HCV RNA negative strands by PCR (Lanford et al 1995; Lerat et al, 1996) and for HCV proteins with the available antibodies.

As previously discussed for HBV, a main issue for understanding HCV-related carcinogenesis is whether the virus is acting only by inducing CAH and cirrhosis or whether it might also directly modify the cellular phenotype. Only little information is presently available, but there are two pieces of evidence which would favour the hypothesis of a direct effect of some HCV isolates: we have reported rare but well characterized HCCs developed on livers with minimal histological lesions and which, despite detailed analysis, showed persistence of HCV RNA in the tumours as the only identified risk factor (De Mitri et al, 1995); this study has demonstrated that, in some cases, HCC might be associated with HCV in the absence of CAH. In vitro, it has been shown recently that expression of a region of the NS3 viral protein induces a transformed phenotype in NIH 3T3 cells (Sakamuro et al, 1995). Although these data are still preliminary, they will be important to follow up. With this view, the impact of HCV genotypes in the risk of developing HCC is an important issue to analyse. A number of recent studies point to the severity of HCV type 1-associated liver lesions, including HCC. Cross-sectional analyses, indeed, have shown a higher relative prevalence of HCV 1 in patients with cirrhosis than in those with moderate CAH; these findings are, however, difficult to interpret because the molecular epidemiology of HCV is presently changing with the recent introduction, at least in France and Italy, of other types, such as HCV 3, by intravenous drug users; in these conditions the duration of HCV infection will differ from one type to the other markedly influence the risk of cirrhosis (review by Bréchot, Falk Symposium 1995, in press; Bukh et al, 1995; Nousbaum et al, 1995). There is still evidence for a more aggressive course of type 1-induced CAH:

1. After liver transplantation, re-infection of the liver graft by HCV 1 induces a more rapidly progressive CAH than do other HCV types, and this is not related to epidemiological factors or to the level of viraemia (Féray et al, 1995; Gane et al, 1996).
2. In recent prospective studies on the risk of developing HCC in patients with HCV-related cirrhosis, infection by genotype 1 has emerged as an independent risk factor (Yamauchi et al, 1994; Silini et al, 1995); along the same lines, HCV 1b was the most prevalent type among the patients we reported with HCV-associated HCC in the absence of cirrhosis (De Mitri et al, 1995). Clearly, these are still indirect pieces of evidence but, altogether, they are consistent with a particular profile of HCV 1 infection; in vitro studies are now mandatory to analyse, comparatively, the different biological properties of various HCV isolates.

Interactions between HBV, HCV and alcohol

HBV and HCV can interact with chronic alcoholic consumption, and there is circumstantial evidence of a high prevalence of HBV and HCV infection in alcoholics. The high prevalence of anti-HCV in alcoholics with cirrhosis (40–50%), relative to those with minimal liver damage (about 20%) suggests that HCV infection might be involved in the development of cirrhosis in some of these patients. This might also account for the high prevalence of anti-HCV (50%) in alcoholics with HCC (Parés et al, 1990; Mendenhall et al 1991; Nalpas et al, 1991; Colombo, 1992; Nalpas et al, 1992). In contrast, there is no evidence of a role for HBV in the development of alcoholic cirrhosis because the prevalence of anti-HBs and anti-HBc, although higher than in the general population, does not significantly differ with regard to the presence or absence of cirrhosis (diagnosed in about 20% of cases). However, there is evidence of a role for HBV in liver cancers in alcoholics because the prevalence of serological HBV markers is significantly increased in these patients (about 50%) and the tumours frequently contain HBV DNA sequences (Attali et al, 1981; Saunders et al 1983; Nalpas et al, 1985; Poynard et al, 1991; Nalpas, 1994). A recent study conducted in France showed that most of HBsAg-negative liver cancer tissues (from alcoholics and non-alcoholics) contained HCV RNA (7/22), HBV DNA (7/22), or both (4/22) (Paterlini et al, 1993). Similar results have been obtained in the USA (Gerber et al, 1992; Liang et al, 1992) and in Spain (Ruiz, et al., 1992) (Table 4). Primary liver cancer in low-endemic areas thus shows a strong association with both viral infections, a fact that has important implications for prevention campaigns.

Co-infection by HBV and HCV might influence liver carcinogenesis at two levels: there is in vivo evidence for decreased replication of both HBV DNA and HCV RNA in patients infected by the two viruses. In vitro expression of the HCV capsid also diminishes encapsidation of the HBV pre-genome. In addition, it is plausible that HBV and HCV genomes might

Table 4. Association of HCC to HCV and HBV.

	HBsAg negative		
	Serum	Liver	
HBV DNA	11/22	37/63	Paterlini et al (1993)
	12/54	NT	Ruiz et al (1992)
	24/105	14/38	Liang et al (1992)
	NT	5/12	Gerber et al (1992)
	4/31	9/31	Sheu et al (1992)
	ND	8/12	Unsal et al (1994)
	3/22	11/22	Remesh et al (1994)
HCV RNA	11/22	5/5 (HCV ⊕)	Paterlini et al (1993)
	42/68	NT	Ruiz et al (1992)
	40/90	7/9 (HCV ⊕)	Liang et al (1992)
	NT	11/20	Gerber et al (1992)
	17/31	18/31	Sheu et al (1992)

act synergistically in the carcinogenic process, but this has not been demonstrated.

SUMMARY

The data presented indicate that viral agents (namely, HBV and HCV) are major environmental aetiological factors for human primary liver cancer. It is important to elucidate the molecular mechanisms further because HCC is one of the few examples of virus-related human cancers. In addition, the available evidence points to the possibility of at least partial prevention of the tumour by large-scale vaccination.

Acknowledgements

The author wishes to thank Patrizia Paterlini for her help in the reviewing the manuscript and Fathia Ouadda for her editing.

REFERENCES

Alberti A, Trevisan A & Fattovich G (1984) The role of hepatitis B virus replication and hepatocytes membrane expression in the pathogenesis of HBV-related hepatic damage. *Hepatology* **12:** 134–143.
Attali P, Thibault N, Buffet C et al (1981) Les marqueurs du virus B chez les alcooliques chroniques. *Gastroenterologic Clinique et biologique* **5:** 1095.
Baginski I, Chemin I, Bouffard P et al (1991) Detection of polyadenylated RNA in hepatitis B virus-infected peripheral blood mononuclear cells by polymerase chain reaction. *Journal of Infectious Diseases* **163:** 996–1000.
Bannasch P, Enzmann H, Hacker HJ et al (1989) Comparative pathobiology of hepatic pre-neoplasia. In Bannasch P, Keppler D & Weber G (eds) *Liver Cell Carcinoma* pp 55–78. Dordrecht: Kluwer Academic.
Bartenschlager R, Ahlborn-Laake L, Yazargil K et al (1995) Substrate determinants for cleavage in cis and in trans by the hepatitis C virus NS3 proteinase. *Journal of Virology* **69:** 198–205.
Benn J & Schneider RJ (1994) Hepatitis B virus HBx protein activates Ras-GTP complex formation ans establishes a Ras, MAP kinase signaling cascade. *Proceedings of the National Academy of Sciences of the USA* **91:** 10 350–10 354.
Benn J & Schneider RJ (1995) Hepatitis B virus HBx protein deregulates cell cycle checkpoint controls. *Biochemistry* **92:** 11 215–11 219.
Berger I & Shaul Y (1987) Integration of hepatitis B virus: analysis of unoccupied sites. *Journal of Virology* **61:** 1180–1186.
Blum H, Stowring L, Figus A, et al (1983) Detection of hepatitis B virus DNA in hepatocytes, bile duct epithelium, and vascular elements by in situ hybridization. *Proceedings of the National Academy of Sciences of the USA* **81:** 6685–6688.
Blum HE, Offensperger WB, Walter S et al (1987) Hepatocellular carcinoma and hepatitis B virus infection: molecular evidence for monoclonal origin and expansion of malignantly transformed hepatocytes. *Journal of Cancer Research and Clinical Oncology* **113:** 466–472.
Bowcock A, Pinto M, Bey E et al (1985) The PLC/PRF/5 human hepatoma cell line. II. Chromosomal assignment of hepatitis B virus integration sites. *Cancer Genetics and Cytogenetics* **18:** 19–26.
Bowyer S, Dusheiko G, Schoub B & Kew M (1987) Expression of the hepatitis B virus genome in chronic hepatitis B carriers and patients with hepatocellular carcinoma. *Proceedings of the National Academy of Sciences of the USA* **84:** 847–850.
Bréchot C (1987) Hepatitis B virus (HBV) and hepatocellular carcinoma. HBV DNA status and its implications. *Journal of Hepatology* **4:** 269–279.

Bréchot C, Pourcel C, Louise A et al (1980) Presence of integrated hepatitis B virus DNA sequences in cellular DNA of human hepatocellular carcinoma. *Nature* **286:** 533–535.

Bréchot C, Hadchouel J, Scotto M et al (1981) State of hepatitis B virus DNA in hepatocytes of patients with HbsAg positive and HbsAg negative liver diseases. *Proceedings of the National Academy of Sciences of the USA* **78:** 3906–3910.

Bréchot C, Hadchouel M, Scotto J et al (1981) Detection of hepatitis B virus DNA in liver and serum: a direct appraisal of the chronic carrier state. *Lancet* **ii:** 765–768.

Bréchot C, Lugassy C, Dejean A et al (1984) Hepatitis B virus DNA in infected human tissues. In Vyas G Dienstag JL & Hoofnagle J (eds) *Viral Hepatitis and Liver Disease* pp 395–409. New York.

Bréchot C, Degos F, Lugassy C et al (1985) Hepatitis B virus DNA in patients with chronic liver disease and negative test for hepatitis B surface antigen. *New England Journal of Medicine* **312:** 270–276.

Buendia MA (1992) Hepatitis. B viruses and hepatocellular carcinoma. *Advances in Cancer Research* **59:** 167–226.

Buendia MA (1994) Animal models for hepatitis B viruses and liver cancer. In Christian B (ed.) *Primary Liver Cancer: Etiological and Progression Factors* pp 211–224. Paris: CRC Press.

Buendia MA, Paterlini P, Tiollais P & Bréchot C (1994) Liver cancer and hepatitis B virus. In Bréchot C (ed.) *Viral Hepatitis. Scientific Basis and Clinical Management* pp 137–164. Edinburgh: Churchill Livingstone.

Bukh J, Miller RH & Purcell RH (1995) Genetic heterogeneity of hepatitis C virus: quasispecies and genotypes. *Seminars in Liver Disease* **15:** 41–63.

Burrell J, Gowans E & Rowland R (1984) Correlation between liver histology and markers of hepatitis B virus replication in infected patients: a study by 'in situ hybridization'. *Hepatology* **4:** 20–24.

Carman W, Thomas H & Domingo E (1993) Viral genetic variation: hepatitis B virus as a clinical example. *Lancet* **341:** 349–353.

Chakraborty PR, Ruiz Opazo H, Shouval D & Shafritz DA (1980) Identification of integrated hepatitis B virus DNA and expression of viral RNA in an HBsAg-producing human hepatocellular carcinoma cell line. *Nature* **286:** 531–533.

Chang MH, Chen PJ, Chen JY et al (1991) Hepatitis B virus integration in hepatitis B virus-related hepatocellular carcinoma in childhood. *Hepatology* **13:** 316–320.

Chang PC, Hu CP, Chen SH et al (1995) Deletion of integrated hepatitis B virus genome and cellular flanking sequences in hepatocellular carcinoma cells in BALB/c mice. *Hepatology* **21:** 1504–1509.

Chazouillères O, Mamish D, Kim M et al (1994) 'Occult' hepatitis B virus as source of infection in liver transplant recipients. *Lancet* **343:** 142–146.

Chen C, Diani A, Brown P et al (1986) Detection of hepatitis B virus DNA in hepatocellular carcinoma. *Hepatology* **67:** 1868.

Chisari FV (1995) Hepatitis B virus transgenic mice: insights into the virus and the disease. *Hepatology* **22:** 1316–1325.

Chisari FV, Klopchin K, Moriyama T et al (1989) Molecular pathogenesis of hepatocellular carcinoma in hepatitis B virus transgenic mice. *Cell* **59:** 1145–1156.

Choo K-B, Liu M-S, Chang P-C et al (1986) Analysis of six distinct integrated hepatitis B virus sequences cloned from the cellular DNA of a human hepatocellular carcinoma. *Virology* **154:** 405–408.

Chu CM, Sheen IS, Liaw YF (1994) The role of hepatitis C virus in fulminant viral hepatitis in an area with endemic hepatitis AB. *Gastroenterology* **107:** 189–195.

Colombo M (1992) Hepatocellular carcinoma. *Journal of Hepatology* **15:** 225–236.

Colombo M & Romeo R (1994) Human primary liver cancer and hepatitis C virus in Western countries and Africa. In Bréchot C (ed.) *Primary Liver Cancer: Etiological and Progressive Factors* pp 49–56. Boca Raton, FL: CRC Press.

Colombo M, De Franchis K, Del Nino E et al (1991) Hepatocellular carcinoma in Italian patients with cirrhosis. *New England Journal of Medicine* **325:** 675–680.

Coursaget P, Le Cann P, Leboulleux D et al (1991) Detection of hepatitis B virus DNA by polymerase chain reaction in HBsAg negative Senegalese patients suffering from cirrhosis of primary liver cancer. *FEMS Microbiology Letters* **67:** 35–38.

Dazza MC, Meneses LV & Girard PM et al (1991) Polymerase chain reaction for detection of hepatitis B virus DNA in HBsAg seronegative patients with hepatocellular carcinoma from Mozambique. *Annals of Tropical Medicine and Parasitology* **85:** 277.

De Mitri S, Poussin K, Baccarini P et al (1995) HCV-associated liver cancer without cirrhosis. *Lancet* **345:** 413–415.

De Thé H, Chomienne C, Lanotte M et al (1990) The t(15;17) translocation of acute promyelocytic leukemia fuses the retinoic acid receptor alpha gene to a novel transcribed locus. *Nature* **347:** 558–561.

De Thé H, Lavau C, Marchio A et al (1991) The PML-RAR-alpha fusion mRNA generated by the t(15,17) translocation in acute promyelocytic leukaemia encodes a functionally altered retinoic acid receptor. *Cell* **66:** 675–684.

Dejean A & De Thé H (1990) Hepatitis B virus as an insertional mutagen in a human hepatocellular carcinoma. *Molecular Biology and Medicine* **7:** 213–222.

Dejean A, Lugassi C, Zafrani S et al (1984a) Detection of hepatitis B virus DNA in pancreas, kidney and skin of two human carriers of the virus. *Journal of General Virology* **65:** 651–655.

Dejean A, Sonigo P, Wain-Hobson S & Tiollais P (1984b) Specific hepatitis B virus integration in hepatocellular carcinoma DNA through a viral 11 base pair direct repeat. *Proceedings of the National Academy of Sciences of the USA* **81:** 5350–5354.

Dejean A, Bougueleret L, Grzeschik KH & Tiollais P (1986) Hepatitis B virus DNA integration in a sequence homologous to v-erbA and steroid receptor genes in a hepatocellular carcinoma. *Nature* **322:** 70–72.

Desdouets C, Sobczak-Thépot J, Murphy M & Bréchot C (1995). Cyclin A: function and expression during cell proliferation. In Meijer L, Guidet S & Lim Tung HY (eds) *Progress in Cell Cycle Research.* pp 115–123. New York: Plenum Press.

Doria M, Klein N, Lucito R & Schneider RJ (1995) The hepatitis B virus HBx protein is a dual specificity cytoplasmic activator of Ras and nuclear activator of transcription factors. *EMBO Journal* **15:** 4747–4757.

Duvoux C, Pawlotsky JM, Bastie M et al (1995) HCV replication levels are low in end-stage HCV-related cirrhosis. *Journal of Hepatology* **23:** 110.

Edman JC, Gray P, Valenzuela P et al (1980) Integration of hepatitis B virus sequences and their expression in a human hepatoma cell. *Nature* **286:** 535–537.

Elfassi E, Romet-Lemonne JL, Essex M et al (1984) Evidence of extrachrosomal forms of hepatitis B viral DNA in a bone marrow culture obtained from a patient recently infected with hepatitis B virus. *Proceedings of the National Academy of Sciences of the USA* **81:** 3526–3528.

Etiemble J, Degott C, Renard CA et al (1994) Liver-specific expression and high oncogenic efficiency of a c-myc transgene activated by woodchuck hepatitis virus insertion. *Oncogene* **9:** 727–737.

Failla C, Tomei L & De Francesco R (1994) Both NS3 and NS4A are required for poteolytic processing of hepatitis C virus nonstructural proteins. *Journal of Virology* **68:** 3753–3760.

Farshid M & Tabor E (1992) Expression of oncogenes and tumor suppressor genes in human hepatocellcular carcinoma and hepatoblastoma cell lines. *Journal of Medical Virology* **38:** 235–239.

Feitelson MA, Zhu M, Duan L-X & London WT (1993) Hepatitis B x antigen and p53 are associated *in vitro* and in liver tissues from patients with primary hepatocellular carcinoma. *Oncogene* **8:** 1109–1117.

Féray C, Gigou M, Samuel D et al (1993) Hepatitis C virus RNA hepatitis B virus DNA in serum and liver of patients with fulminant hepatitis. *Gastroenterology* **104:** 549–555.

Féray C, Gigou M, Samuel D et al (1995) Influence of the genotypes of hepatitis C virus on the severity of recurrent liver disease after liver transplantation. *Gastroenterology* **108:** 1088–1096.

Fischer M, Runkel L & Schaller H (1994) HBx protein of hepatitis B virus interacts with the C-terminal portion of a novel human proteasome alpha-subunit. *Virus Genes* **10:** 99–102.

Fourel G, Tiollais P & Buendia MA (1990a) Nucleotide sequence of the woodchuck N-myc gene (WN-mycl). *Nucleic Acids Research* **18:** 4918.

Fourel G, Trépo C, Bougueleret L et al (1990b) Frequent activation of N-myc genes by hepadnavirus insertion in woodchuck liver tumors. *Nature* **347:** 294–298.

Fourel G, Couturier J, Wei et al (1994) Evidence for long-range oncogene activation by hepadnavirus insertion. *EMBO Journal* **13:** 2526–2534.

Fournier J-G, Kessous A, Richer et al (1982) Detection of hepatitis B viral RNAs in human liver tissues by in situ hybridization. *Biology of the Cell* **43:** 225–228.

Fowler M, Thomas H & Monjardino J (1986) Cloning and analysis of integrated hepatitis B virus DNA of the adr suntype derived from a human primary liver cell carcinoma. *Journal of General Virology* **61:** 771–775.

Freytag von Loringhoven A, Koch S, Hofschneider PH & Koshy R (1985) Co-transcribed 3′ host sequences augment expression of integrated hepatitis B virus DNA. *EMBO Journal* **4:** 249–255.

Fujimoto Y, Hampton LL, Wirth PJ et al (1994) Alterations of tumor suppressor genes and allelic losses in human hepatocellular carcinomas in China. *Cancer Research* **54**: 281–285.

Galloway DA & McDougall JK (1983) The oncogenic potential of herpes simplex virus: evidence for a 'hit and run' mechanism. *Nature* **302**: 21–24.

Galun E, Offensperger WB, von Weizsäcker F et al (1992) Human non-hepatocytes support hepadnaviral replication and virion production. *Journal of General Virology* **73**: 173–178.

Gane EJ, Naoumov NV, Mondelli MU (1996) A longitudinal analysis of hepatitis C virus replication following liver transplantation. *Gastroenterology* (in press).

Garcia M, De Thé H, Tiollais P et al (1993) A hepatitis B virus pre-S-retinoic acid receptor béta chimera transforms erythrocytic progenitor cells in vitro. *Cell Biology* **90**: 89–93.

Georgi-Geisberger P, Berns H, Loncarevic IF et al (1992) Mutations on free and integrated hepatitis B virus DNA in a hepatocellular carcinoma: footprints of homologous recombination. *Oncology* **49**: 386–395.

Gerber MA, Shieh YSC, Shim K-S et al (1992) Detection of replicative hepatitis C virus sequences in hepatocellular carcinoma. *American Journal of Pathology* **141**: 1271–1277.

Gerin J, Cote P, Korba B et al (1991) Hepatitis B virus and liver cancer: the woodchuck as an experimental model of hepadnavirus-induced liver cancer. In Hollinger FB, Lemon SM & Margolis H (eds) *Viral Hepatitis and Liver Disease*. pp 556–559. Baltimore: Williams and Wilkins.

Graef E, Caselmann W, Wells J & Koshy K (1995) Enzymatic properties of over exposed HBV-mevalonate fusion proteins and mevalonate kinase proteins in the human hepatoma cell line PLC/PRF/5. *Virology* **208**: 696–703.

Grakoui A, Wychowski C, Lins et al (1993) Expression and identification of hepatitis of hepatitis C virus polyprotein cleavage products. *Journal of Virology* **67**: 1385–1395.

Gretch D, Corey L, Wilson J et al (1994) Assessment of hepatitis virus RNA levels by quantitative competitive RNA polymerase chain reaction: High-titer viremia correlates with advanced stage of disease. *Journal of Infectious Diseases* **169**: 1219–1225.

Hadchouel M, Scotto J, Huset C et al (1985) Presence of HBV DNA in spermatozoa—a possible vertical transmission of HBV via the germ line. *Journal of Medical Virology* **16**: 61–66.

Hadziyannis SJ, Lieberman HM, Karvountzis GG & Shafritz DA (1983) Analysis of liver disease, nuclear HBsAg, viral replication, and hepatitis B virus DNA, in liver and serum of HBeAg Vs. anti-Hbe positive carriers of hepatitis B virus. *Hepatology* **3**: 656–662.

Hagen TM, Huang S, Curnutte J et al (1994) Extensive oxidative DNA damage in hepatocytes of transgenic mice with chronic active hepatitis destined to develop hepatocellular carcinoma. *Medical Sciences* **91**: 12 808–12 812.

Hahm B, Han DS, Back SH et al (1995) NS3–4A of hepatitis C virus is a chymotrypsin-like protease. *Journal of Virology* **69**: 2534–2539.

Haruna Y, Hayashi N, Katayama K et al (1991) Expression of X protein and hepatitis B virus replication in chronic hepatitis. *Hepatology* **13**: 417–421.

Hatada I, Tokino T, Ochiya T & Matsubara K (1988) Co-amplification of integrated hepatitis B virus DNA and transforming gene hst-1 in a hepatocellular carcinoma. *Oncogene* **3**: 537–540.

Henkler F, Waseem N, Golding MHC et al (1995) Mutant p53 but not hepatitis B virus X protein is present in hepatitis B virus-related human hepatocellular carcinoma. *Cancer Research* **55**: 6084–6091.

Hildt E, Urban S, Lauer U et al (1993) ER-localization and functional expression of the HBV transactivator MHBs. *Oncogene* **8**: 3359–3367.

Hino O, Kitagawa T, Koike K et al (1984) Detection of hepatitis B virus DNA in hepatocellular carcinomas in Japan. *Hepatology* **4**: 90–95.

Hino O, Shows TB & Rogler CE (1986) Hepatitis B virus integration site in hepatocellular carcinoma at chromosome 17;18 translocation. *Proceedings of the National Academy of Sciences of the USA* **83**: 8338–8342.

Hino O, Ohtake K & Rogler CE (1989) Features of two hepatitis B virus (HBV) DNA integrations suggest mechanisms of HBV integration. *Journal of Virology* **63**: 2638–2643.

Hino O, Tabata S & Hotta Y (1991) Evidence for increased in vitro recombination with insertion of human hepatitis B virus DNA. *Proceedings of the National Academy of Sciences of the USA* **88**: 9248–9252.

Hino O, Kitagawa T, Nomura K et al (1992) Comparative molecular pathogenesis of hepatocellular carcinomas. In Klein-Szanto AJP, Anderson MW, Barrett JC & Slaga TJ (eds) *Comparative Molecular Carcinogenesis*. pp 173–185. Baltimore: Wiley-Liss.

Hirowatari Y, Hijikata M, Tanji Y & Shimotohno K (1995) Expression and processing of putative nonstructural proteins of hepatitis C virus in insect cells using baculovirus vector. *Virus Research* **35:** 43–61.

Hsia CC, Axiotis CA, Di Bisceglie A et al (1992) Mutations of p53 gene in hepatocellular carcinoma: roles of hepatitis B virus and aflatoxin contamination in the diet. *Journal of the National Cancer Institute* **84:** 1638–1641.

Huang SN & Chisari FV (1995) Strong, sustained hepatocellular proliferation precedes hepatocarcinogenesis in hepatitis B surface antigen transgenic mice. *Hepatology* **21:** 620–626.

Kam W, Rall LB, Smuckler EA et al (1982) Hepatitis B viral DNA in liver and serum of asymptomatic carriers. *Proceedings of the National Academy of Sciences of the USA* **79:** 7522–7526.

Kato N, Sekiya H, Ootsuyama Y et al (1993) Humoral immune response to hypervariable region 1 of the putative envelope glycoprotein (gp70) of hepatitis C virus. *Journal of Virology* **67:** 3923–3930.

Kekulé A, (1994) Hepatitis B virus transactivator proteins: the 'trans' hypothesis of liver carcinogenesis. In Bréchot (ed.) *Primary Liver Cancer: Etiological and Progression Factors* pp 191–210. Boca Raton, FL: CRC Press.

Kekulé AS, Lauer U, Weiss L et al (1993) Hepatitis B virus transactivator HBx uses a tumor promoter signalling pathway. *Nature* **361:** 742–745.

Kekulé AS, Lauer U, Meyer M et al (1990) The pre-S2/S region of integrated hepatitis B virus DNA encodes a transcriptional transactivator. *Nature* **343:** 457–461.

Kew M (1989) Role of cirrhosis in hepatocarcinogenesis. In Bannasch P, Keppler D & Weber CC (eds) *Liver Cell Carcinoma.* pp 37–45. Dordrecht: Kluwer Academic.

Kew MC & Popper H (1984) Relationship between hepatocellular carcinoma and cirrhosis. *Seminars in Liver Disease* **4:** 136–146.

Kim C-M, Koike K, Saito I et al (1991) HBx gene of hepatitis B virus induces liver cancer in transgenic mice. *Nature* **351:** 317–320.

Kiyosawa K, Sodeyama T, Tanaka E, et al (1990) Interrelationship of blood transfusion, non-A, non-B hepatitis hepatocellular carcinoma: analysis by detection of antibody to hepatitis C virus. *Hepatology* **12:** 671–675.

Koch S, Freytag von Loringhoven A, Hofschneider PH & Koshy R (1984a) Amplification and rearrangement in hepatoma cell DNA associated with integrated hepatitis B virus DNA. *EMBO Journal* **3:** 2185–2189.

Koch S, Freytag von Loringhoven A, Kahmann R et al (1984b) The genetic organization of integrated hepatitis B virus DNA in the human hepatoma cell line PLC/PRF/5. *Nucleic Acids Research* **12:** 6871–6876.

Koike K (1995) Hepatitis B virus HBx gene and hepatocarcinogenesis. *Intervirology* **38:** 134–142.

Koike K, Kobayashi M, Mizusawa H et al (1983) Rearrangement of the surface antigen gene of hepatitis B virus integrated in the human hepatoma cell lines. *Nucleic Acids Research* **11:** 5391–5402.

Koike K, Moriya H, Yotsuyanagi H et al (1994a) Induction of cell cycle progression by hepatitis B virus HBx gene expression in quiescent mouse fibroblasts. *Journal of Clinical Investigation* **94:** 44–49.

Koike K, Moriya K, Iino S et al (1994b) High-level expression of hepatitis B virus HBx gene and hepatocarcinogenesis in transgenic mice. *Hepatology* **19:** 810–819.

Korba BE, Wells F & Tennant BC et al (1987) Lymphoid cells in the spleens of woodchuck hepatitis virus-infected woodchucks are a site of active viral replication. *Journal of Virology* **61:** 1318–1324.

Korba BE, Cote PJ & Gerin JL (1988a) Mitogen-induced replication of woodchuck hepatitis virus in cultured peripheral blood lymphocytes. *Science* **241:** 1213–1216.

Korba BE, Gowans EJ & Wells FV et al (1988b) Systemic distribution of woodchuck hepatitis virus in the tissue of experimentally infected woodchucks. *Virology* **165:** 172–181.

Korba BE, Cote PJ & Wells FV et al (1989a) Natural history of woodchuck hepatitis virus infections during the course of experimental viral infection: Molecular virologic features of the liver and lymphoid tissues. *Journal of Virology* **63:** 1360–1370.

Korba BE, Wells FV & Baldwin B et al (1989b) Hepatocellular carcinoma in woodchuck hepatitis virus-infected woodchucks: presence of viral DNA in tumor tissue from chronic carriers and animals serologically recovered from acute infections. *Hepatology* **9:** 461–470.

Koretz RL, Abbey H, Coleman E & Gitnick G (1993) Non-A, non-B post-transfusion hepatitis: looking back in the second decade. *Annals of Internal Medicine* **119:** 110–115.

Koshy R & Wells J (1991) Deregulation of cellular gene expression by HBV transactivators in hepato-carcinogenesis. *Advances in Applied Biotechnology* **13:** 159–170.

Koshy R, Koch S & Freytag von Loringhoven A et al (1983) Integration of hepatitis B virus DNA: evidence for integration in the single-stranded gap. *Cell* **34:** 215–223.

Koshy R, Meyer M & Kékulé A et al (1991) Altered functions of hepatitis B virus proteins as a consequence of viral DNA integration may lead to hepatocyte transformation. In Hollinger FB, Lemon SM & Margolis H (eds) *Viral Hepatitis and Liver Disease*. pp 566–572. Baltimore: Williams & Wilkins.

Kurosaki M, Enomoto N, Sakamoto N et al (1995) Detection and analysis of replicating hepatitis C virus RNA in hepatocellular carcinoma tissues. *Journal of Hepatology* **22:** 527–535.

Lanford RE, Chavez D, Vonchisari F & Sureau C (1995) Lack of detection of negative-strand hepatitis C virus RNA in peripheral blood mononuclear cells and other extrahepatic tissues by the highly strand-specific rTth reverse transcriptase PCR. *Journal of Virology* **69:** 8079–8083.

Lauer U, Weib L, Lipp M et al (1994) The hepatitis B virus PreS2/S^T Transactivation utilizes AP-1 and transcription factors for transactivation. *Hepatology* **19:** 23–31.

Lee TH, Finegold MJ, Shen R-F et al (1990) Hepatitis B virus transactivator X protein is not tumori-genic in transgenic mice. *Journal of Virology* **64:** 5939–5947.

Lee TH, Elledge SJ & Butel JS (1995) Hepatitis B virus X protein interacts with a probable cellular DNA repair protein. *Journal of Virology* **69:** 1107–1114.

Lerat H, Berby F, Trabaud MA et al (1996) Specific detection of hepatitis C virus minus strand RNA in hematopoietic cells. *Journal of Clinical Investigation* **97:** 845–851.

Levine AJ (1993) The tumor suppressor genes. *Annual Review of Biochemistry* **62:** 623–651.

Liang T, Baruch Y & Ben-Porath E (1991) Hepatitis B virus infection in patients with idiopathic liver disease. *Hepatology* **13:** 1044–1051.

Liang T, Jeffers L, Cheinquer H et al (1992) Viral etiology of hepatocellular carcinoma in United States. *Hepatology* **16:** 128A.

Liang TJ, Jeffers L, Rajender K et al (1993) Fulminant or subfulminant non-A, non-B viral hepatitis: the role of hepatitis CE viruses. *Gastroenterology* **104:** 556–562.

Lin C, Pragai BM & Grakoui AEA (1994) Hepatitis C virus NS3 serine proteinase: trans-cleavage requirements and processing kinetics. *Journal of Virology* **68:** 8147–8157.

Loncarevic I, Schrantz P, Zentgraft H et al (1990a) Replication of hepatitis B virus in a hepatocellular carcinoma. *Virology* **174:** 158–168.

Loncarevic IF, Zentgraf H & Schröder CH (1990b) Sequence of a replication competent hepatitis B virus genome with a preX open reading frame. *Nucleic Acids Research* **18:** 4940.

London WT & Blumberg BS (1982) Acellular model of the role of hepatitis virus in the pathogenesis of primary hepatocellular carcinoma. *Hepatology* **2:** 105–145.

Lugassy C, Bernuau J, Thiers V et al (1987) Sequences of hepatitis B virus DNA in the serum and liver of patients with acute benign and fulminant hepatitis. *Journal of Infectious Diseases* **155:** 64–71.

Magrin S, Craxi A & Fabiano C (1994) Hepatitis C viremia in chronic liver disease: relationship to interferon-alpha or corticosteroid treatment. *Hepatology* **19:** 273–279.

Marion PL, Oshiro LS, Regnery DC et al (1980) A virus in beechey ground squirrels that is related to hepatitis B virus of humans. *Proceedings of the National Academy of Sciences of the USA* **77:** 2941–2945.

Mason A, Yoffe B, Noonan C et al (1992) Hepatitis B virus DNA in peripheral-blood mononuclear cells in chronic hepatitis B after HBsAg clearance. *Hepatology* **16:** 36–41.

Matsubara K (1991) Chromosomal changes associated with hepatitis B virus DNA integration and hepatocarcinogenesis. In McLachlan A (ed.) *Molecular Biology of the Hepatitis B Virus* pp 245–256. Boca Raton, FL: CRC Press.

Matsubara K & Tokino T (1990) Integration of hepatitis B virus DNA and its implications for hepato-carcinogenesis. *Molecular Biology and Medicine* **7:** 243–260.

Matsumoto H, Yoneyama T, Mitamura K et al (1988) Analysis of integrated hepatitis B virus DNA and cellular flanking sequences cloned from a hepatocellular carcinoma. *International Journal of Cancer* **42:** 1–6.

Matsuura Y & Miyamura T (1993) The molecular biology of hepatitis C virus. *Virology* **203:** 297–304.

Mendenhall CL, Seeff L, Diehl AM et al (1991) Antibodies to hepatitis B virus and hepatitis C virus in alcoholic hepatitis and cirrhosis: their prevalence and clinical relevance. *Hepatology* **14:** 581–589.

Meyer M, Caselman W, Schlüter V et al (1992a) Hepatitis B virus transactivator MHBst: activation of NF-KB, selective inhibition by antioxidants and integral membrane localization. *EMBO Journal* **11:** 2991–3001.

Meyer M, Wiedorn KH & Hofschneider PH (1992b) Chromosome 17:7 translocation is associated with hepatitis B virus DNA integration in human hepatocellular carcinoma DNA. *Hepatology* **15:** 665.

Michalak TI, Pasquinelli C, Gui ot S & Chisari FV (1994) Hepatitis B virus persistence after recovery from acute hepatitis. *Journal of Clinical Investigation* **93:** 230–239.

Miller RH & Robinson WS (1986) Common evolutionary origin of hepatitis B virus and retroviruses. *Proceedings of the National Academy of Sciences of the USA* **83:** 2531–2535.

Mizusawa H, Taira M, Yaginuma K et al (1985) Inversely repeating integrated hepatitis B virus DNA and cellular flanking sequences in the human hepatoma-derived cell line huSP. *Proceedings of the National Academy of Sciences of the USA* **82:** 208–212.

Mondelli M, Naumov N & Eddleston A (1984) The immunopathogenesis of liver cell damage in chronic infection. In Chisari F (ed.) *Advances in Hepatitis Research.* pp 144–151. New York: Masson.

Monjardino JP, Fowler MJF & Thomas HC (1983) Defective hepatitis B virus DNA molecules detected in a stable integration pattern in a hepatoma cell line, and in induced tumours and derived cell lines. *Journal of General Virology* **64:** 2299–2303.

Morgan D, Pecararo G, Rosenberg I & Defendi V (1990) Human papillomavirus type 6b DNA is required for initiation but not maintenance of transformation of C127 mouse cells. *Journal of Virology* **64:** 969–976.

Murakami Y, Hayashi K, Hirohashi S & Sekiya T (1991) Aberrations of tumor suppressor p53 and retinoblastoma genes in human hepatocellular carcinomas. *Cancer Research* **51:** 5520–5525.

Nagaya T, Nakamura T, Tokino T et al (1987) The mode of hepatitis B virus DNA integration in chromosomes of human hepatocellular carcinoma. *Genes and Development* **1:** 773–782.

Nakamura T, Tokino T, Nagaya T & Matsubara K (1988) Microdeletion associated with the integration process of hepatitis B virus DNA. *Nucleic Acids Research* **16:** 4865–4873.

Nalpas B (1994) Alcohol and hepatocellular carcinoma. In Brechot C (ed.) *Primary Liver Cancer: Etiological and Progression Factors.* pp 231–248. Boca Raton, FL: CRC Press.

Nalpas B, Berthelot P, Thiers V et al (1985) Hepatitis B virus multiplication in the absence of usual serological markers—a study of 146 alcoholics. *Journal of Hepatology* **1:** 89–97.

Nalpas B, Driss F, Pol S et al (1991) Association between HCV and HBV infection in hepatocellular carcinoma and alcoholic liver disease. *Journal of Hepatology* **12:** 70.

Nalpas B, Thiers V, Pol S et al (1992) Hepatitis C viremia and anti-HCV antibodies in alcoholics. *Journal of Hepatology* **14:** 381–384.

Naumova AK & Kisselev LL (1990) Biological consequences of interactions between hepatitis B virus and human nonhepatic cellular genomes. *Biomedical Sciences* **1:** 233–238.

Nishida N, Fukuda Y, Kokuryu H et al (1993) Role and mutational heterogeneity of the p53 gene in hepatocellular carcinoma. *Cancer Research* **53:** 368–372.

Nousbaum JB, Pol S, Nalpas B et al (1995) Hepatitis C virus types 1b (II) infection in France and Italy. *Annals of Internal Medicine* **122:** 161–168.

Ohkoshi S (1991) Detection of HBV DNA in non-A, non-B hepatic tissues using the polymerase chain reaction assay. *Gastroenterology Japan* **26:** 728.

Omata M (1990) Significance of extrahepatic replication of HBV. *Hepatology* **12:** 364–366.

Parés A, Barrera JM, Caballeria J et al (1990) Hepatitis C virus antibodies in chronic alcoholic patients: association with severity of liver injury. *Hepatology* **12:** 1295–1299.

Pasquinelli C, Lauré F, Chatenaud L et al (1986) Hepatitis B virus DNA in mononuclear blood cells. *Journal of Hepatology* **3:** 95–103.

Pasquinelli C, Garreau F, Bougueleret L et al (1988) Rearrangement of a common cellular DNA domain on chromosome 4 in human primary liver tumors. *Journal of Virology* **62:** 629–632.

Paterlini P & Bréchot C (1994) Hepatitis B virus and primary liver cancer in hepatitis B surface antigen-positive and negative patients. In Bréchot C (ed.) *Primary Liver Cancer: Etiological and Progression Factors.* pp 167–190. Boca Raton, FL: CRC Press.

Patelini P, Gerken G, Nakajima E et al (1990) Polymerase chain reaction to detect hepatitis b virus DNA and RNA sequences in primary liver cancers from patients negative for hepatitis B surface antigen. *New England Journal of Medicine* **323:** 80–85.

Paterlini P, Gerken G, Khemeny F et al (1991) Primary liver cancer in HBsAg negative patients: a study of HBV genome using the polymerase chain reaction. In Vyas G, Dienstag JL & Hoofnagle JC (eds) *Viral Hepatitis and Liver Disease,* pp 222–226. Baltimore: Williams & Wilkins.

Paterlini P, Driss F, Pisi E et al (1993) Persistence of hepatitis B and hepatitis C viral genomes in primary liver cancers from HBsAg negative patients: a study of a low endemic area. *Hepatology* **17:** 20–29.

Paterlini P, Poussin K, De Mitri S et al (1994) Rate of persistence, structure, and expression of HBV genome in HCC developing in HBsAg-negative patients. In Nishioka K, Suzuki H, Mishiro S & Odat C (eds) *Viral Hepatitis and Liver Disease.* pp 757–762. Tokyo: Springer Verlag.

Pontisso P, Poon MC, Tiollais P & Bréchot C (1984) Detection of HBV DNA in mononuclear blood cells. *British Medical Journal* **288:** 1563–1566.

Poynard T, Aubert A, Lazizi Y et al (1991) Independent risk factors for hepatocellular carcinoma in French drinkers. *Hepatology* **13:** 896.

Preisler-Adams S, Schlayer HJ, Peters T et al (1993) Sequence analysis of hepatitis B virus DNA in immunologically negative infection. *Archives of Virology* **133:** 385–396.

Quade K, Saldanha J, Thomas H & Monjardino J (1992) Integration of hepatitis B virus DNA through a mutational hot spot within the cohesive region in a case of hepatocellular carcinoma. *Journal of General Virology* **73:** 179–182.

Ramesh R, Panda SK, Jameel S & Rajasambandam P (1994) Mapping of the hepatitis B virus genome in hepatocellular carcinoma using PCR and demonstration of a potential trans-activator encoded by the frequently detected fragment. *Journal of General Virology* **75:** 327–334.

Raimondo G, Burk R, Lieberman H et al (1988) Interrupted replication of hepatitis B virus in liver tissue of HBsAg carriers with hepatocellular carcinoma. *Virology* **166:** 103–112.

Robinson WS (1990) Hepadnaviridae and their replication. In Fields BN, Knipe DM, Chanock RM, Hirsch MS, Melnick JL, Monath TP & Roizman B (eds) *Fields Virology.* pp 2137–2169. New York: Raven Press.

Rogler CE & Summers J (1982) Novel forms of woodchuck hepatitis virus DNA isolated from chronically infected woodchuck liver nuclei. *Journal of Virology* **44:** 852–863.

Rogler CE, Sherman M, Su CY et al (1985) Deletion in chromosome 11p associated with a hepatitis B integration site in hepatocellular carcinoma. *Science* **230:** 319–322.

Romet-Lemonne JL, McLane MF, Elfassi E et al (1983) Hepatitis B virus infection in cultured human lymphoblastoid cells. *Science* **221:** 667–669.

Rossner MT (1992) Hepatitis B virus X-gene product: a promiscuous transcriptional activator (review). *Journal of Medical Virology* **36:** 101–117.

Ruiz J, Sangro B, Cuende JI et al (1992) Hepatitis B and C viral infections in patients with hepatocellular carcinoma. *Hepatology* **16:** 637–641.

Sakamuro D, Furukawa T & Takegami T (1995) Hepatitis C virus nonstructural protein NS3 transforms NIH 3T3 cells. *Journal of Virology* **69:** 3893–3896.

Santolini E, Migliaccio G & La Monica N (1994) Biosynthesis and biochemical properties of the hepatitis C virus core protein. *Journal of Virology* **68:** 3631–3641.

Saunders J, Wodak A, Morgan-Capner P et al (1983) Importance of markers of hepatitis B virus in alcoholic liver disease. *British Medical Journal* **286:** 1851.

Schlüter V, Meyer M, Hofschneider PH et al (1994) Integrated hepatitis B virus X and 3′ truncated preS/S sequences derived from human hepatomas encode functionally active transactivators. *Oncogene* **9:** 1–10.

Scotto J, Hadchouel M, Wain-Hobson S et al (1985) Hepatitis B virus DNA in Dane particles: evidence for the presence of replicative intermediates. *Journal of Infectious Diseases* **151:** 610–617.

Seef LB, Buskell-Bales Z, Wright EC et al (1992) Long-term mortality after transfusion-associated non-A, non-B hepatitis. *New England Journal of Medicine* **327:** 1906–1911.

Sell S (1993) The role of determined stem-cells in the cellular lineage of hepatocellular carcinoma. *International Journal of Developmental Biology* **37:** 189–201.

Sell S, Hunt JM, Dunsford HA & Chisari FV (1991) Synergy between hepatitis B virus expression and chemical hepatocarcinogens in transgenic mice. *Cancer Research* **51:** 1278–1285.

Shafritz DA, Shouval D, Sherman H et al (1981) Integration of hepatitis B virus DNA into the genome of liver cells in chronic liver disease and hepatocellular carcinoma. *New England Journal of Medicine* **305:** 1067–1073.

Shaul Y, Ziemer M, Garcia PD et al (1984) Cloning and analysis of integrated hepatitis virus sequences from a human hepatoma cell line. *Journal of Virology* **51:** 776–787.

Shaul Y, Garcia PD, Schonberg S & Rutter WJ (1986) Integration of hepatitis B virus DNA in chromosome-specific satellite sequences. *Journal of Virology* **59:** 731–734.

Sheu JC, Huang GT, Shih LN et al (1992) Hepatitis C and B viruses in hepatitis B surface antigen-negative hepatocellular carcinoma. *Gastroenterology* **103:** 1322–1327.

Shih C, Burke K, Chou MJ et al (1987) Tight clustering of human hepatitis B virus integration sites in hepatomas near a triple-stranded region. *Journal of Virology* **61**: 3491–3498.

Shimoda T, Shikata T, Karasawa T & Tsukagoshi S (1981) Light microscopic localization of hepatitis B virus antigens in the human pancreas. *Gastroenterology* **81**: 898–1005.

Silini E, Bono F, Cividini A, et al (1995) Differential distribution of hepatitis C virus genotypes in patients with and without liver function abnormalities. *Hepatology* **21**: 285–290.

Slagle BL, Zhou YZ & Butel JS (1991) Hepatitis B virus integration event in human chromosome 17p near the p53 gene identifies the region of the chromosome commonly deleted in virus-positive hepatocellular carcinomas. *Cancer Research* **51**: 49–54.

Smith KT & Campo MS (1988) 'Hit and run' transformation of mouse C127 cells by bovine papillomavirus type 4: the viral DNA is required for the initiation but not for maintenance of the transformed phenotype. *Virology* **64**: 39–47.

Sullivan DE & Gerber MA (1994) Conservation of hepatitis C virus 5′ untranslated sequences in hepatocellular carcinoma and the surrounding liver. *Hepatology* **19**: 551–553.

Tabor E, Farshid M, Di Bisceglie A & Hsia CC (1992) Increased expression of transforming growth factor-alpha after transfection of a human hepatoblastoma cell line with the hepatitis B virus. *Journal of Medical Virology* **37**: 271–273.

Takada S & Koike K (1990) Trans-activation function of a 3′ truncated X gene-cell fusion product from integrated hepatitis B virus DNA in chronic hepatitis tissues. *Proceedings of the National Academy of Sciences of the USA* **87**: 5628–5632.

Takada S, Gotoh Y, Hayashi S et al (1990) Structural rearrangement of integrated hepatitis B virus DNA as well as cellular flanking DNA is present in chronically infected hepatic tissues. *Journal of Virology* **64**: 822–828.

Takada S, Yaginuma K, Arii M et al (1992a) Molecular biology of hepatitis B virus and hepatocellular carcinoma. In Koike K (ed.) *Primary Liver Cancer in Japan*. pp 75–87. Tokyo: Springer Verlag.

Takada S, Takase S, Enomoto N et al (1992b) Clinical backgrounds of the patients having different types of hepatitis C virus genomes. *Journal of Hepatology* **14**: 35–40.

Takada S, Kido H, Fukutomi A et al (1994) Interaction of hepatitis B virus X protein with a serine protease, tryptase TL, as an inhibitor. *Oncogene* **9**: 341–348.

Tanaka Y, Esumi M & Shikata T (1988) Frequent integration of hepatitis B virus DNA in non-cancerous liver tissue from hepatocellular carcinoma patients. *Journal of Medical Virology* **26**: 7–14.

Tanji Y, Hijikata M, Satoh S et al (1995) Hepatitis C virus-encoded nonstructural protein NS4A has versatile functions in viral protein processing. *Journal of Virology* **69**: 1575–1581.

Tarao K, Shimizu A, Ohkawa S et al (1992) Developement of hepatocellular carcinoma associated with increases in DNA synthesis in the surrounding cirrhosis. *Gastroenterology* **103**: 595–600.

Tatzelt J, Fechteler K, Langenbach P & Doerfler W (1993) Fractionated nuclear extracts from hamster cells catalyse cell-free recombination at selective sequences between adenovirus DNA and a hamster preinsertion site. *Genetics* **90**: 7356–7360.

Tokino T & Matsubara K (1991) Chromosomal sites for hepatitis B virus integration in human hepatocellular carcinoma. *Journal of Virology* **65**: 6761–6764.

Tokino T, Fukushige S, Nakamura T et al (1987) Chromosomal translocation and inverted duplication associated with integrated hepatitis B virus in hepatocellular carcinomas. *Journal of Virology* **61**: 3848–3854.

Tong MJ, El-Farra NS, Reikes AR et al (1995) Clinical outcomes after transfusion-associated hepatitis C. *New England Journal of Medicine* **332**: 1463–1466.

Toshkov I, Chisari FV & Bannasch P (1994) Hepatic preneoplasia in hepatitis B virus transgenic mice. *Hepatology* **20**: 1162–1172.

Transy C, Fourel G, Robinson WS et al (1992) Frequent amplification of c-myc in ground squirrel liver tumors associated with past or ongoing infection with a hepadnavirus. *Proceedings of the National Academy of Sciences of the USA* **89**: 3874–3878.

Tremolada F, Casarin C, Alberti A et al (1992) Long-term follow-up of non-A, non-B (type C) post-transfusion hepatitis. *Journal of Hepatology* **16**: 273–281.

Truant R, Antunovic J, Greenblatt J et al (1995) Direct interaction of the hepatitis B virus HBx protein with p53 leads to inhibition by HBx of p53 response element-directed transactivation. *Journal of Virology* **69**: 1851–1859.

Ueda H, Ohkoshi S, Harris CC & Jay G (1995) Synergism between the HBx gene and aflatoxin B-1 in the development of murine liver cancer. *International Journal of Oncology* **7**: 735–740.

Unsal H, Yakicier C, Marçais C et al (1994) Genetic heterogeneity of hepatocellular carcinoma. *Proceedings of the National Academy of Sciences of the USA* **91:** 822–826.

Urano Y, Watanabe K, Lin C et al (1991) Interstitial chromosomal deletion within 4q11-q13 in a human hepatoma cell line. *Cancer Research* **51:** 1460–1464.

Wang HP & Rogler CE (1988) Deletions in human chromosome arms 11p and 13 p in primary hepatocellular carcinomas. *Science* **48:** 72.

Wang HP & Rogler CE (1991) Topoisomerase I-mediated integration of hepadnavirus DNA in vitro. *Journal of Virology* **65:** 2381–2392.

Wang Y, Chen P, Wu X et al (1990) A new enhancer element, ENII, identified in the X gene of hepatitis B virus. *Journal of Virology* **64:** 3977–3981.

Wang W, London T & Feitelson M (1991a) Hepatitis B x antigen in hepatitis B virus carrier patients with liver cancer. *Cancer Research* **51:** 4971–4977.

Wang W, London WT, Lega L & Feitelson MA (1991b) HBxAg in the liver from carrier patients with chronic hepatitis and cirrhosis. *Hepatology* **14:** 29–37.

Wang W-P, Myers RL & Chiu I-M (1991c) Single primer-mediated polymerase chain reaction: application in cloning of two different 5'-untranslated sequences of acidic fibroblast growth factor mRNA. *DNA and Cell Biology* **10:** 771–777.

Wang J, Zindy F, Chenivesse X et al (1992a) Modification of cyclin A expression by hepatitis b virus DNA integration in a hepatocellular carcinoma. *Oncogene* **7:** 1653–1656.

Wang JT, Sheu JC, Lin JT et al (1992b) Detection of replicative form of hepatitis C virus RNA in peripheral blood mononuclear cells. *Journal of Infectious Diseases* **166:** 1167–1169.

Wright ML, Hsu H, Donegan E et al (1991) Hepatitis C virus not found in fulminant non-A, non-B hepatitis. *Annals of Internal Medicine* **115:** 111–112.

Yaginuma K, Kobayashi M, Yoshida E & Koike K (1985) Hepatitis B virus integration in hepatocellular carcinoma DNA: duplication of cellular flanking sequences at the integration site. *Proceedings of the National Academy of Sciences of the USA* **82:** 4458–4462.

Yaginuma K, Kobayashi H, Kobayashi M et al (1987) Multiple integration site of hepatitis B virus DNA in hepatocellular carcinoma and chronic active hepatitis tissues from children. *Journal of Virology* **61:** 1808–1813.

Yamauchi M, Nakahara M, Hisato N et al (1994) Different prevalence of hepatocellular carcinoma between patients with liver cirrhosis due to genotype II and III of hepatitis C virus. *International Hepatology Communications* **2:** 328–332.

Yanagi M, Kaneko S, Unoura M et al (1990) Hepatitis C virus in fulminant hepatic failure. *New England Journal of Medicine* **324:** 1895.

Yasui H, Hino O, Ohtake K et al (1992) Clonal growth of hepatitis B virus integrated hepatocytes in cirrhotic liver nodules. *Cancer Research* **52:** 6810–6814.

Yeh S-H, Chen P-J, Chen H-L et al (1994) Frequent genetic alterations at the distal region of chromosome 1p in human hepatocellular carcinomas. *Cancer Research* **54:** 4188–4192.

Yoffe B, Noonan C, Melnick J & Hollinger F (1986) Hepatitis B virus DNA in mononuclear cells and analysis of cell subsets for the presence of replicative intermediates of viral DNA. *Journal of Infectious Diseases* **153:** 471–477.

Yoffe B, Burns DK, Bhatt HS & Combes B (1990) Extrahepatic hepatitis B virus DNA sequences in patients with acute hepatitis B infection. *Hepatology* **12:** 187–192.

Zerial M, Salinas J, Filipski J & Bernardi G (1986) Genomic localization of hepatitis B virus in a human hepatoma cell line. *Nucleic Acids Research* **14:** 8373–8385.

Zhang XK, Egan JO, Huang DP et al (1992) Hepatitis B virus DNA integration and expression of an Erb B-like gene in human hepatocellular carcinoma. *Biochemical and Biophysical Research Communications* **188:** 344–351.

Zhou YZ, Butel JS, Li PJ et al (1987) Integrated state of subgenomic fragments of hepatitis B virus DNA in hepatocellular carcinoma from mainland China. *Journal of National Cancer Institute* **79:** 223–231.

Ziemer M, Garcia P, Shaul Y & Rutter WJ (1985) Sequence of hepatitis B virus DNA incorporated into the genome of a human hepatoma cell line. *Journal of Virology* **53:** 885–892.

Zoulim F, Saputelli J & Seeger C (1994) Woodchuck hepatitis virus X protein is required for viral infection in vivo. *Journal of Virology* **68:** 2026–2030.

10

Liver transplantation in virus-induced chronic liver disease

ALESSANDRA COLANTONI
NICOLA DE MARIA
STEFANO FAGIUOLI
DAVID H. VAN THIEL

Orthotopic liver transplantation (OLTx) is the therapy of choice for patients with end-stage liver disease for whom there is no other medical or surgical alternative treatment. The development of surgical techniques and immunosuppression over the preceding three decades as well as the more recent recognition of transplantation medicine as a subspeciality in hepatology, has enabled most active liver transplant centres to achieve 1-year survival rates up to 85–90%.

Chronic viral hepatitis caused by HBV, HCV, HDV or non-A, non-B, non-C virus infection is the most frequent indication for OLTx world-wide. Transplant candidates having liver disease related to any of these hepatitis viruses account for more than 30% of all adult transplants (Fagiuoli et al, 1993). Typically, individuals transplanted for end-stage chronic viral liver disease have overt evidence of liver failure and one or more clinical complications of their liver disease, as shown in Table 1.

Unfortunately for a large number of patients who have received an OLTx for viral hepatitis, disease recurrence has been almost universal, and in many it has led to either accelerated disease progression to cirrhosis, occasionally with hepatic cancer over a 2–5 year period; or a unique form of subacute hepatic failure termed 'fibrosing cholestatic hepatitis'. Prior to

Table 1. The main biochemical and clinical variables that state the need for OLTx in patients with chronic viral liver disease.

Biochemical	Clinical
Albumin < 2.5 g/dl	Hepatic encephalopathy
Prothrombin time > 5 seconds above normal	Intractable ascites
Bilirubin < 15 mg/dl	Hepato-renal syndrome
	Recurrent spontaneous bacterial peritonitis
	Recurrent variceal bleeding
	Hepatocellular carcinoma

Baillière's Clinical Gastroenterology—
Vol. 10, No. 2, July 1996
ISBN 0–7020–2094–X
0950–3528/96/020375 + 14 $12.00/00

Copyright © 1996, by Baillière Tindall
All rights of reproduction in any form reserved

OLTx, the HBV or HCV replicative status of the patient needs to be assessed. The incidence of viral hepatitis recurrence in liver allografts depends on multiple factors, including the specific viral agent (HBV, HCV, HDV), the patient's serological status and the clinical presentation of the disease at the time of OLTx. The high rate of disease recurrence and its more rapid course in transplant recipients is a direct consequence of two factors: (1) the high viral load experienced by the allograft liver arising from the serum and extrahepatic sites of infection in the graft recipient, and (2) the requirement for life-long immunosuppression that is gluco-corticoid-based in order to prevent allograft rejection. Both factors inhibit host defence mechanisms directed at viral infections. The latter also enhances the rate of viral replication by interacting with a replication promoter site within the genome. Efforts to prevent or treat viral hepatitis in liver allografts recipients are of great interest to transplant physicians and surgeons.

LIVER TRANSPLANTATION FOR HEPATITIS B VIRUS INFECTION

HBV-related end-stage liver disease is a world-wide problem of great magnitude. It is estimated that more than 300 million individuals are affected by some form of HBV-related chronic liver disease around the world. OLTx is the only therapy for patients with end-stage liver disesase for whom conventional medical treatment is no longer effective. OLTx for end-stage liver disease secondary to HBV infection has evolved rapidly during the last two decades. Initially, HBV-related chronic liver disease was considered an ideal indication for OLTx because no other therapy existed, and it was assumed that the virus infected only the liver. The latter assumption was wrong and, as a result, viral infection of the allograft was common, leading to significantly reduced graft and patient survival rates. As this experience accumulated, HBV infection became an absolute contra-indication for OLTx in many centres. With a closer examination of the accumulated OLTx results for HBV-related disease it became clear that subgroups of individuals with HBV have a good outcome after transplantation. These include those who are HBV DNA-negative using dot blot hybridization assay, and those with either con-founding HDV infection or fulminant HBV disease. Each of these groups either has low levels of HBV DNA or is DNA-negative, and as a result recurrent HBV infection is usual (Samuel et al, 1991a; Van Thiel et al, 1994b; Lake, 1995).

The precise source of allograft infection following successful transplant surgery remains unclear. Most believe that it occurs as a consequence of ongoing viraemia with direct infection of the liver graft from virus in the plasma. However, Feray et al (1990) have identified liver allograft recipients who were HBV DNA-negative in plasma and in the resected liver but who were HBV DNA-positive in circulating peripheral mono-nuclear cells and subsequently developed overt allograft viral hepatitis.

Extrahepatic sites of viral infection and replication have been described in individuals with HBV disease; these extrahepatic foci of infection may be responsible for the allograft infection as a consequence of immuno-suppression-induced viral reactivation in OLTx recipients (Omata, 1990; Yoffe et al, 1990).

Pathogenesis of graft re-infection

HBV DNA sequences have been demonstrated in spleen, thymus, lymph nodes, pancreas, kidneys, thyroid gland, testis, adrenal glands and mono-nuclear blood cells (Feray et al, 1990; Yoffe et al, 1990). Due to the specific hepatotrophic activity of HBV, viral DNA replication seems to have no pathological effect in these extrahepatic sites. However, these sites can act as a viral reservoir in which DNA replication can either be enhanced or triggered as a result of immunosuppression in a liver transplant recipient (Omata, 1990).

High-dose corticosteroids given in the immediate post-OLTx period can interact with the glucocorticoid-responsive enhancer region of the HBV genome, resulting an overproduction of HBV particles (Tur-Kaspa et al, 1988). In addition, cyclosporin A has been shown to enhance viral repli-cation and to enhance the severity of chronic HBV infection in both animal and in vitro models of HBV disease (Cote et al, 1991). The result-ing exaggerated viral replication, with massive accumulation of viral proteins in the hepatocytes, may result in a direct cytopathic liver injury occurring in addition to the usual immune-mediated mechanism of HBV toxicity. This combination of pathogenic mechanisms has been postulated to be the basis for fibrosing cholestatic hepatitis (Davies et al, 1991; Lau et al, 1992).

Re-infection risk and viraemia

Viral load, as defined by the presence of HBV DNA (or HBeAg positivity) in the serum pre-OLTx, is the strongest predictor of HBV recurrence after transplantation. The largest series of recipients transplanted for HBV-related chronic liver disease show that 3-year survival rates after OLTx are reduced significantly in HBV DNA-positive recipients as compared with recipients transplanted for other disease indications who are HBV DNA-negative (Samuel et al, 1993). Pooled data obtained from many different series show that more than 95% of HBV DNA-positive patients have evidence of HBsAg positivity following OLTx whereas those who are HBV DNA-negative prior to OLTx become HBsAg positive in as few as 10% of cases (Table 2) (Mora et al, 1990; Muller et al, 1991; Samuel et al, 1991a, Todo et al, 1991; O'Grady et al, 1992; Burra et al, 1993; Ranjan et al, 1993; Samuel et al, 1993; Konig et al, 1994; Terrault et al, 1994). Most importantly, the 3–5 years' survival post-transplant is reduced in indi-viduals transplanted for HBV-related chronic liver disease who have a recurrence, having a survival of only 50%, whereas the survival of those without HBV recurrence is 83%.

Table 2. Recurrence of HBV infection and survival after OLTx in patients receiving short-term HBIg or no treatment.

	HBIg (no/short-term)		HBIg (long-term)	
	Re-infection rate	3-year survival	Re-infection rate	3-year survival
HBV DNA(+)	93/96 (96%)	40%	44/54 (81%)	50%
HBV DNA(−)	33/49 (67%)	50%	25/98 (25%)	80%
HBV/HDV	13/27 (48%)	50%	7/68 (10%)	80–90%

Data pooled from several series.

Chronic active hepatitis with cirrhosis and delta co-infection

The situation for those co-infected with HBV and HDV appears paradoxical in that co-infection in a non-transplant setting is known to produce more rapid disease progression and to be more resistant to interferon therapy than is isolated HBV infection alone. Post-transplant, the reverse situation is true. This paradox can be explained, however, when it is recalled that HDV infection down-regulates HBV replication and the risk of disease recurrence relates directly to the viral carriage rate at the time of OLTx. Transplantation of individuals co-infected with HBV and HDV results in the demonstration of HDV infection of the liver allograft early post-OLTx in the absence of HBV markers (in either the serum or liver) or graft dysfunction. This unique form of HDV infection probably arises either from HDV encoated in HBsAg present in the blood or from extrahepatic reservoirs. The clinical course of isolated HDV infection post-OLTx is indolent and resolves spontaneously unless the HBV infection also recurs. Histological hepatitis and diffuse spreading of HDV within the liver occurs only in the presence of active HBV replication. These observations suggest that HDV in OLTx recipients can replicate in the absence of HBV; is not directly cytopathic and requires the presence of active HBV replication to induce clinical liver damage (David et al, 1993).

Overall, patients with HDV co-infection have a more favourable outcome after OLTx. The early studies of OLTx with the use of short-term HBIg prophylaxis protocols for combined HBV/HDV end-stage liver disease were discouraging (Ottobrelli et al, 1991; Samuel et al, 1991b). Subsequent studies of OLTx for combined HBV/HDV liver disease in recipients treated with long-term passive prophylaxis have shown both a reduced graft re-infection rate (10%) and improved survival (up to 88% at 3 years) (Table 2) (David et al, 1993; Samuel et al, 1993; Samuel et al, 1995; Villamil et al, 1995).

Prophylaxis of re-infection: use of hepatitis B immune globulin (HBIg)

The very high rate of disease recurrence in liver transplant recipients transplanted for HBV-related liver disease has led to attempts at both active immunoprophylaxis with pre-operative anti-HBV vaccination (Lauchart et al, 1987a) and peri- and post-operative passive immunoprophylaxis with hepatitis B immune globulins (Lauchart et al, 1987b).

Although HBIg have been effective in preventing HBV re-infection in liver transplant recipients affected by HBV-related fulminant hepatic failure, HBV-related cirrhosis with confounding HDV co-infection as well as HBV DNA-negative HBV-related cirrhosis, the results of passive immunoprophylaxis in HBV DNA-positive individuals have been controversial: most series showed little, if any, reduction in re-infection rates in viraemic patients treated with protocols targetting an anti-HBs titre above 100 IU/l (Lauchart et al, 1987b; Samuel et al, 1993). By contrast, groups targeting an anti-HBs titre above 500 IU/l have shown a dramatic reduction or no HBV re-infection in viraemic patients treated with their high-dose long-term HBIg protocols (Belle et al, 1994; McGory et al, 1994; Lake, 1995; Pruett, 1995). These results clearly indicate that the ideal doses and duration of the HBIg treatment in viraemic patients have not been fully established. It appears that higher doses during the peri- and immediate post-transplant period are critical for a good outcome, and targetting the anti-HBs titre above 500 IU/l increases the likelihood of long-term disease-free survival. It remains to be determined how long HBIg therapy needs to be continued post-OLTx. This latter question is important for several reasons. First, the use of HBIg adds at least $20–30 000 to the annual cost of post-OLTx care. Second, at least in the United States, the only HBIg preparations commercially available contain small amounts of mercury as an antiseptic. The continuous administration of HBIg with trace amounts of mercury over years is likely to lead to mercury toxicity as a post-OLTx morbidity. Current protocols of HBIg therapy vary from centre to centre but the most frequently used one is as follows: 10 000 U of HBIg is given while the patient is anhepatic and the same dose is repeated daily for 10 days followed by a monthly intramuscular dose of 1500 U which is continued indefinitely. The use of anti-HBV vaccine, at least at standard doses, in HBV-infected individuals has not been shown to be useful in producing HBV immunity (Lauchart et al, 1987a; Muller et al, 1991).

Clinical spectrum of HBV infection in liver allograft

The clinical course of recurrent HBV infection in liver allografts is accelerated as compared with the course of disease observed in non-immunosuppressed individuals. Post-transplant recurrence of HBV infection is almost always associated with histological abnormalities. Cirrhosis has been reported to occur within 2–3 years and even as early as 8 months after OLTx (Van Thiel et al, 1994b; Lake, 1995). The histological spectrum of HBV infection in the liver allografts ranges from indolent infection to an aggressive chronic hepatitis. Demetris et al were the first to report on the histological findings of individuals with recurrent HBV infection. Thirty-four of 45 cases (75%) transplanted for HBV disease developed a recurrent infection. Chronic active hepatitis or cirrhosis was found in 27 cases (79%), submassive necrosis in 3 (9%) and minimal histological changes or normal findings only in 4 (12%) (Demetris et al, 1990).

Overall, recurrent type B hepatitis in liver allografts resembles the original HBV infection except for its rapid evolution. The rapid evolution of post-OLTx HBV disease is probably the result of the immunosuppressive therapy that is required to prevent graft rejection. Occasionally, a new picture of HBV-related liver injury can be can be recognized histologically in liver allografts. This syndrome is termed fibrosing cholestatic hepatitis. It occurs in up to 25% of the cases with recurrent HBV infection. It is characterized by serpiginous periportal fibrosis, canalicular and cellular cholestasis and hepatocellular ballooning. Little or no cellular infiltrate is present in the hepatic lobule and portal areas. HBsAg and HBcAg are expressed strikingly within the hepatocytes, with more than 90% of the cells demonstrating these antigens: the ballooning appears to be a consequence of uncontrolled HBsAg synthesis and retention by the infected cells (Demetris et al, 1990; Davies et al, 1991; Lau et al, 1992). It is believed by many that, in the situation of uncontrolled viral replication occurring in an immunosuppressed individual, HBV becomes directly cythopathogenic. The combination of uncontrolled viral replication and direct viral cyto-toxicity are thought to account for the unique histological pattern of fibrosing cholestatic hepatitis. The clinical course of this syndrome resembles late-onset hepatic failure rather than a chronic hepatitis, resulting in the need for retransplantation within a few months of OLTx. Subsequent transplants in individuals with fibrosing cholestatic hepatitis do even more poorly, with an even more rapid down-hill course. Thus, repeat OLTx is not recommended for such cases.

TREATMENT OF HBV INFECTION

Pre-OLTx

Historically, IFN has not been widely used in cases waiting for OLTx because it can produce an exacerbation of disease activity that has the potential to be life-threatening in an HBsAg-positive decompensated potential transplant recipient. In two clinical studies on patients with advanced chronic liver disease, who were treated with interferon, a transient HBV clearance occurred but persisted for only as long as IFN was being administered (Hoofnagle et al, 1993; Marcellin et al, 1994). The difficulty associated with matching the period of HBV DNA negativity achieved with IFN with the availability of a graft and the IFN-related side-effects, makes this therapy unlikely to be acceptable to most physicians, surgeons and patients.

Among other antiviral agents that can be utilized in the treatment of patients with HBV prior to OLTx, a nucleoside analogue, $2',3'$-dideoxy-$3'$-thiacytidine (lamivudine), has been shown to induce rapid hepatitis B viral DNA suppression in an animal model and is currently under clinical evaluation world-wide (Tyrrel et al, 1993; De Man et al, 1995; Grellier et al, 1995). If these promising preliminary results are confirmed by current ongoing European and American trials, the use of lamivudine in cases of chronic hepatitis B is likely to revolutionize existing concepts about OLTx for HBV DNA-positive individuals.

Recently, granulocyte–macrophage colony stimulating factor (GM-CSF) has been reported to enhance NK-cell and macrophage proliferation, resulting in an increased likelihood of viral clearance with the use of interferon (IFN). HBV DNA levels in blood have been shown to decline with GM-CSF therapy (Martin et al, 1993). IFN and GM-CSF may act synergistically to reduce HBV carriage rates.

Post-OLTx

The antiviral agents acyclovir and ganciclovir, both being nucleoside analogues, have been used with little or no long-term effectiveness in cases of HBV disease. The latter agent has reduced HBV levels but rarely eliminates viral carriage. However, repetitive cycles of ganciclovir, have been shown to reduce HBV carriage and to incite a remission in cases of chronic type B hepatitis (Gish et al, 1994).

The more recent agents, famciclovir and especially lamivudine, appear to be more promising. Both agents markedly reduce HBV viral carriage rates. Famciclovir, an analogue of ganciclovir, prevents DNA elongation by inhibiting DNA polymerase activity. Its use in liver transplant recipients with HBV recurrence has been reported (Boker et al, 1994; Kruger et al, 1994).

Foscarnet, a novel antiviral agent that inhibits viral specific DNA polymerase, has been shown to reduce serum HBV DNA levels in both an animal model and recurrent HBV infection in humans (Locarnini et al, 1993).

Lamivudine has shown to produce HBV clearance from the serum in the most cases reported to date. Unfortunately, the effect of lamivudine appears to be transient and persists only as long as the agent is being administered (De Man et al, 1995). This suggests that life-long lamivudine therapy may be required. Toxic reactions to lamivudine, consisting of myopathy and a sensorimotor neuropathy, have been reported and may be more likely to occur with chronic and potentially life-long use.

All these nucleoside analogue agents are targeted to specific steps that are essential for hepatitis B virus replication. In most treated OLTx recipients, a marked but transient suppression of HBV DNA has been shown, suggesting that there is a basis for such an approach.

The role of interferon in HBV disease in the peri-transplant situation is likely to evolve a consequence of the introduction of lamivudine. Following OLTx, concerns about the potential for inducing allograft rejection with IFN have limited its use. Fortunately, the reported empirical use of IFN in liver allograft recipients has not been associated with enhanced allograft rejection rates (Wright et al, 1992). However, the use of IFN in allograft recipients has not been particularly useful either. Although rare cases of viral clearance with its use have been reported (Hopf et al, 1991; Neuhaus et al, 1991; Wright et al, 1992a; Gurakar et al, 1994a; Villamil et al, 1994), this remains the exception rather than the rule. The combined use of lamivudine to reduce viral carriage rates followed by the addition of IFN to produce viral clearance in individuals with low viral loads has not yet been investigated but would appear to be a fruitful area of clinical investigation.

Re-transplantation

The results of re-transplantation for recurrent HBV disease have been disappointing (Crippin et al, 1994). In one series of seven patients who received a second liver allograft for HBV recurrence, the mortality was 85% within 100 days of re-transplantation (Todo et al, 1991). The European experience, based on 19 recipients of a second allograft, showed a 68% total mortality rate soon after OLTx (Samuel et al, 1993). A review of the United States experience on 20 cases of re-transplantation for HBV recurrence revealed a 95% total mortality (Crippin et al, 1994). The mean time to death or re-transplantation (third OLTx) in both the last two studies was about 4 months. The faster rate of both HBV recurrence and histological disease occurrence suggests the presence of an even more aggressive type of HBV infection following re-transplantation for HBV-related end-stage liver disease whose pathogenic mechanisms are yet to be clarified. The conventional HBIg prophylactic protocols have proven to be ineffective in preventing such a discouraging outcome. However, in a series of seven patients re-transplanted for HBV recurrence and treated with very high doses of HBIg (in order to maintain an anti-HBs titre above 500 IU/l), the recurrence rate was 15%, with all patients alive at a mean follow-up of 24 months (Kiyasu et al, 1994, Pruett, 1995). These preliminary results are consistent with what was observed in the transplantation of HBV DNA-positive individuals: if one can maintain HBIg serum levels high enough to 'neutralize' circulating HBsAg, graft re-infection may be prevented, even in patients with a very high viral load.

LIVER TRANSPLANTATION FOR HEPATITIS C VIRUS INFECTION

The presence of detectable anti-HCV (Kuo et al, 1989) and the recent introduction of the polymerase chain reaction (PCR) for the detection of HCV RNA have demonstrated that HCV is responsible for most cases of non-A, non-B hepatitis. It has been estimated that 600 million subjects world-wide are affected by HCV. Annually, in the United States 150 000 individuals are infected by HCV, 50–70% of whom become chronic and half develop cirrhosis. HCV disease accounts for an even greater number of transplants than does HBV disease. In fact, currently, HCV infection represents the leading cause of cirrhosis requiring OLTx in the United States, where 15–40% of adult OLTx candidates at each centre are transplanted for hepatitis C-related disease. The indications for OLTx for HCV disease are essentially identical to those for HBV disease. Specifically, the individual should have life-threatening disease for which no alternative therapy exists, and have one or more complications of chronic liver disease and the associated portal hypertension (Table 1).

Re-infection risk and clinical spectrum of HCV infection in liver allograft

HCV disease can recur like HBV but it does so at a rate different from that of HBV disease. HCV infection recurrence rates are as great as those experienced for HBV. In fact, almost all the patients transplanted for HCV-related chronic hepatitis experience a recurrent HCV infection. No correlation has been found between the level of viraemia before transplantation and the risk of recurrence of HCV infection in liver allograft recipients principally because the recurrence rate is essentially universal (Pons, 1995). Severe or multiple rejection episodes may result in an earlier onset of recurrent HCV infection (Sheiner, personal communication, Toronto, Canada). In addition to recurrence of disease, de novo HCV infections following OLTx in previously HCV-negative individuals have been reported to occur in up to 35% of cases transplanted at some centres (Wright et al, 1992). Thus, in the absence of other identifiable causes, HCV is the most common cause of chronic hepatitis post-OLTx (Poterucha et al, 1992). Despite recurrence of disease, the overall short-term survival rates for both graft and patients are good, ranging from 87 to 100% at 2 years. However, in post-OLTx, HCV disease, longer-periods of follow-up document a reduced survival rate comparable to what is seen in cases of HBV disease.

The magnitude and significance of HCV infection in immunosuppressed individuals is grossly underestimated using anti-HCV tests. Compared with HCV RNA by PCR, anti-HCV tests are associated with a large number of false-negative results, particularly with ELISA tests. Even recombinant immunoblot assay (RIBA) tests, which are considered more specific than ELISA, show a low sensitivity in the post-transplant setting: data from reported series show that from 25 to 83% of recipients with 'indeterminate' results on RIBA-2 are actually HCV RNA-positive. Moreover, 9–46% of patients with RIBA-2-negative tests are HCV RNA-positive. It is therefore essential to utilize the determination of HCV RNA (possibly both in serum and tissue) to monitor HCV recurrence or 'de novo' infection in transplant recipients (Lau et al, 1993).

Clinical spectrum of HCV infection in liver allograft

Disease recurrence develops slower, over 3–5 years rather than 1–3 years, and as a result has only recently become recognized. In most patients with recurrent HCV infection, hepatic injury is mild, although chronic active hepatitis develops in 50% of cases after an average of 7 months post-OLTx (Konig et al, 1994; Shah et al, 1992). Among 43 patients with recurrent HCV disease following successful OLTx, Ferrel et al (1992) reported that 51% of the subjects had histological hepatitis, 41% of whom had a mild form of the disease; 9% of the patients had cirrhosis or fibrosis.

A clinical diagnosis of recurrent hepatitis is difficult because it mimics rejection, ischaemia and biliary obstruction as well as other forms of hepatic infection. Serial biopsy specimens with persistent lobular pathology and HCV RNA quantification are requested to document the presence of hepatitis C (Ferrel et al, 1992; Mateo et al, 1993). Several groups have reported a clinical and histological picture of fibrosing cholestatic hepatitis in cases of HCV disease post-OLTx that mirrors the situation in cases of HBV infection. This syndrome is characterized by a very high titre of HCV carriage, progressive disease with poor results for both graft and patient survival.

The initial reports that recurrent HCV disease in liver allograft recipients is often inconsequential may not survive the test of time. With prolonged post-OLTx follow-up, clinically severe recurrent disease is becoming a major concern. Worse yet, the extensive experience at the University of Pittsburgh reported by Drs Rakela and Fung (personal communication, Reston, Virginia) demonstrates that the long-term costs are substantial. Specifically, they reported greater graft and patient losses at 4–5 years following OLTx for HCV than they have experienced for cases of HBV in their institution.

The pathogenetic mechanism of graft injury in recipients with HCV recurrence is poorly understood. As it is for HBV infection, circulating virions at the time of transplantation are the most likely source of HCV infection of the graft. Genotypic analysis of HCV infection before and after OLTx demonstrated a high degree of homology, suggesting graft infection by the original viral strain (Feray et al, 1992). HCV RNA replicative intermediates have been found in PBMC of OLTx recipients in whom both serum and liver tested negative for HCV RNA.

Quantification of HCV RNA levels demonstrates that post-OLTx serum viraemia is up to 16-fold higher than pre-transplantation (Chazouilleres et al, 1994). The high viraemic levels associated with hepatocyte injury and the low degree of inflammation suggest the presence of a direct cytopathic mechanism. However, the fact that only slightly more than half of HCV RNA-positive liver transplant recipients develop histological hepatitis, and that there is no correlation between levels of viraemia and degree of hepatic injury, postulate the existence of a different pathogenetic mechanism of damage.

Treatment of HCV re-infection

IFN is the only agent commercially available for the treatment of HCV disease. It has been used in both pre- and post-OLTx. When used for pre-OLTx little or no benefit is evident unless high doses are used (Gurakar et al, 1994b). The use of high doses requires the concomitant use of either G-CSF of GM-CSF to maintain WBC counts at levels enabling the IFN to be given (Gurakar et al, 1994b). Preliminary reports of the use of such combinations have been made. The optimism of the initial report may need to be tempered as the time post-OLTx for the patients in the initial study continues to accumulate.

The use of IFN in OLTx recipients appears to reduce the serum ALT level and clinical signs and symptoms of disease in only a few patients (Wright et al, 1992b). It does not reduce the rate of disease progression—except in a very few, who clear HCV as a consequence of its use (van Thiel et al, 1994a). The most promising therapy that currently exists consists of a combination of IFN plus ribavirin (Bizollon et al, 1994; Gane et al, 1995). This combination post-OLTx appears to reduce the signs and symptoms of viral liver disease better than is achievable with IFN alone. The rate at which viral clearance is achieved after short-term therapy with this combination in allograft recipients, however, remains to be reported. Unfortunately, unlike the situation with HBV, no oral nucleoside analogues or hepatitis C immunoglobulin preparations that are effective at reducing the rate of recurrent HCV disease in liver allograft are now available

SUMMARY

The current status of liver transplantation (OLTx) for chronic viral hepatitis is reviewed. The major issues addressed include the rate of recurrence of disease, its severity and natural history, and the potential for therapy. These issues vary markedly for each type of viral hepatitis. The development of new antiviral agents for clinical use may change the current restriction on liver transplantation for hepatitis B virus (HBV)-related liver disease such that it begins to challenge hepatitis C virus (HCV) as the principal indication for OLTx world-wide.

REFERENCES

Angus P, Bowden G, McCaughan G et al (1993) Hepatitis B (HBV) pre-core mutant infection is associated with severe recurrent disease following liver transplantation (abstract). *Hepatology* **18:** 70A.
Belle SH, Beringer KC, Detre KM et al (1994) Trends in liver transplantation in the United States. In Terasaki PI & Cecka JM (eds) *Clinical Transplant 1993*, pp 19–36. Los Angeles: UCLA Press.
Bizollon T, Ducerf C & Sciarrino E (1994) Ribavirin and interferon treatment for hepatitis C recurrence following orthotopic liver transplantation. *Journal of Hepatology* **21:** S58.
Boker KHW, Ringe B, Kruger M et al (1994) Prostaglandin E plus famciclovir. A new concept for the treatment of severe hepatitis B after liver transplantation. *Transplantation* **57:** 1706.
Burra P, Pontisso P, Rossaro L et al (1993). HBV-DNA detected by PCR in serum and liver during the follow-up of HBsAg positive transplanted patients (abstract). *Hepatology* **18:** 326A.
Burton LK, Alexander JL, Goldstein RM et al (1993) Should any patient who is hepatitis B surface antigen-positive be transplanted? (abstract). *Hepatology* **18:** 70A.
Chazouilleres O, Kim M, Combs C et al (1994) Quantitation of hepatitis C virus RNA in liver transplant recipients. *Gastroenterology* **106:** 994–999.
Cote PJ, Korba BE, Steinberg H et al (1991) Cyclosporin A modulates the course of woodchuck hepatitis virus infection and induces chronicity. *Journal of Immunology* **146:** 3138–3144.
Crippin J, Foster B, Carlen S et al (1994) Retransplantation in hepatitis B—a multicenter experience. *Transplantation* **54:** 823–826.
David E, Rathier J, Pucci A et al (1993) Recurrence of hepatitis D (delta) in liver transplants: histopathological aspects. *Gastroenterology* **104:** 1122–1128.
Davies SE, Portmann BC, O'Grady JG et al (1991) Hepatic histological findings after transplantation for chronic hepatitis B infection, including a unique pattern of fibrosing cholestatic hepatitis. *Hepatology* **13:** 150–157.

De Man RA, Niesters HJM, Fevery J et al (1995) Evaluation by limiting dilution PCR of HBV-DNA decrease in a double-blind randomized six-month trial of Lamivudine for chronic Hepatitis B: implications for the application in liver transplant recipients. Presentation at American Association for the study of liver diseases, Single topic Symposium, Liver Transplantation for chronic viral hepatitis: Reston, Virginia, March, 1995.

Demetris AJ, Todd S, van Thiel DH et al (1990) Evolution of hepatitis B virus liver disease after hepatic replacement. Practical and theoretical considerations. *American Journal of Pathology* **137:** 667–676.

Fagiuoli S, Shah G, Wright HI et al (1993) Types, causes and therapies of hepatitis occurring in a liver allograft. *Digestive Disease and Science* **38:** 449–456.

Feray C, Zignego AL, Samuel D et al (1990) Persistent hepatitis B virus infection of mononuclear blood cells without concomitant liver infection. The liver transplantation model. *Transplantation* **49:** 1155–1158.

Feray C, Samuel D, Thiers V et al (1992) Reinfection of liver graft by hepatitis C virus after liver transplantation. *Journal of Clinical Investigation* **89:** 1361–1365.

Ferrel LD, Wright TL, Roberts J et al (1992) Hepatitis C viral infection in liver transplant recipients. *Hepatology* **16:** 865–876.

Fung JJ, Rakela J, Pinna A et al (1995) Liver transplantation for hepatitis B: What have we learned and what does the future hold? *Liver Transplantation and Surgery* **1:** 274–280.

Gane EJ, Tibbs CJ, Ramage JK et al (1995) Ribavirin therapy for hepatitis C infection following liver transplantation. *Transplantation International* **8:** 61–64.

Gish RG, Keeffe EB, Fang JWS et al (1994) Gancyclovir treatment of recurrent hepatitis B virus infection in orthotopic liver transplant recipients (abstract). *Gastroenterology* **106:** A899.

Grellier L, Brown D, Berenek P et al (1995) Lamivudine prophylaxis: a new strategy for prevention of hepatitis B reinfection in liver transplantation for hepatitis B DNA positive cirrhosis. Presentation at American Association for the study of liver diseases, Single topic Symposium, Liver Transplantation for chronic viral hepatitis: Reston, Virginia, March, 1995.

Gurakar A, Fagiuoli S, Hassanein T et al (1994a) Prophylactic interferon-alpha therapy following liver transplantation: does it prevent allograft infection? *European Journal of Gastroenterology and Hepatology* **6:** 429–432.

Gurakar A, Gavaler JS, Fagiuoli S et al (1994b) The use of GM-CSF to enhance hematologic parameters of patients with cirrhosis and hypersplenism. *Journal of Hepatology* **21:** 582–586.

Hoofnagle JH, Di Bisceglie AM, Waggoner JG et al (1993) Interferon-alpha for patients with clinically apparent cirrhosis due to hepatitis B. *Gastroenterology* **104:** 1116–1121.

Hopf U, Neuhaus P, Lobeck H et al (1991) Follow-up of recurrent hepatitis B and delta infection in liver allograft recipients after treatment with recombinant interferon-alpha. *Journal of Hepatology* **13:** 339–346.

Kiyasu PK, Ishitani MB, McGory RW et al (1994) Prevention of hepatitis B recurrence after a second liver transplant—the role of maintenance polyclonal HBIg therapy. *Transplantation* **57:** 823–826.

Konig V, Hopf U, Neuhaus P et al (1994) Long-term follow-up of hepatitis B virus infected recipients after orthotopic liver transplantation. *Transplantation* **58:** 553–559.

Kruger M, Tillmann HL, Trautwein C et al (1994) Treatment of hepatitis B virus reinfection after liver transplantation with famciclovir (abstract). *Hepatology* **20:** 130A.

Kuo G, Choo QL, Alter HJ et al (1989) An assay for circulating antibodies to a major etiologic virus of human non-A, non-B hepatitis. *Science* **244:** 3–5.

Lake J (1995) Should liver transplantation be performed for patients with chronic hepatitis B? *Liver Transplantation and Surgery* **1:** 260–265.

Lau JYN, Bain VG, Davies SE et al (1992) High-level expression of hepatitis B viral antigens in fibrosing cholestatic hepatitis. *Gastroenterology* **102:** 956–962.

Lau JY, Davis GL, Kniffen J et al (1993) Significance of serum hepatitis C virus RNA levels in chronic hepatitis. *Lancet* **341:** 1501–1504.

Lauchart W, Muller R & Pichlmayer R (1987a) Immunoprophylaxis of hepatitis B virus reinfection in recipients of human allografts. *Transplantation Proceedings* **19:** 2387–2389.

Lauchart W, Muller R & Pichlmayer R (1987b) Long-term immunoprophylaxis of hepatitis B virus reinfection in recipients of human allografts. *Transplantation Proceedings* **19:** 4051–4053.

Locarnini S, Bowden DS, Angus P et al (1993) Pathogenesis and chemotherapy of severe B virus recurrence following liver transplantation (abstract). International Symposium on Viral Hepatitis and Liver Disease, Tokyo.

McGory R, Ishitani W, Oliveira C et al (1994) Pharmacokinetics of hepatitis B immune globulin in patients with orthotopic liver transplantation secondary to chronic hepatitis B virus induced cirrhosis (abstract). *Hepatology* **20:** 130A.

Marcellin B, Samuel D, Areias J et al (1994) Pretransplantation treatment and recurrence of hepatitis B virus infection after liver transplantation for hepatitis B-related end stage liver disease. *Hepatology* **19:** 6–12.

Martin J, Bosch O, Moraleda G et al (1993) Pilot study of recombinant human granulocyte–macrophage colony-stimulating factor in the treatment of chronic hepatitis B. *Hepatology* **18:** 775–780.

Mateo R, Demetris A, Sico E et al (1993) Early detection of de novo hepatitis C infection in patients after liver transplantation by reverse transcriptase polymerase chain reaction. *Surgery* **114:** 442–448.

Mora NP, Klintmalm GB, Poplawski SS et al (1990) Recurrence of hepatitis B after liver transplantation: does hepatitis-B-immunoglobulin modify the recurrent disease? *Transplantation Proceedings* **22:** 1549–1550.

Muller R, Gubernatis G, Farle M et al (1991) Liver transplantation in HBs antigen (HBsAg) carriers. Prevention of hepatitis B virus (HBV) recurrence by passive immunization. *Journal of Hepatology* **13:** 90–96.

Neuhaus P, Steffen R, Blumhardt G et al (1991) Experience with immunoprophyaxis and interferon therapy after liver transplantation in HBsAg positive patients. *Transplantation Proceedings* **23:** 1522–1524.

O'Grady JG, Smith JM, Davies SE et al (1992) Hepatitis B virus reinfection after liver transplantation: serological and clinical implications. *Journal of Hepatology* **14:** 104–111.

Omata M (1990) Significance of extrahepatic replication of hepatitis B virus. *Hepatology* **2:** 364–366.

Ottobrelli A, Marzano S, Smedile A et al (1991). Patterns of hepatitis delta virus reinfection and disease in liver transplantation. *Gastroenterology* **101:** 1649–1655.

Pons JA (1995) Role of liver transplantation in viral hepatitis. *Journal of Hepatology* **22 (supplement 1):** 146–153.

Poterucha JJ, Rakela J, Lumeng L et al (1992) Diagnosis of chronic hepatitis C after liver transplantation by the detection of viral sequences with polymerase chain reaction. *Hepatology* **15:** 42–45.

Pruett TL (1995) HBIg immunoprophylaxis in the United States: IV studies. Presentation at American Association for the study of liver diseases, Single topic Symposium, Liver Transplantation for Chronic Viral Hepatitis: Reston, Virginia, March, 1995.

Ranjan D, Tennyson GS, Poplawski SC et al (1993) Improved survival in hepatitis B surface antigen positive liver transplant recipient (abstract). *Hepatology* **18:** 342A.

Samuel D, Bismuth A, Mathieu D et al (1991a) Passive immunoprophylaxis after liver transplantation in HBsAg positive patients. *Lancet* **337:** 813–815.

Samuel D, Bismuth A, Serres C et al (1991b) HBV infection after liver transplantation in HBsAg positive patients: experience with long-term immunoprophylaxis. *Transplantation Proceedings* **23:** 1492–1494.

Samuel D, Muller R, Alexander G et al (1993) Liver transplantation in European patients with the hepatitis B surface antigen. *New England Journal of Medicine* **329:** 1842–1847.

Samuel D, Zignego AL, Raynes M et al (1995) Long-term clinical and virological outcome after liver transplantation for cirrhosis caused by chronic delta hepatitis. *Hepatology* **21:** 333–339.

Shah G, Demetris AJ, Gavaler JS et al (1992) Incidence, prevalence and clinical course of hepatitis C following liver transplantation. *Gastroenterology* **103:** 323–329.

Terrault N, Ascher NL, Hahn J et al (1994) Prophylactic therapy is the most important factor determining recurrence in hepatitis B surface antigen positive patients undergoing liver transplantation (abstract). *Hepatology* **20:** 138A.

Todo S, Demetris AJ, Van Thiel et al (1991) Orthotopic liver transplantation for patients with hepatitis B virus-related liver diseases. *Hepatology* **13:** 619–626.

Tur-Kaspa R, Shaul Y, Moore DD et al (1988) The glucocorticoid receptor recognizes a specific nucleotidic sequence in hepatitis B virus DNA causing increased activity of the HBV enhancer. *Virology* **167:** 630–633.

Tyrrel DLJ, Mitchell MC, DeMan RA et al (1993) Phase II trial with lamivudine for chronic hepatitis B (abstract). *Hepatology* **18:** 112A.

Van Thiel DH, Baddour N, Fagiuoli S et al (1994a) Interferon-alpha treatment of viral hepatitis in patients with liver allografts treated either with FK 506 or Cyclosporine A. *European Journal of Gastroenterology and Hepatology* **6:** 787–791.

Van Thiel DH, Wright HI & Fagiuoli S (1994b) Liver transplantation for hepatitis B virus-associated cirrhosis: a progress report. *Hepatology* **20:** 20S–23S.

Villamil FG, Petrovic LM, Podesta LG et al (1994) Interferon alpha-2b therapy for recurrent hepatitis B virus infection following liver transplantation. *Hepatology* **20:** 1679 (abstract).

Villamil FG & Vierling JM (1995) Recurrence of viral hepatitis after liver transplantation: insights into management. *Liver Transplantation and Surgery* **1 (supplement 1):** 89–99.

Wright HI, Gavaler JS, Van Thiel DH et al (1992a) Preliminary experience with alpha-2b-interferon therapy of viral hepatitis in liver allograft recipients. *Transplantation* **53:** 121–124.

Wright TL, Donegan E, Hsu HH et al (1992b) Recurrent and acquired hepatitis C viral infection in liver transplant recipients. *Gastroenterology* **103:** 317–322.

Yoffe B, Burns DK, Bhatt HS et al (1990) Extrahepatic hepatitis B virus DNA sequences in patients with acute hepatitis B infection. *Hepatology* **12:** 187–192.

Index

Note: Page numbers of article titles are in **bold** type.

389